Plunkett's
PROCEDURES FOR THE **MEDICAL**
ADMINISTRATIVE ASSISTANT

Heather Ramsay, BA, MEd (DE)
Learning Manager, Medical Support Services
Holland College
Charlottetown, PE

Marie Rutherford, Dipl., in Nursing, BA
Faculty, Office Administration-Medical/Health Services
Georgian College
Barrie, ON

ELSEVIER

PLUNKETT'S PROCEDURES FOR THE MEDICAL ADMINISTRATIVE ASSISTANT,
FIFTH EDITION

ISBN: 978-1-77172-196-7

Notice

Practitioners and researchers must always rely on their own experience and knowledge in evaluating and using any information, methods, compounds, or experiments described herein. Because of rapid advances in the medical sciences, in particular, independent verification of diagnoses and drug dosages should be made. To the fullest extent of the law, no responsibility is assumed by Elsevier, authors, editors, or contributors for any injury and/or damage to persons or property as a matter of products liability, negligence, or otherwise, or from any use or operation of any methods, products, instructions, or ideas contained in the material herein.

Library of Congress Control Number: 2019952356

VP Education Content: Kevonne Holloway
Content Strategist, Canada Acquisitions: Roberta A. Spinosa-Millman
Director, Content Development: Laurie Gower
Content Development Specialist: Sandy Matos
Publishing Services Manager: Shereen Jameel
Project Manager: Umarani Natarajan
Design Direction: Amy Buxton

Printed in the United States of America

Last digit is the print number: 9 8 7 6 5 4 3 2

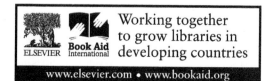

Plunkett's

PROCEDURES FOR THE **MEDICAL ADMINISTRATIVE ASSISTANT**

To the hardworking students across our great country of Canada. May our work instill inspiration and ignite a passion for the exciting and diverse career of medical office administration. Your dedication will bring rewards you cannot yet imagine.

Thank you to my family and friends for their patience and encouragement. To my colleagues, past and present, thank you for your dedication to the advancement of health care and the medical office profession. Your influences are lasting and cherished.

Heather Ramsay

To health care students who have not yet realized the potential and importance of the career you have chosen, this book was written for you. We believe the content will shape your learning and enhance your focus as you embark on your new professional path.

To all health care professionals who have dedicated their lives to this wonderful profession, thank you.

Finally, to all my former patients who have taught me lasting and meaningful lessons, thank you.

Marie Rutherford

Preface

The dynamic health care field and the technology that supports it are constantly advancing. Instructional publications are revised to ensure that current standards reflect evolving changes. You are embarking on an exciting career as a medical administrative assistant, one that will present everyday challenges as well as many opportunities for change and career advancement. *Plunkett's Procedures for the Medical Administrative Assistant,* fifth edition, will provide you with the learning outcomes you require to be a successful contributor to health care and to a health care team.

The medical office is a diverse environment that requires in-demand skills and knowledge. The medical administrative assistant must be knowledgeable of office procedures, various computer programs, medical transcription, terminology, and anatomy; in addition, he or she must demonstrate excellent interpersonal communication, professional conduct, and the ability to manage stress. The focus of this text is on office procedures in a medical office, complementary care office, and hospital environment.

The text covers foundational learning and office procedures essential for a medical administrative assistant to know. Topics include electronic medical records, appointment scheduling and suggested patient flow methodologies; records management; accounting; health care billing; hospital records, reports, and requisitioning; meeting organization; ordering procedures; and medical legal issues. In addition, we have included appropriate formats for letters, memos, and forms. On the accompanying Evolve site, we have provided practice questions, exercises, checklists, forms, and templates.

In addition, there are four useful appendices. Appendix A offers a quick reference to common abbreviations used in the health care field. Appendix B lists laboratory tests and general ordering indications as well as the expected turnaround times. Appendix C provides an overview of commonly prescribed drugs, including brand and generic names. Appendix D lists names of recommended resource tools such as medical dictionaries, handbooks, and other books on health care to which you can refer.

The assignments in the text attempt to simulate tasks that would be encountered in a medical environment. Dr. J.E. Plunkett will be the physician who assigns the majority of your tasks. The originating author, Lorna Plunkett, based the first edition on Dr. Plunkett, who was her husband's Uncle Elmer. In 1931, after graduating from Queen's University and spending nine months at the Mayo Clinic in Minneapolis, he set up his medical practice at 278 O'Connor Street

in Ottawa. He was a dedicated surgeon and physician until his untimely demise in 1952. The inscript on the letterhead used for the assignments was taken from one of his prescription pad pages on which his wife, Marion, had written a recipe. All other names and the associated medical information are fictitious.

We have also provided information on 15 fictitious patients. You will notice throughout the book that some exercises and examples deal with these patients. This was intended to provide a patient database to be used as needed.

New to the Fifth Edition

The fifth edition of *Plunkett's Procedures for the Medical Administrative Assistant* presents a colourful new design with *Did You Know?* and *Critical Thinking* highlights throughout. As much as possible, efforts have been made to provide a pan-Canadian perspective throughout the text. Each chapter introduces updated and expanded information on original topics. New material related to procedures, health-related laws, and technological advancements, including electronic medical records, are incorporated. Chapter reorganization brings legal topics and important association descriptions to the forefront in an effort to reinforce their influence throughout the text. Chapter highlights include the following:

Chapter 1–Explores the personal qualities, skills, and knowledge requirements of a medical administrative assistant. Areas of employment are introduced.

Chapter 2–Associations that influence how medical administrative assistants approach their work are outlined. Common medico-legal problems are discussed.

Chapter 3–Explores reception duties and contemporary scheduling methodologies. Clinical skills are introduced, as is the concept of electronic medical records (EMR).

Chapter 4–Features and organization of patient charts are outlined, and alphabetical, subject, and numerical filing rules are highlighted.

Chapter 5–Telephone equipment and etiquette as well as types of calls are explained. Modern eCommunication tools, including telehealth networks, are introduced.

Chapter 6–Traditional and electronic methods of preparing, sending, and receiving mail are included. Letter, memo, and punctuation styles are examined.

Chapter 7–A primary focus on provincial and territorial health plans, including the key topics of eligibility, portability, fee schedules, claims submission, and remittance advice.

Uninsured services, third-party billing, and workers' compensation boards are explored.

Chapter 8–Enhanced focus reflective of automated accounting processes and tools, along with an added overview of payroll preparation, including source deductions and remittance procedures.

Chapter 9–Key components of supply chain management are introduced and examined. Emphasis is placed on safety (WHMIS), along with vaccination and medication handling protocol.

Chapter 10–Examination of, and the developmental importance of, an office procedures manual is highlighted. Key considerations are reflected, as is the content formulation.

Chapter 11–Introduces meeting structure and further defines categories of meetings. Specific documentation attributes including notices, agenda, and minutes are presented, along with event management components.

Chapter 12–Hospital record composition and the diverse hospital environment are explored. Specific types of reports generated in a hospital setting are presented. The various roles of the medical administrative assistant in a hospital setting are also outlined.

Chapter 13–Best practices for preparing resumes, cover letters, and other employment documents are offered, along with information on job search techniques and employment opportunities.

Acknowledgements

The preparation of the fifth edition has been a challenging and rewarding process. We would like to acknowledge the work of Lorna Plunkett, whose work is still a prominent feature in the book, as well as the previous edition's author, Elsbeth McCall. Their foundational work allowed us to build upon the content for the new edition.

We want to thank the following for letting us tap into their knowledge and expertise to make this text the best we could for the students and instructors who will be using it. Thanks goes to Yukon Medical Association; Government of Yukon, Health and Social Services; Lauren Romano, Lead Product Trainer at QHR Technologies; and Mike Eburne, Senior Creative Strategist at QHR Technologies.

Thanks also to the following organizations for the permission to print the many forms that appear in the text:
Canada Post
Canadian Centre for Occupational Health and Safety
Canadian Medical Association
Canadian Medical Protective Association
Dean et Fils, Inc.
eHealth Saskatchewan
International Association of Administrative Professionals

Manitoba Health Services Commission
Nova Scotia Department of Health
Ontario Medical Association
Ontario Ministry of Health and Long-Term Care
Peterborough Regional Health Centre (formerly Peterborough Civic Hospital and St. Joseph's Hospital)
Public Works and Government Services Canada
Régie de l'assurance maladie du Québec (RAMQ)
Scotia Bank/The Bank of Nova Scotia
Worker's Compensation Board (WCB) Alberta, Manitoba, PEI
Workplace Safety and Insurance Board (WSIB) Ontario

As we approached the revision for the fifth edition, we couldn't have done so without the support of the Elsevier Inc. team. Special thanks to our Content Strategist, Roberta Spinosa-Millman, for her support throughout. Thanks to our Content Development Specialist, Sandy Matos, for her guidance and support through the development process. Special thanks to the artists who recreated many of the figures for this edition, as well as to the members of the production and permissions group for their work on the fifth edition.

We would also like to acknowledge and thank the reviewers of the book for their feedback and suggestions.

Reviewers

The following instructors provided feedback for this edition:

Denise Cacchioni, BSc, DC
Faculty of Commerce and Business Administration
Douglas College
New Westminster, British Columbia

Sheena M. Graves, RN
Office Administration Department
Faculty of Commerce and Business
Douglas College
New Westminster, British Columbia

Avis Hardy, RN, MSN (retired)
Medical Instructor
Saskatoon Business College
Saskatoon, Saskatchewan

Donna Harper, CHUC, PID, MOA
Canadian Health Care Academy
Surrey, British Columbia

Ann Knowlton
Director of Academic Studies
Crossroads Truck & Career Academy of
Trades, Business and Health Care
Ottawa, Ontario

Dr. Harminder Mathur, PID, DGO, MBBS
Instructor, Health Sciences
Stenberg College
Surrey, British Columbia

Amy Pytlowany, BSc
Faculty Head, Medical Office Assisting
triOS College Business Technology Healthcare
Mississauga, Ontario

Darlene J. Vail, MOA, MLT
Instructor of Medical Office Administration
Algonquin Careers Academy
Mississauga, Ontario

Contents

About the Authors

Heather Ramsay

Heather Ramsay is a faculty member in the Medical Support Services (MSS) program at Holland College, Prince Edward Island. Heather graduated from this same diploma program in 1993 before she went on to earn a Bachelor of Arts (psychology and sociology) degree from the University of Prince Edward Island. She then began her journey into health care administration, working as a medical secretary, medical transcriptionist, and medical office manager over the course of her career. With an offer to assist in the development of a new medical office administration program, Heather made the move into education and teaching at a private career college before moving to Holland College, the community college of Prince Edward Island. In 2015, Heather received a Master of Education degree from Athabasca University and, subsequently, a certificate of adult education equivalency while teaching in the MSS program. Over the course of her teaching career, Heather has been involved in curriculum development and delivery of all MSS program courses, including medical office procedures, medical terminology and anatomy, and medical transcription. She has also taught these same courses via distance education as a sessional instructor. Heather's greatest hope is that her students develop a passion for medical office administration and use this passion to foster continuous improvement in the delivery of health care services.

Heather resides in Prince Edward Island with her husband, Paul. She has a keen interest in fitness and nutrition and holds a diploma in natural nutrition. She also enjoys cooking and baking as well as boating on the beautiful waterways of Prince Edward Island.

Marie Rutherford

Marie Rutherford is a faculty member in the office administration program at Georgian College in Barrie, Ontario, with a specialty focus in health services. She commenced her career path working as a medical office assistant in a one-physician practice; soon realizing her devotion to health care, she returned to college to complete a nursing program. After several years of working in various health care practices and hospital settings in both administrative and nursing roles, she was led to transition her knowledge to a teaching career that has spanned more than 20 years. She began with course deliveries covering anatomy and medical office procedures in a private career college, then moved to Georgian College in 1999. In early 2000, she returned to school again to continue degree studies on a part-time basis. In the post-secondary educational setting, she found a place to combine her passion for health care and her love of continual learning in one complete package. In her faculty role, she held the position of program coordinator, and she has led three program teams through curriculum development and design. Looking to enhance her teaching skills, Marie has continued her studies recently by attending an Instructional Design and Technology program at a local university.

Marie resides in Barrie, Ontario, with her husband. Her interests include reading, travelling, and caring for her furry friends. Keeping fit and active is important for Marie because it enhances her quality of life.

1

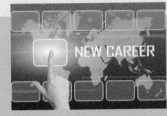

Source: © CanStock Photo Inc./Mazirama

Your Future as a Medical Administrative Assistant

This chapter provides an orientation to the role and responsibilities of a medical administrative assistant. You will discover the sought-after personal and professional qualities of those who choose this career, while exploring the broad scope of employment opportunities. The importance of establishing and maintaining a client-focused approach to all work activities is outlined. This commitment to service reaches far beyond the frontline and includes preserving confidentiality, practicing privacy, and fostering excellent team communication. These topics, along with ideas for self-care, are introduced in this chapter.

CHAPTER OUTLINE

Introduction

Becoming a Member of the Health Care Team

Career Qualifications

Responsibilities and Duties

Client Service

Stress Management

Career Opportunities

LEARNING OBJECTIVES

After reading this chapter, you will be able to:

1. Understand personal qualities required for employment in a medical environment
2. Understand the skill and knowledge requirements for the medical administrative assistant
3. Understand the professional appearance for a medical administrative assistant
4. Understand the importance of client service
5. Understand the importance of stress management
6. Understand the scope of career opportunities

KEY TERMS

Confidentiality: The dictionary defines confidential as "entrusted with secrets." In the medical field this term applies to patient identification as well as patient information, diagnosis, prognosis, and medical records access (manual and electronic).

Medical administrative assistant: A health care professional with training in scheduling, office records management, medical billing, medical transcription, and general office procedures who performs administrative and/or clinical duties in a medical office environment.

Medical transcriptionist: An individual who produces a keyed copy of dictated medical office notes and hospital reports.

Superior keyboarding and proofreading skills are required, along with an excellent understanding of anatomy, terminology, and pharmacological terms and references.

Speech recognition editor: A medical transcriptionist who proofreads and edits medical documentation that has been dictated through a speech recognition program. They convert the rough-draft text created by the speech recognition program into accurate and complete documents.

Privacy: In health care, privacy relates to how the personal information of patients is collected, disclosed, used, maintained, and accessed.

Introduction

A position as a health care professional is exciting and rewarding. You are embarking on a career path that will allow you, as a medical administrative assistant, to join this stimulating specialty. Historically, medicine has been a mysterious but intriguing subject; the news media frequently affords it headline status because innovations in the control of serious illnesses are happening every day. As a medical administrative assistant, you will play a valuable role in this complex system of administration, science, technology, innovation, and collaboration. Although your program of study will provide you a point of entry to the health care industry, you will be required to upgrade your skills and education to maintain your efficiency and knowledge. The changes in health care are constant, and an early commitment to professional development will assist you in becoming a valuable member of a health care team.

Becoming a Member of the Health Care Team

It is important to remember that the medical environment is a team environment (see Fig. 1.1). The types of professionals that you work with every day will depend largely on your working environment. Because health care is so diverse, so are its team structures. If you work in a private physician's office, your team structure may include only the physician, you, and any supporting housekeeping and maintenance personnel. In a larger collaborative clinic, your team can be much more diverse and include the housekeeping staff, building maintenance staff, supply service personnel, nurses and nurse practitioners, physicians, allied health professionals, and other medical administrative assistants. A hospital setting is larger still, and the team consists of not only the staff working directly with you on your floor or in your department but also the rest of the hospital departments and staff, including the volunteers.

Regardless of team structure or size, everyone plays an important role and is reliant on one another to deliver the best possible patient care. The team will rely on you as the medical administrative assistant to possess, maintain, and build on the skills, attributes, and abilities described in the following paragraphs.

Career Qualifications

The job turnover rate in your chosen career is surprisingly low and the opportunities diverse. This would indicate that medical administrative assistants derive a great deal of satisfaction from their positions. It also indicates that those seeking employment in this field must have superior personal qualifications and professional skills.

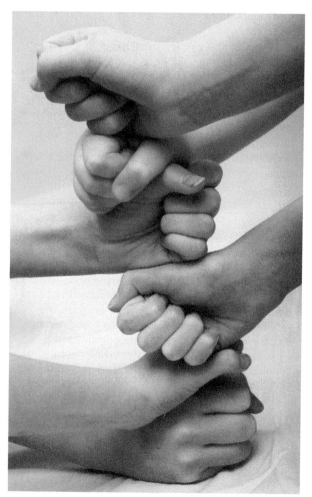

• **Fig. 1.1** The medical administrative assistant works with a whole team of health care professionals. (istockphoto.com/LisaValder)

DID YOU KNOW?

The Canada Job Bank reports that approximately 19,000 new medical administrative assistant jobs will be available between 2017 and 2026. That will bring the total number of medical administrative assistants in Canada to over 67,000.

Source: Canada Job Bank (2018). Administrative Assistant, Medical in Canada: Outlook. Retrieved from https://www.jobbank.gc.ca/marketreport/outlook-occupation/25791/ca

CRITICAL THINKING

If there are qualities in Box 1.1 that you do not recognize in yourself, what can you do to advance or develop these desired qualities?

Personal Qualities

If you think about why you have chosen this profession, you likely recognize that you possess many of the qualities listed in Box 1.1.

Skill and Knowledge Requirements

The medical office environment can be extremely busy and cause many stressful moments for the medical administrative assistant. At all times, you need to present a calm, professional appearance. Having the ability to prioritize your workload and manage multiple demands is essential. You must also master the additional job-related skills and knowledge as listed in Box 1.2.

• BOX 1.1 Personal Qualities of a Medical Administrative Assistant

Pleasing personality
Genuine interest in people and in helping
Ability to assume responsibility and maintain professional discipline
Ability to remain calm under pressure
Respect for and discretion around the privacy of others
Empathy, compassion, and patience
Honesty and reliability
Professional attitude that includes equitable treatment and respect for all
Dedication and loyalty
Understanding and helpfulness
Openness to change and lifelong learning

DID YOU KNOW?

Most employers of medical administrative assistants require the completion of a one- to two-year college program in the career area. They may also require advanced courses in areas such as medical transcribing or health information management.

DID YOU KNOW?

The average recommended two-handed touch-typing speed for medical administrative assistants is 50 to 60 net words per minute. A higher speed of 70+ net words per minute is recommended for medical transcriptionists.

Personal Appearance

Professional attitude, skills, and knowledge are complemented by a professional personal appearance, and a professional appearance is often related to levels of confidence and trust. In health care, dress code recommendations are also closely tied into employee and patient safety. You can effectively cultivate your professional image by following the professional dress and hygiene policies of your institution. The policies may include rules or guidelines relating to the items in Box 1.3. If a formal policy is not available for your institution, take the professional initiative to ask your employer for recommendations, and seek feedback on your choices.

CRITICAL THINKING

Your new office (or college program) has a clearly defined dress code. You notice that a coworker (or classmate) is not following the policy. You feel as if he or she is getting away with disregarding the policy, so you also break code. You immediately receive a warning that breaking policy is not acceptable, and you are provided with the reasons why. What do you do?

Responsibilities and Duties

The skills and knowledge discussed in Box 1.2 are required to fulfill the responsibilities and perform the daily tasks of a medical administrative assistant. These daily tasks vary

---

• BOX 1.2 Job-Related Skills of a Medical Administrative Assistant

Effective written and verbal communication skills
Good organizational ability and efficiency
Fast and accurate keyboarding skills
Sound understanding of medical terminology and anatomy
Knowledge of clinical tests, procedures, and basic pharmacology
Exceptional attention to detail
Excellent word processing, transcription, and speech recognition skills
Knowledge of basic computer programs applications, including speech recognition
Knowledge of electronic medical records and billing systems
Ability to manage multiple and competing demands
Ability to work efficiently on an individual basis and as part of a team
Excellent problem-solving abilities and critical thinking skills

---

• BOX 1.3 Professional Appearance Guidelines

Suitable footwear for your workplace
Limitations on fragrances due to allergies
Type, colour, and fit of uniforms or scrubs
Definition of appropriate professional dress
Recommendations related to hair, makeup, jewellery, tattoos, and piercings
Guidelines related to occupational hygiene

---

and are largely dependent on the area of employment you choose. However, most positions will require the performance of some or all of the following duties:

1. Frontline reception that includes greeting patients, answering the telephones, responding to electronic communications, and communicating messages to patients and staff
2. Scheduling, confirming, rescheduling, and cancelling appointments
3. Preparing and stocking examination rooms
4. Recording patient information on a variety of forms
5. Creating and maintaining confidential and accurate patient files (electronic and paper)
6. Taking inventory and ordering paper and medical supplies
7. Maintaining financial journals and accounts for third-party or uninsured billing
8. Maintaining petty cash and performing basic banking duties
9. Data entry and submission of medical billings to a ministry of health
10. Organizing meetings and creating meeting documentation including notices, agendas, and minutes
11. Establishing and maintaining policy and procedures manuals
12. Preparing and sending diagnostic samples to their appropriate laboratories
13. Establishing and maintaining filing systems
14. Creating, proofreading, mailing, and sorting office communications
15. Communicating with nonpatient clients and partners such as the physician's colleagues, pharmaceutical representatives, and local or national association members

As you explore the remainder of this text, each of these duties will be expanded upon, and you will gain a better understanding of your future as a medical administrative assistant.

CRITICAL THINKING

Review Box 1.2, Job-Related Skills of a Medical Administrative Assistant. See how many of the skills you can relate to the list of duties and responsibilities in the previous paragraph.

Client Service

Never underestimate the importance of first impressions! You are the voice of your doctor's practice. You are the first person to greet the patients when they visit the doctor. Many people judge the physician's practice by their first impression.

In addition to having a professional appearance, it is important to be friendly and to greet patients with a pleasant voice and expression (see Fig. 1.2). Remember that people who visit the doctor's office are usually under stress. It is your responsibility to help put them at ease. Be sure to acknowledge patients as quickly as possible. If the physician is behind schedule, inform the patients when they arrive that there is a delay.

Your level of client service and active engagement in the patient-care process also impact your employer and patients in less obvious ways. What you do behind the scenes in your workplace can greatly affect the outcome of the patient experience and the level of trust a patient feels for the physician and the health care team. For instance, physicians have a legal obligation to provide their patients with the best possible care, and this includes avoiding negligent and unprofessional actions. These unprofessional actions involve a physician, or an agent of a physician, not providing acceptable standards of care, competence, or skill in attending to a patient, resulting in the patient suffering harm or injury (Canadian Medical Protective Association, 2016). As a team member, you can assist the physician and other health care providers in avoiding unprofessional actions by providing excellent client service beyond the front line. Box 1.4 highlights some essential tips for ensuring excellent standards of care and service.

Although it seems less obvious, how you treat other employees within your organization (internal customers),

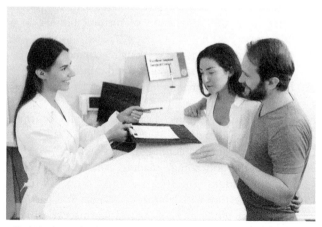

• **Fig. 1.2** A good attitude goes a long way in patient and staff relationships. (istockphoto.com/vadimguzhva)

• **BOX 1.4** **Client Service Beyond the Front Line**

Facilitating constant and effective communication between team members

Ensuring all necessary equipment, materials, and supplies are available and ready

Creating effective patient information materials based on up-to-date protocols

Understanding your professional limitations in providing care instructions

Undergoing proper training before accepting tasks beyond your scope of practice

Employing effective scheduling techniques

Ensuring excellent records management practices are in place

Confirming safety protocols are in place and well communicated

your health authority, or partnering health authorities can impact patient care. The relationships you have with other departments and facilities should be cooperative, communicative, and geared toward benefiting patients. Maintaining a level of professionalism, courtesy, and competence when booking appointments, requesting information, or providing advice will foster positive results. On the other hand, being difficult or unprofessional with departments or service providers that your patients and employer rely on may cause delays and increased stress for everyone involved.

Confidentiality

Throughout your career as a medical administrative assistant, you will encounter many "secrets." You will hear, read, and observe things that are extremely confidential. It is your responsibility to ensure that the details of a patient's medical situation are not passed on to others without consent. If a patient is attending your office for medical treatment, they are assuming that the reason for their visit will remain the knowledge of that office and any other medical offices or health facilities required for their care (e.g., a pharmacy, a laboratory, a consultant). However, you must have a patient's written consent to share information with anyone outside of that circle of care (e.g., a third-party insurance company). A breach of confidentiality can result in termination of employment and potential physical or emotional harm to a patient.

Confidentiality is a subject that ties in closely with our ability to be discreet. When patients approach your work area, it is important that you use a softer voice while conversing with them. Do not discuss their illness or reason for seeing the doctor in a voice that may be heard by others in the waiting area. If your conversations with patients may be overheard by others, move to an area where you can talk privately. If you have a questionnaire that needs to be filled out, have the patients do it themselves and be available for assistance if it is needed. Some other practical tips are listed in Box 1.5.

Privacy

Although the terms *privacy* and *confidentiality* are sometimes used interchangeably, each is quite unique in practice. Whereas confidentiality relates to an ethical obligation

• BOX 1.5 Tips for Maintaining Confidentiality

Divert your computer screen or use a privacy filter
Turn files or other papers upside down when patients
  approach your desk
Make sure there are no files or reports left in examination rooms
Employ proper filing and records management techniques to
  avoid reporting errors
Be cautious and discreet when leaving voice mail messages

of a medical practitioner and his or her staff to keep the medical situations of their patients private, privacy is a legal right related to how personal information is collected, used, maintained, and accessed. As a medical administrative assistant, you must become familiar with the privacy laws in your province to serve your clients appropriately (Chapter 2 provides information about privacy law).

All medical administrative assistants must be cautious when collecting personal patient information. If your office does not need the information to provide care to the patient, it should not be collected. For instance, a social insurance number is not needed to provide health care in Canada.

If you are not directly involved in the patient's care, you should not be accessing his or her records. Accessing records for unwarranted reasons is called "snooping," and it is not acceptable. For instance, if you work at a hospital and know your neighbour was admitted, you cannot legally access that neighbour's record if you are not directly involved in his or her care. Electronic health records are regularly audited, so "snooping" can easily be tracked and lead to loss of employment, penalties, and fines.

DID YOU KNOW?

A Canadian student was fined $25,000 for snooping in personal health records during a health care practicum experience.

Finally, be careful what information you disclose during patient care, even when the patient has implied third-party consent. For instance, a patient may have agreed to a specialist consultation. Information collected by your employer that is related to this medical issue will understandably be shared with the consultant. However, information unrelated to the referral should not be shared—this is disclosing or using patient information in an inappropriate way.

Stress Management

The health care environment is very busy and demanding, often creating stressful situations for the medical administrative assistant. Although you will not be able to predict all difficult or stressful situations in such a dynamic atmosphere, you can avoid the undue stresses that come from being disorganized or having poor time management. Organize and prioritize your routine daily tasks in a way that will allow you to more effectively deal with the inevitable interruptions. For instance, if you have trouble staying on task or multitasking, make a standardized list of your non-urgent daily duties and check off each item as you accomplish it (see Fig. 1.3). Having a list frees up space in your mind to deal with other demands and therefore relieves some of the stress of the day. Also make sure you understand the overall goals of the health care team you are working with—you are

Daily Tasks	M	T	W	T	F	S	S
Place any unfiled reports in today's patients' charts	✓						
Provide physician with today's patient list/schedule	✓						
Listen to voice mail messages and respond as required	✓						
Open mail and route or file as required	✓						
Transcribe pending letters or reports	✓						
Send (or call for) required patient referrals	✓						
Collect and file reports reviewed by physician	✓						
Complete outgoing patient calls as required	✓						
Sterilize instruments and stock examination rooms	✓						
Pull patient charts for the next office day	✓						
Pack up lab materials for delivery to the hospital or lab	✓						

• Fig. 1.3 Daily Tasks Checklist Sample

an important part of making everyone's day run smoothly. In addition to your list of regular daily tasks, each day will bring a unique set of goals that need to be accomplished for the team. A daily to-do list will keep you on track in a less stressful manner. For instance, you may be responsible for inputting and submitting the office billing on Thursday of each week, you may be responsible for making deposits to the bank on Wednesday of each week, or you may be responsible for arranging monthly team meetings. All the individual tasks related to these duties should be noted on daily to-do lists in order of priority. You can also build on the practise of making checklists for each of these individual tasks to ensure you do not miss any steps in the processes you are required to perform. These practices will assist in relieving undue stresses that present themselves.

Unfortunately, stressful situations cannot always be avoided or predicted. If you encounter a difficult patient, remain calm and in control. Try to move the patient to a private area, and be an active listener—let the patient express their frustrations, try to be reassuring, express your understanding of the problem, and clarify any misinformation or misunderstandings about the situation. Their anger is not usually directed at you and is usually caused by anxiety, so do not become defensive or argumentative, and maintain eye contact with them. Additional professional development in non-violent crisis prevention intervention and suicide prevention, or both, may be helpful for dealing with these kinds of situations. Your local mental health association may be helpful in directing your search for either or both of these courses.

It is equally important to get enough physical exercise, rest, and relaxation and to eat nutritious meals—all essential ingredients for a reduced stress level. Many employers now offer workplace wellness programs that address each of these needs so that employee burnout and stress can be minimized. If you work for a small employer who does not offer such programs, take the initiative to gauge the team's interest in informal workplace wellness challenges. The Government of Canada also works to promote fair and safe workplaces through a number of free initiatives. There are free webinars, checklists, guidelines, and advice for all Canadian employers and employees. Its publication *Psychological Health in the Workplace* provides practical strategies for dealing with workplace stress, which are outlined in Table 1.1.

Career Opportunities

The employment opportunities for medical administrative assistants are diverse. Some of the main areas of employment are single- or multi-doctor clinics, hospitals, primary care clinics or networks, long-term care facilities, or other community or public health departments.

Clinics

There are many clinic types and sizes across Canada. They range from single-doctor enterprises to collaborative care clinics that offer services from general practitioners, specialist

TABLE 1.1	Practical Strategies for Improving Psychological Health and Safety
Level of Intervention	**Strategies**
Employee	• Be supportive of peers who are experiencing stress • Come to work with a positive attitude • Ask for help and offer help in situations of workplace abuse • Report any incidence of workplace abuse, violence, or harassment • Take rest during designated breaks and holidays • Achieve work–life balance • Achieve a healthy lifestyle by eating well and exercising
Manager or Supervisor	• Clearly outline employee responsibilities • Be able to recognize early indicators of workplace stress • Accommodate employees who need flexible work arrangements • Provide training on workplace psychological health • Recognize employee contributions • Be accessible and actively promote employee participation in team-building exercises • Lead by modelling respectful workplace behaviours • Keep up to date on psychological health policies

Adapted from Wang, S., & Karpinski, E. (2016). *Psychological Health in the Workplace*. Prepared by Labour Program: Fair, Safe and Productive Workplaces. Employment and Social Development Canada. Retrieved from https://www.canada.ca/en/employment-social-development/services/health-safety/reports/psychological-health.html

physicians, and non-physician specialists. The size and type of the clinic will impact the type of jobs available and the daily tasks you will perform, along with the working atmosphere. For instance, if you choose to work in a single-doctor practice, your range of duties will be very broad; you may be considered the clinic manager and have a close relationship with the doctor and the patients. However, if you work in a multi-doctor or collaborative practice, you will share the work amongst several team members. You may be asked to perform one main task for the team, such as scheduling the clinic, or you may be asked to rotate through the system doing various tasks based on the clinic's needs. You may even be considered for additional training in areas such as performing noninvasive clinical procedures, venipuncture, blood pressure monitoring, or performing electrocardiograms.

Hospitals

Employment opportunities exist at all stages of hospital care, from the admission of the patient to the discharge, or in the management of documents in the medical records

• BOX 1.6   Job Opportunities in Hospitals

Admissions clerk for emergency, inpatient, or outpatient departments
Nursing unit clerk (also called health unit coordinator, ward clerk, or unit secretary)
Health records clerk or secretary
Medical transcriptionist or speech recognition editor
Booking clerk or secretary for outpatient clinics, operating rooms, laboratories, or diagnostic imaging departments
Medical administrative assistant in laboratory, imaging, pharmacy, and other departments

department. In addition to inpatient services, most hospitals provide outpatient and ambulatory treatment and have added wellness and health teaching to their programs. Examples of job opportunities in the hospital atmosphere are found in Box 1.6.

Long-Term and Specialized Care Facilities

In addition to clinics and acute- or emergency-care hospitals, there are many facilities that serve more well-defined sections of the population. These public and private sector opportunities include positions in long-term care homes or communities, psychiatric hospitals or mental health services, addiction services, and public health agencies. Positions in these areas include nursing unit clerks, medical administrative assistants, and health information managers or records clerks.

Other Medical Office Administration Jobs

Although hospitals and clinics may be thought of as the more traditional areas of employment for medical administrative assistants, there are many other areas to consider when you begin your job search. Some of these opportunities may require additional training or, on the other hand, may not require all the skills you developed during your training. However, all positions play a vital role in delivering quality health care. Some companies to consider are outlined in Box 1.7.

• BOX 1.7   Additional Health Care–Related Opportunities

Provincial laboratories
Provincial and federal health care plan offices
Practitioners' offices (optometrists, chiropractors, massage therapists, naturopaths, podiatrists)
Dentists' offices
Veterinarian hospitals and offices
Home care organizations
Medical supply companies
Medical foundations
Insurance companies
Medical, nursing, and research departments of universities and colleges
Pharmaceutical companies
Occupational health and safety and workers' compensation boards
Law offices managing personal injury claims
Online medical transcription companies

Summary

You are now aware of the many skills, abilities, personal qualities, and professional requirements of medical administrative assistants. You are aware that confidentiality and privacy are key issues when providing client care. You have discovered that the Canadian health care system offers a wide range of opportunities for trained medical administrative assistants and that the employment outlook for the industry is healthy. You are now on your way to discovering how to carry out the responsibilities and duties of your new career. As you work through the remainder of this text, note the topics that interest you the most and recognize your strengths. Doing so will assist you during your job search at the conclusion of your program of study.

Assignments

Assignment 1.1

Set up a personal file (portfolio) to begin collecting evidence of your achievements, challenges, academic documents, and other relevant data. This will allow you to maintain a record of documents to be used within this program and throughout your career, for example, letters of reference, performance evaluations, work-related "thank you" letters, diplomas/certificates, educational transcripts, and copies of successfully completed projects/assignments.

Assignment 1.2

Write a short essay (one to two pages) stating why you have chosen a career as a medical administrative assistant. Outline the personal qualities you possess that will enable you to be an effective health care professional. Be prepared to defend your ideas.

Assignment 1.3

Take a few moments to complete the rating sheet (Fig. 1.4; also available on the Evolve website). Be as objective and honest as you can. Reflect on your answers and consider how your personal choices may affect the first impression you make to employers and patients. Keep the sheet in your portfolio to be used in Assignment 13.2.

Assignment 1.4

Do you currently possess all the skills and personal qualities required for a health care environment? Perhaps you have some of the skills and some of the personal qualities but not at the level necessary to secure the position you are seeking.

To assess your current skills and personal qualities as they relate to a position as a medical administrative assistant,

RATING SHEET
A FIRST IMPRESSION

Place a check mark (✔) in the space that best describes your personal attributes.

Facial Expression

☐ Happy Smile   ☐ Serious Outlook   ☐ Blank Expression

Voice

☐ Loud Tone   ☐ Soft Spoken   ☐ Well Modulated

Communication Ability

☐ Control Conversation   ☐ Shy and Withdrawn   ☐ Outgoing and Friendly

Language Skills

☐ Adequate   ☐ Excellent   ☐ Poor

Hair Style

☐ Acceptable for Business   ☐ Unacceptable   ☐ Just Acceptable

Make-up

☐ Accentuated   ☐ Light   ☐ Heavy

Nails

☐ Manicured   ☐ Suitable   ☐ Rough

Clothes

☐ High Fashion   ☐ Comfortable   ☐ Sloppy

Hygiene

☐ Excellent   ☐ Good   ☐ Needs Improvement

OVERALL FIRST IMPRESSION

☐ Excellent   ☐ Acceptable   ☐ Poor

• **Fig. 1.4** Rating Sheet

complete the skills and personal qualities inventory sheet found on the Evolve website.

Be as objective as possible as you assess your skills and qualities; retain your inventory sheet in your portfolio for use in Assignment 13.4.

Topics for Discussion

1. Relate a health care experience you have had
   a. When a first impression in health care was positive. What qualities or skills of the health care professionals or others involved made it positive?
   b. When a first impression in health care was negative. What qualities or skills could the health care professional or others involved improve upon?
   c. How do you think that you as a medical administrative assistant will respond in a similar situation?
2. List 10 areas within health care where medical administrative assistants are required. Given your current knowledge of health care opportunities, where do you think your skills and qualities might best be put to use?
3. Some physicians prefer that their medical administrative assistants wear a uniform. Discuss pros and cons of wearing or not wearing uniforms.

4. Discuss how confidentiality could be breached and how such a breach can be avoided.
5. Why is it important to know the members of the team you are working with?
6. Patient care or client services provided by the medical administrative assistant extend well beyond the first impression. Choose an item or items from Box 1.4 and discuss how performing the task, or not performing the task, will impact patient care.
7. Attending to the needs of the physician and the patients is the main priority in a medical office atmosphere. However, you still have many other important tasks to complete during each day. Discuss some strategies for keeping your stress levels in check when you have so many competing demands on your time.

References

Canadian Medical Protective Association. (2016). *Medical-legal handbook for physicians in Canada, version 8.2.* Retrieved from https://www.cmpa-acpm.ca/en/advice-publications/handbooks.

Wang, S., & Karpinski, E. (2016). *Psychological health in the workplace. Prepared by labour program: Fair, safe and productive workplaces. Employment and social development canada.* Retrieved from https://www.canada.ca/en/employment-social-development/services/health-safety/reports/psychological-health.html.

2

Health Associations and the Law

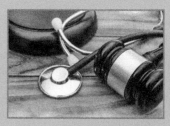

This chapter will introduce historical figures and symbols that influence and represent medical associations and the practice of modern medicine. You will explore key ethical and legal considerations for health care professionals and discover which Canadian associations, organizations, and governing bodies develop, implement, and monitor medical law.

You will learn about associations that focus on the development and maintenance of administrative standards across a variety of health care specialties. These associations provide medical administrative assistants with opportunities for career development and encourage the use of tools and processes that assist employers in upholding their legal obligations.

CHAPTER OUTLINE

Introduction

Historical Figures and Symbols

Associations

Legal Considerations

LEARNING OBJECTIVES

After reading this chapter, you will be able to:

1. Possess a greater awareness of who Hippocrates was, what the Oath of Hippocrates is, and what the significant medical symbols are.
2. Understand the existence of codes of ethics.
3. Describe the associations and organizations of importance.
4. Understand the rules and regulations pertaining to the practice of medicine.
5. Understand the various statutes that pertain to the medical environment.
6. Describe reporting procedures.
7. Recognize the various types of medico-legal problems.
8. Describe the restrictions necessary to ensure patient confidentiality.
9. Understand the minimum standards for medical records maintenance.

KEY TERMS

ARMA Canada: ARMA Canada is a division of ARMA International, the World's leading information management association.

Association for Healthcare Documentation Integrity (AHDI): AHDI is a professional association for medical transcriptionists and the publisher of the AHDI *Book of Style*.

Caduceus: A medical symbol that depicts two snakes encircling a staff that is topped with two wings, signifying peace and healing. The staff was given to the Greek god Hermes, messenger to the gods, by his half-brother Apollo (Rodgers, 2017).

Association of Administrative Professionals (AAP): AAP is a national professional association for administrative professionals from a variety of backgrounds.

Canadian Medical Association (CMA): CMA is a national association that unites physician members on health and medical matters and provides ethical guidance to Canadian physicians through its CMA Code of Ethics publication (Canadian Medical Association [CMA] and Joule Inc., 2000).

Canadian Medical Protective Association (CMPA): CMPA is a not-for-profit organization that provides advice and assistance to physicians when medico-legal difficulties arise. It also provides valuable resources related to risk management and safe medical care for health care professionals (Canadian Medical Protective Association [CMPA], n.d.).

Canadian Health Information Management Association (CHIMA): CHIMA is "the certifying body and national association that represents leadership and excellence in health information management" (Canadian Health Information Management Association [CHIMA], 2018, para 1).

Fraud: A deception deliberately practised to secure unfair or unlawful gain.

Hippocrates: Hippocrates is known as the Father of Medicine.

International Association of Administrative Professionals (IAAP): IAAP is a professional association for administrative assistants from all backgrounds, including health care.

Mandatory: Required or commanded by authority.

National Association for Health Unit Coordinators (NAHUC): NAHUC provides support, certification, and standards of practice for health unit coordinators.

Negligence: Failure to exercise the degree of care considered reasonable under the circumstances, resulting in an unintended injury to another party.

Power of Attorney (POA): A specific individual chosen by you to act on your behalf should you become unable to do so.

Royal College of Physicians and Surgeons of Canada: The national professional association that sets the educational standards and oversees the medical education of Canadian physicians.

Staff of Aesculapius: A medical symbol that depicts a single snake encircling a staff that signifies the art of healing. Aesculapius was the son of Apollo; he was known as the Greek god of medicine.

Statutes: Established laws or rules; laws enacted by a legislature.

World Health Organization (WHO): The WHO is the authority guiding international health within the United Nations.

Introduction

Learning about the history of a topic often helps our understanding of it; the history of medicine is no different. Although science and technology have progressed rapidly, some teachings and symbols have persisted over time and continue to influence the practising physicians and policymakers of today. These days, policies, guidelines, laws, and standards are communicated to medical professionals through associations. As a medical administrative assistant, you have a responsibility to recognize the associations that influence your physician's practice, and you need to make the effort to understand the rules and regulations they present. The policies and laws of these associations will influence how you approach your everyday responsibilities, such as record keeping, reporting of incidents, maintaining confidentiality, and respecting privacy. In addition to physician-focused associations, there is a broad range of associations geared toward the professional development and certification of administrative professionals. Being an active member of an association can elevate and broaden your skill set, which, in turn, will positively influence your physician's medical practice.

Historical Figures and Symbols

The earliest medical teachings were highly spiritual and theological undertakings that largely observed illness as punishment for moral carelessness or for deviating from superstitious beliefs. Over time, practitioners began to incorporate more scientific and modern practices; however, the influence of early historical and mythical figures and symbols still has connections to modern practice.

Hippocrates is known as the Father of Medicine (see Fig. 2.1). He was born on the island of Cos between 470 and 460 B.C. and belonged to the family that claimed descent from the mythical Aesculapius, son of Apollo. There was already a long medical tradition in Greece before his day, and thus he is supposed to have inherited his knowledge chiefly through his predecessor, Herodicus; he enlarged his education by extensive travel. Though the evidence is unsatisfactory, he is said to have taken part in the efforts to halt the great plague that

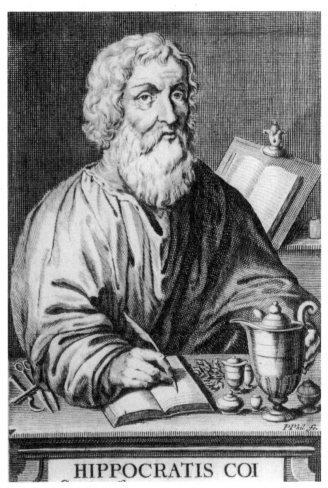

• **Fig. 2.1** Hippocrates is known as the Father of Medicine. (Source: Young, A. P. (2003). *Kinn's The Administrative Medical Assistant: An Applied Learning Approach* [5th ed], [p. 17: Figure 2-2]. St. Louis: Elsevier/Saunders.)

devastated Athens at the beginning of the Peloponnesian war. He died at Larissa between 380 and 360 B.C.

One of the works attributed to Hippocrates is the famous Hippocratic Oath (see Box 2.1). Today doctors still swear the oath, which is an ethical and moral declaration of how they intend to practise medicine. The oath does not represent any legal obligation itself, but it is

I SWEAR by Apollo the physician, and Aesculapius, and Health, and All-heal, and all the gods and goddesses, that, according to my ability and judgment, I will keep this Oath and this stipulation—to reckon him who taught me this Art equally dear to me as my parents, to share my substance with him, and relieve his necessities if required; to look upon his offspring in the same footing as my own brothers, and to teach them this art, if they shall wish to learn it, without fee or stipulation; and that by precept, lecture and every other mode of instruction, I will impart a knowledge of the Art to my own sons, and those of my teachers, and to disciples bound by stipulation and oath according to the law of medicine, but to none others.

I will follow that system of regimen which, according to my ability and judgment, I consider for the benefit of my patients, and abstain from whatever is deleterious and mischievous.

I will give no deadly medicine to anyone if asked, nor suggest any such counsel; and in like manner I will not give to a woman a pessary to produce abortion. With purity and with holiness I will pass my life and practise my Art.

I will not cut persons laboring under the stone, but will leave this to be done by men who are practitioners of this work. Into whatever houses I enter, I will go into them for the benefit of the sick, and will abstain from every voluntary act of mischief and corruption; and, further, from the seduction of females or males, of freemen and slaves. Whatever, in connection with my professional service, or not in connection with it, I see or hear, in the life of men, which ought not to be spoken of abroad, I will not divulge, as reckoning that all such should be kept secret. While I continue to keep this Oath unviolated, may it be granted to me to enjoy life and the practice of the art, respected by all men, in all times. But should I trespass and violate this Oath, may the reverse be my lot.

At the time of being admitted as a member of the medical profession:

I SOLEMNLY PLEDGE to consecrate my life to the service of humanity

I WILL GIVE to my teachers the respect and gratitude that is their due

I WILL PRACTISE my profession with conscience and dignity

THE HEALTH OF MY PATIENT will be my first consideration

I WILL RESPECT the secrets that are confided in me, even after the patient has died

I WILL MAINTAIN by all the means in my power, the honour and the noble traditions of the medical profession

MY COLLEAGUES will be my sisters and brothers

I WILL NOT PERMIT considerations of age, disease or disability, creed, ethnic origin, gender, nationality, political affiliation, race, sexual orientation, social standing or any other factor to intervene between my duty and my patient

I WILL MAINTAIN the utmost respect for human life

I WILL NOT USE my medical knowledge to violate human rights and civil liberties, even under threat

I MAKE THESE PROMISES solemnly, freely and upon my honour

Source: World Medical Association, Inc. (2018). *Declaration of Geneva*. Retrieved from https://www.wma.net/policies-post/wma-declaration-of-geneva/wma_declaration-of-geneva_a4_en/

Hippocrates. Hippocrates is believed to have studied medicine at a healing temple built in Aesculapius' honour on the island of Cos.

DID YOU KNOW?

The Canadian Medical Association uses the staff of Aesculapius as its official symbol. Eight of its branches (Alberta, Manitoba, New Brunswick, Newfoundland and Labrador Nova Scotia, Ontario, Saskatchewan, and Yukon), the World Health Organization, and the Royal College of Physicians and Surgeons of Canada have also adopted the staff as their symbol.

the basis for more modern-day codes and charters that physicians answer to. The Declaration of Geneva (see Box 2.2), published by the World Medical Association, builds upon the Hippocratic oath and is known as its modern-day version. It is now the oath more commonly sworn by physicians as they enter medical practice (World Medical Association, Inc., 2018). The Declaration of Geneva was last published in 2006 and is currently undergoing revision.

Two symbols are used in many areas of health care and allied health care to indicate a relationship to medicine. You will notice that many of the associations discussed in this chapter have some form of the symbols representing their organization. There is debate about the history and significance of each symbol; however, they both remain popular in various forms.

The staff of Aesculapius (see Fig. 2.2), also called *the rod of Aesculapius,* is a medical icon that depicts a single snake encircling a staff and signifies the art of healing. Aesculapius was the son of Apollo and was referred to as *the god of medicine*. One version of the story that relates Aesculapius to this symbol says he speared a snake to protect a child in his care. The dead snake was brought back to life with a leaf that he ultimately used to heal the child. Because of his influence and powers of healing, you will find Aesculapius mentioned prominently in the first line of the Oath of

Another mythological staff, the caduceus (see Fig. 2.2), belonged to Apollo but was given to his half-brother Hermes to assist him in his job as messenger of the gods. One story says that Hermes used the staff to break up a fight and bring peace between two snakes. However, Hermes' job was not related to medicine, so there is a lack of clarity around how this became a medical symbol. It is likely that the symbol's connection to Apollo is responsible for its relationship to medicine (Rodgers, 2017).

Associations

The range of health care–related associations and organizations across Canada is extensive. There are associations of direct significance to medical administrative assistants for professional development and continued education, and there are those that relate more directly to physicians but indirectly influence you as a representative of your physician—we will focus on these two types. In addition

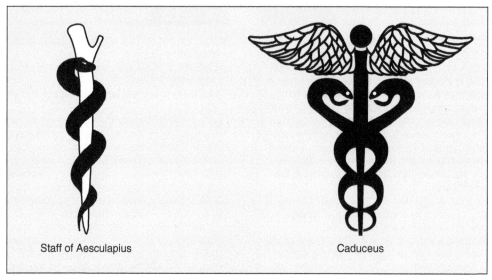

Staff of Aesculapius   Caduceus

• **Fig. 2.2** Staff of Aesculapius and the caduceus. (Source: Young, A. P. [2003]. *Kinn's The Administrative Medical Assistant: An Applied Learning Approach* [5th ed], [p. 17: Figure 2-1]. St. Louis: Elsevier/Saunders.)

to these, there are associations relating to hospitals, nurses, physiotherapists, nursing homes, health records administrators, and so on. It is important to recognize that many of the associations outlined will have connections, similar goals, partnerships, or impacts on each other in some way. They may uphold similar laws, rules, or regulations, or may work together within Canada's health care system.

Contact information for all physicians; health care associations; provincial, territorial, and federal departments of health; and Canadian health care associations can be found in both print and online versions of the *Canadian Medical Directory* available from Scott's Directories.

Canadian Medical Association

The Canadian Medical Association (CMA) is a national organization that unites physician members on health matters and deals with the federal government on these matters. It has 12 provincial medical association branches, and these provincial branches may have municipal or regional medical association branches (Box 2.3). An important function of CMA is providing ethical guidance to Canadian physicians through its CMA Code of Ethics publication. This code of ethics outlines the responsibilities of physicians to patients, to the profession, and to themselves (Fig. 2.3). Although the wording is quite different, it is easy to compare its focus to that of the Oath of Hippocrates. Like the Oath, the Code is not considered law; however, actions that deviate from the responsibilities outlined in it could certainly lead to legal complications for physicians. CMA reviews the Code regularly to determine whether updates are required. Its most recent review was in March 2018, and it was determined that no changes were required.

Another important publication of CMA is the Physicians' Charter. The Charter complements CMA policies and the CMA Code of Ethics. The goal of Canadian physicians, in partnership with their patients, is to provide the best health care possible. The Physicians' Charter (see Fig. 2.4)

• **BOX 2.3** **Provincial and Territorial Medical Associations**

- Canadian Medical Association (www.cma.ca)
- Doctors of British Columbia (https://www.doctorsofbc.ca)
- Alberta Medical Association (www.albertadoctors.org)
- Saskatchewan Medical Society (www.sma.sk.ca)
- Doctors Manitoba (http://www.docsmb.org)
- Ontario Medical Association (www.oma.org)
- Québec Medical Association (www.amq.ca)
- New Brunswick Medical Society (www.nbms.nb.ca)
- Doctors of Nova Scotia (www.doctorsns.com)
- Medical Society of Prince Edward Island (http://mspei.org)
- Newfoundland and Labrador Medical Association (www.nlma.nl.ca)
- Northwest Territories Medical Association (http://www.hss.gov.nt.ca/en/services/professional-licensing/physicians)
- Yukon Medical Association (www.yukondoctors.ca)

expresses what Canadian physicians need to achieve this goal and fulfill their responsibilities as outlined in the Code.

DID YOU KNOW?

The CMA first published its Code of Ethics in 1868. It is updated every 5 to 6 years and undergoes major revisions every 20 years.

Source: Canadian Medical Association. (2018). Advocacy. Retrieved from https://www.cma.ca/En/Pages/code-of-ethics.aspx

Royal College of Physicians and Surgeons of Canada

The Royal College of Physicians and Surgeons of Canada is a national professional association that sets the educational standards and oversees the medical education of Canadian physicians (2018). It protects the health of Canadians by helping physicians build and maintain skills, knowledge, and expertise in their chosen specialties.

CMA CODE OF ETHICS AND PROFESSIONALISM

The CMA Code of Ethics and Professionalism articulates the ethical and professional commitments and responsibilities of the medical profession. The Code provides standards of ethical practice to guide physicians in fulfilling their obligation to provide the highest standard of care and to foster patient and public trust in physicians and the profession. The Code is founded on and affirms the core values and commitments of the profession and outlines responsibilities related to contemporary medical practice.

In this Code, ethical practice is understood as a process of active inquiry, reflection, and decision-making concerning what a physician's actions should be and the reasons for these actions. The Code informs ethical decision-making, especially in situations where existing guidelines are insufficient or where values and principles are in tension. The Code is not exhaustive; it is intended to provide standards of ethical practice that can be interpreted and applied in particular situations. The Code and other CMA policies constitute guidelines that provide a common ethical framework for physicians in Canada.

In this Code, medical ethics concerns the virtues, values, and principles that should guide the medical profession, while professionalism is the embodiment or enactment of responsibilities arising from those norms through standards, competencies, and behaviours. Together, the virtues and commitments outlined in the Code are fundamental to the ethical practice of medicine.

Physicians should aspire to uphold the virtues and commitments in the Code, and they are expected to enact the professional responsibilities outlined in it.

Physicians should be aware of the legal and regulatory requirements that govern medical practice in their jurisdictions.

A. VIRTUES EXEMPLIFIED BY THE ETHICAL PHYSICIAN

Trust is the cornerstone of the patient–physician relationship and of medical professionalism. Trust is therefore central to providing the highest standard of care and to the ethical practice of medicine. Physicians enhance trustworthiness in the profession by striving to uphold the following interdependent virtues:

Compassion

A compassionate physician recognizes suffering and vulnerability, seeks to understand the unique circumstances of each patient and to alleviate the patient's suffering, and accompanies the suffering and vulnerable patient.

Honesty

An honest physician is forthright, respects the truth, and does their best to seek, preserve, and communicate that truth sensitively and respectfully.

Humility

A humble physician acknowledges and is cautious not to overstep the limits of their knowledge and skills or the limits of medicine, seeks advice and support from colleagues in challenging circumstances, and recognizes the patient's knowledge of their own circumstances.

Integrity

A physician who acts with integrity demonstrates consistency in their intentions and actions and acts in a truthful manner in accordance with professional expectations, even in the face of adversity.

Prudence

A prudent physician uses clinical and moral reasoning and judgement, considers all relevant knowledge and circumstances, and makes decisions carefully, in good conscience, and with due regard for principles of exemplary medical care.

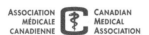

ASSOCIATION MÉDICALE CANADIENNE   CANADIAN MEDICAL ASSOCIATION

• **Fig. 2.3** Example of a code of ethics. (Source: *The Canadian Medical Association Code of Ethics.* [Update 2018]. Reprinted by permission of the Canadian Medical Association.)

B. FUNDAMENTAL COMMITMENTS OF THE MEDICAL PROFESSION

Commitment to the well-being of the patient

- Consider first the well-being of the patient; always act to benefit the patient and promote the good of the patient.
- Provide appropriate care and management across the care continuum.
- Take all reasonable steps to prevent or minimize harm to the patient; disclose to the patient if there is a risk of harm or if harm has occurred.
- Recognize the balance of potential benefits and harms associated with any medical act; act to bring about a positive balance of benefits over harms.

Commitment to respect for persons

- Always treat the patient with dignity and respect the equal and intrinsic worth of all persons.
- Always respect the autonomy of the patient.
- Never exploit the patient for personal advantage.
- Never participate in or support practices that violate basic human rights.

Commitment to justice

- Promote the well-being of communities and populations by striving to improve health outcomes and access to care, reduce health inequities and disparities in care, and promote social accountability.

Commitment to professional integrity and competence

- Practise medicine competently, safely, and with integrity; avoid any influence that could undermine your professional integrity.
- Develop and advance your professional knowledge, skills, and competencies through lifelong learning.

Commitment to professional excellence

- Contribute to the development and innovation in medicine through clinical practice, research, teaching, mentorship, leadership, quality improvement, administration, or advocacy on behalf of the profession or the public.
- Participate in establishing and maintaining professional standards and engage in processes that support the institutions involved in the regulation of the profession.
- Cultivate collaborative and respectful relationships with physicians and learners in all areas of medicine and with other colleagues and partners in health care.

Commitment to self-care and peer support

- Value personal health and wellness and strive to model self-care; take steps to optimize meaningful co-existence of professional and personal life.
- Value and promote a training and practice culture that supports and responds effectively to colleagues in need and empowers them to seek help to improve their physical, mental, and social well-being.
- Recognize and act on the understanding that physician health and wellness needs to be addressed at individual and systemic levels, in a model of shared responsibility.

Commitment to inquiry and reflection

- Value and foster individual and collective inquiry and reflection to further medical science and to facilitate ethical decision-making.
- Foster curiosity and exploration to further your personal and professional development and insight; be open to new knowledge, technologies, ways of practising, and learning from others.

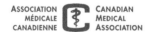

ASSOCIATION MÉDICALE CANADIENNE   CANADIAN MEDICAL ASSOCIATION

• **Fig. 2.3, cont'd.**

CMA PHYSICIAN'S CHARTER

C. PROFESSIONAL RESPONSIBILITIES

Physicians and patients

Patient-physician relationship

The patient–physician relationship is at the heart of the practice of medicine. It is a relationship of trust that recognizes the inherent vulnerability of the patient even as the patient is an active participant in their own care. The physician owes a duty of loyalty to protect and further the patient's best interests and goals of care by using the physician's expertise, knowledge, and prudent clinical judgment.

In the context of the patient–physician relationship:

1. Accept the patient without discrimination (such as on the basis of age, disability, gender identity or expression, genetic characteristics, language, marital and family status, medical condition, national or ethnic origin, political affiliation, race, religion, sex, sexual orientation, or socioeconomic status). This does not abrogate the right of the physician to refuse to accept a patient for legitimate reasons.

2. Having accepted professional responsibility for the patient, continue to provide services until these services are no longer required or wanted, or until another suitable physician has assumed responsibility for the patient, or until after the patient has been given reasonable notice that you intend to terminate the relationship.

3. Act according to your conscience and respect differences of conscience among your colleagues; however, meet your duty of non-abandonment to the patient by always acknowledging and responding to the patient's medical concerns and requests whatever your moral commitments may be.

4. Inform the patient when your moral commitments may influence your recommendation concerning provision of, or practice of any medical procedure or intervention as it pertains to the patient's needs or requests.

5. Communicate information accurately and honestly with the patient in a manner that the patient understands and can apply, and confirm the patient's understanding.

6. Recommend evidence-informed treatment options; recognize that inappropriate use or overuse of treatments or resources can lead to ineffective, and at times harmful, patient care and seek to avoid or mitigate this.

7. Limit treatment of yourself, your immediate family, or anyone with whom you have a similarly close relationship to minor or emergency interventions and only when another physician is not readily available; there should be no fee for such treatment.

8. Provide whatever appropriate assistance you can to any person who needs emergency medical care.

9. Ensure that any research to which you contribute is evaluated both scientifically and ethically and is approved by a research ethics board that adheres to current standards of practice. When involved in research, obtain the informed consent of the research participant and advise prospective participants that they have the right to decline to participate or withdraw from the study at any time, without negatively affecting their ongoing care.

10. Never participate in or condone the practice of torture or any form of cruel, inhuman, or degrading procedure.

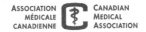

ASSOCIATION MÉDICALE CANADIENNE   CANADIAN MEDICAL ASSOCIATION

• **Fig. 2.4** Physicians' Charter from the Canadian Medical Association. (Source: Reprinted by permission of the Canadian Medical Association.)

Decision-making

Medical decision-making is ideally a deliberative process that engages the patient in shared decision-making and is informed by the patient's experience and values and the physician's clinical judgment. This deliberation involves discussion with the patient and, with consent, others central to the patient's care (families, caregivers, other health professionals) to support patient-centred care.

In the process of shared decision-making:

11. Empower the patient to make informed decisions regarding their health by communicating with and helping the patient (or, where appropriate, their substitute decision-maker) navigate reasonable therapeutic options to determine the best course of action consistent with their goals of care; communicate with and help the patient assess material risks and benefits before consenting to any treatment or intervention.

12. Respect the decisions of the competent patient to accept or reject any recommended assessment, treatment, or plan of care.

13. Recognize the need to balance the developing competency of minors and the role of families and caregivers in medical decision-making for minors, while respecting a mature minor's right to consent to treatment and manage their personal health information.

14. Accommodate a patient with cognitive impairments to participate, as much as possible, in decisions that affect them; in such cases, acknowledge and support the positive roles of families and caregivers in medical decision-making and collaborate with them, where authorized by the patient's substitute decision-maker, in discerning and making decisions about the patient's goals of care and best interests.

15. Respect the values and intentions of a patient deemed incompetent as they were expressed previously through advance care planning discussions when competent, or via a substitute decision-maker.

16. When the specific intentions of an incompetent patient are unknown and in the absence of a formal mechanism for making treatment decisions, act consistently with the patient's discernable values and goals of care or, if these are unknown, act in the patient's best interests.

17. Respect the patient's reasonable request for a second opinion from a recognized medical expert.

Physicians and the practice of medicine

Patient privacy and the duty of confidentiality

18. Fulfill your duty of confidentiality to the patient by keeping identifiable patient information confidential; collecting, using, and disclosing only as much health information as necessary to benefit the patient; and sharing information only to benefit the patient and within the patient's circle of care. Exceptions include situations where the informed consent of the patient has been obtained for disclosure or as provided for by law.

19. Provide the patient or a third party with a copy of their medical record upon the patient's request, unless there is a compelling reason to believe that information contained in the record will result in substantial harm to the patient or others.

20. Recognize and manage privacy requirements within training and practice environments and quality improvement initiatives, in the context of secondary uses of data for health system management, and when using new technologies in clinical settings.

21. Avoid health care discussions, including in personal, public, or virtual conversations, that could reasonably be seen as revealing confidential or identifying information or as being disrespectful to patients, their families, or caregivers.

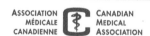

ASSOCIATION   CANADIAN
MÉDICALE   MEDICAL
CANADIENNE   ASSOCIATION

• **Fig. 2.4,** cont'd.

Managing and minimizing conflicts of interest

22. Recognize that conflicts of interest may arise as a result of competing roles (such as financial, clinical, research, organizational, administrative, or leadership).

23. Enter into associations, contracts, and agreements that maintain your professional integrity, consistent with evidence-informed decision-making, and safeguard the interests of the patient or public.

24. Avoid, minimize, or manage and always disclose conflicts of interest that arise, or are perceived to arise, as a result of any professional relationships or transactions in practice, education, and research; avoid using your role as a physician to promote services (except your own) or products to the patient or public for commercial gain outside of your treatment role.

25. Take reasonable steps to ensure that the patient understands the nature and extent of your responsibility to a third party when acting on behalf of a third party.

26. Discuss professional fees for non-insured services with the patient and consider their ability to pay in determining fees.

27. When conducting research, inform potential research participants about anything that may give rise to a conflict of interest, especially the source of funding and any compensation or benefits.

Physicians and self

28. Be aware of and promote health and wellness services, and other resources, available to you and colleagues in need.

29. Seek help from colleagues and appropriate medical care from qualified professionals for personal and professional problems that might adversely affect your health and your services to patients.

30. Cultivate training and practice environments that provide physical and psychological safety and encourage help-seeking behaviours.

Physicians and colleagues

31. Treat your colleagues with dignity and as persons worthy of respect. Colleagues include all learners, health care partners, and members of the health care team.

32. Engage in respectful communications in all media.

33. Take responsibility for promoting civility, and confronting incivility, within and beyond the profession. Avoid impugning the reputation of colleagues for personal motives; however, report to the appropriate authority any unprofessional conduct by colleagues.

34. Assume responsibility for your personal actions and behaviours and espouse behaviours that contribute to a positive training and practice culture.

35. Promote and enable formal and informal mentorship and leadership opportunities across all levels of training, practice, and health system delivery.

36. Support interdisciplinary team-based practices; foster team collaboration and a shared accountability for patient care.

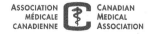

ASSOCIATION MÉDICALE CANADIENNE   CANADIAN MEDICAL ASSOCIATION

• **Fig. 2.4, cont'd.**

Physicians and society

37. Commit to ensuring the quality of medical services offered to patients and society through the establishment and maintenance of professional standards.

38. Recognize that social determinants of health, the environment, and other fundamental considerations that extend beyond medical practice and health systems are important factors that affect the health of the patient and of populations.

39. Support the profession's responsibility to act in matters relating to public and population health, health education, environmental determinants of health, legislation affecting public and population health, and judicial testimony.

40. Support the profession's responsibility to promote equitable access to health care resources and to promote resource stewardship.

41. Provide opinions consistent with the current and widely accepted views of the profession when interpreting scientific knowledge to the public; clearly indicate when you present an opinion that is contrary to the accepted views of the profession.

42. Contribute, where appropriate, to the development of a more cohesive and integrated health system through inter-professional collaboration and, when possible, collaborative models of care.

43. Commit to collaborative and respectful relationships with Indigenous patients and communities through efforts to understand and implement the recommendations relevant to health care made in the report of the Truth and Reconciliation Commission of Canada.

44. Contribute, individually and in collaboration with others, to improving health care services and delivery to address systemic issues that affect the health of the patient and of populations, with particular attention to disadvantaged, vulnerable, or underserved communities.

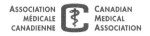

ASSOCIATION MÉDICALE CANADIENNE | CANADIAN MEDICAL ASSOCIATION

• **Fig. 2.4, cont'd.**

Provincial and Territorial Colleges of Physicians and Surgeons

Each province and territory has its own College of Physicians and Surgeons or equivalent licensing authority. Established by provincial and territorial legislation, the Colleges of Physicians and Surgeons are the official bodies that oversee complaints against, licensing, and disciplining of doctors. Physicians must be members to practise medicine in their province or territory. Close liaison is maintained between the provincial and territorial medical associations and the provincial Colleges; however, they are completely

separate and distinct from each other with unique goals and responsibilities.

Physician members of the College who have completed rigorous national examinations in a medical or surgical specialty are called *Royal Fellows*. To keep this distinction, physicians must be enrolled in the College's Maintenance of Certification program (MOC). Anyone can search the membership database on the College's website to determine whether a physician is a fellow. All physicians can apply to be certified by the College without having to become fellows; however, most do.

Family physicians are licensed but not certified by the Royal College of Physicians and Surgeons of Canada. They have their own College called *the College of Family Physicians of Canada*, and they have their own educational requirements. They too can become fellows of their College, but the designation is not earned through examinations; it is obtained by nomination after 10 years of certification with the College. In Québec, the Collège des médecins du Québec (CMQ) certifies both family physicians and specialty physicians.

DID YOU KNOW?

International Medical Graduates (IMGs) must undergo a multistep process to become fully licensed physicians in Canada. Although the process varies by province, IMGs generally take part in a process of approximately seven phases before they can practise independently. Requirements for each province and territory can be obtained from their College of Physicians and Surgeons.

ALBERTA
College of Physicians and Surgeons of Alberta
http://www.cpsa.ca/   Email: memberinquiries@cpsa.ab.ca

2700 Telus Plaza South   Telephone: 780-423-4764
10020-100 Street NW   Public inquiries: 1-800-561-3899
Edmonton, AB T5J 0N3   Physicians-only line: 1-800-320-8624
                               Fax: 780-420-0651

BRITISH COLUMBIA
College of Physicians and Surgeons of British Columbia
https://www.cpsbc.ca/   Email: registration@cpsbc.ca

300-669 Howe Street   Telephone: 604-733-7758
Vancouver, BC V6C 0B4   Toll-free: 1-800-461-3008
                               Fax: 604-733-3503

MANITOBA
College of Physicians and Surgeons of Manitoba
http://cpsm.mb.ca/   Email: TheRegistrar@cpsm.mb.ca

1000 - 1661 Portage Avenue   Telephone: 204-774-4344
Winnipeg, MB R3J 3T7   Fax: 204-774-0750

NEW BRUNSWICK
College of Physicians and Surgeons of New Brunswick
http://cpsnb.org/en/   Email: info@cpsnb.org

1 Hampton Road, Suite 300   Telephone: 506-849-5050 or
Rothesay, NB E2E 5K8   Toll-free: 1-800-667-4641
                               Fax: 506-849-5069

NEWFOUNDLAND AND LABRADOR
College of Physicians and Surgeons of Newfoundland & Labrador
https://www.cpsnl.ca/web/cpsnl   Email: cpsnl@cpsnl.ca

139 Water St, Suite 603   Telephone: 709-726-8546
Saint John's, NL A1C 1B2   Fax: 709-726-4725

NORTHWEST TERRITORIES
Health and Social Services
http://www.hss.gov.nt.ca/en Email: professional_licensing@gov.nt.ca

Government of the   Telephone: 867-920-8058
Northwest Territories   Fax: 867-873-0484
PO Box 1320
Yellowknife, NT X1A 2L9

NOVA SCOTIA
College of Physicians and Surgeons of Nova Scotia
https://cpsns.ns.ca/   Email: registration@cpsns.ns.ca

7071 Bayers Road   Telephone: 902-422-5823
Suite 5005   Toll-free: 1-877-282-7767
Halifax, NS B3L 2C2   Fax: 902-422-5035

NUNAVUT
Department of Health and Social Services
https://www.gov.nu.ca/health Email: info@gov.nu.ca

Government of Nunavut   Telephone: 1-877-212-6438
P.O. Box 1000 Station 200
Iqaluit, Nunavut X0A 0H0

ONTARIO
College of Physicians and Surgeons of Ontario
http://www.cpso.on.ca/   Email: feedback@cpso.on.ca

80 College Street   Telephone: 416-967-2603
Toronto, ON M5G 2E2   General inquiries: 1-800-268-7096
                              Physician inquiries: 416-967-2606

PRINCE EDWARD ISLAND
College of Physicians and Surgeons of Prince Edward Island
http://cpspei.ca/   Email: MelissaMacDonald@cpspei.ca

14 Paramount Drive   Telephone: 902-566-3861
Charlottetown, PE C1E 0C7 Fax: 902-566-3986

QUEBEC
Collège des médecins du Québec
http://www.cmq.org/   Email: info@cmq.org

1250 boulevard René-Lévesque Ouest Telephone: 514-933-4441
Suite 3500   Toll-free: 1-888-MÉDECIN
Montréal, QC H3B 0G2   Fax: 514-933-3112

SASKATCHEWAN
College of Physicians and Surgeons of Saskatchewan
https://www.cps.sk.ca/imis/   Email: cpss@quadrant.net

500-321A-21st Street East   Telephone: 306-244-7355
Saskatoon, SK S7K 0C1   Toll-free: 1-800-667-1668
                              Fax (general): 306-244-0090
                              Fax (registrar): 306-244-2600

YUKON
Yukon Medical Council
http://www.yukonmedicalcouncil.ca/   Email: ymc@gov.yk.ca

c/o Registrar of Medical Practitioners Telephone: 867-667-3774
Box 2703 C-18   Fax: 867-393-6483
Whitehorse, YT Y1A 2C6

• **Fig. 2.5** Provincial and Territorial Colleges of Physicians and Surgeons.

One practical way to identify a physician's membership type is by the professional designation in the signature. As a medical administrative assistant, you may be asked to explain what the abbreviations after a physician's name mean. See Box 2.4 for some common professional designations related to the Colleges. Physicians may use these abbreviations in addition to their Doctor of Medicine (MD) designation (e.g., J. E. Plunkett, MD, FRC(P)SC).

The Canadian Medical Protective Association

The Canadian Medical Protective Association is a mutual defence union of Canadian physicians. Mutual defence means that CMPA and its members have a shared responsibility to each other to practise in a manner consistent with the values of the medical profession. The association was founded in 1901, and its purpose is to provide its members with legal advice and counselling on any matters involving legal action. The association pays all legal costs incurred in the defence of such legal actions as well as any damages that the courts may award to the plaintiff. Members are also assisted with the defence of provincial governing body disciplinary actions, coroner inquests, and so on. Most provincial and territorial CMA branches, including those in Nova Scotia, Prince Edward Island, Yukon, Manitoba, and Saskatchewan, reimburse physicians for some portion of the cost of liability insurance they purchase through CMPA.

Although not their specific intention, the handbooks and articles published by the CMPA are of great value to medical administrative assistants. The publications help assistants gain an understanding of the important topics their employers deal with every day, and they provide information for reducing risk in the workplace. The handbooks contain practical information on topics such as records retention guidelines, age of majority for consent, how to safely deal with electronic information, and overall practice management. Medical administrative assistants can download informational posters for their offices and work with CMPA to create customized posters for topics related to risk management, such as using electronic records or providing informed consent. When using CMPA resources, it is important to make sure the most up-to-date information is being reviewed because the legislation upon which the information is based may change. See Box 2.5 for examples of CMPA handbooks. CMPA handbooks can be found on the association's website at https://www.cmpa-acpm.ca/en/advice-publications/handbooks.

World Health Organization

The World Health Organization (WHO) is the authority guiding international health within the United Nations. In Canada, the WHO collaborates with universities and provincial and federal agencies, such as Health Canada and the Public Health Agency of Canada, to research health trends, determine and report on risk factors, provide guidance and leadership through health emergencies, and set standards of ethical and technical practice for its members. One practical connection between medical administrative assistants and the WHO is through its International Classification of Diseases (ICD)—this publication (Box 2.6) outlines the diagnostic standards and associated diagnostic codes used to determine health trends. Its use is one way provinces and territories contribute health data. For instance, every patient who encounters a physician is assigned a diagnosis, and its diagnostic code is recorded during the billing process. We will further explore the ICD publication in later chapters.

Administrative Professionals' Associations

As mentioned in the introduction, there are associations that are more focused on the specific needs of administrative professionals. Membership can lead to opportunities for professional development, networking, volunteerism, leadership, and specialized designations through certifications (see Box 2.7; e.g., Jane Smith, CAP, CHDS). For a list of benefits related to association membership, see Box 2.8.

Association of Administrative Professionals (AAP)

Association of Administrative Professionals (AAP) is a Canadian chartered nonprofit professional organization founded in April 1951. The AAP is active in encouraging its members to

---

• BOX 2.4   Professional Designations for Doctors

FRCSC or FRC(P)SC: Fellow of the Royal College of Surgeons of Canada
FRCPC or FRCP(S)C: Fellow of the Royal College of Physicians of Canada
DRCPSC: Diplomat of Royal College of Physicians and Surgeons of Canada
FCFP: Fellow of the College of Family Physicians
CCFP: Certification in the College of Family Physicians
MCFP: Member of the College of Family Physicians
CMQ (FM): Collège des médecins du Québec Specialist's Certificate in Family Medicine

---

• BOX 2.5   CMPA Handbooks

Medical-Legal Handbook for Physicians in Canada
Consent: A Guide for Canadian Physicians
Electronic Records Handbook
Data Sharing Principles in Electronic Records Handbook
How Office Staff Can Help Reduce Risk (article)

• BOX 2.6   International Classification of Diseases

"ICD defines the universe of diseases, disorders, injuries and other related health conditions, listed in a comprehensive, hierarchical fashion that allows for: easy storage, retrieval and analysis of health information for evidenced-based decision-making; sharing and comparing health information between hospitals, regions, settings and countries; and data comparisons in the same location across different time periods."

Source: World Health Organization. (2018). *ICD Purposes and Uses.* Retrieved from http://www.who.int/classifications/icd/en/

• BOX 2.7   Designations for Administrative Professionals

CAP: Certified Administrative Professional
CCAP: Canadian Certified Administrative Professional
RHDS: Registered Healthcare Documentation Specialist
CHDS: Certified Healthcare Documentation Specialist
CHUC: Certified Health Unit Coordinator
CHIM: Certified Health Information Manager

---

further their education and enhance their career opportunities by continuously upgrading their skills and professionalism. Association members are encouraged to obtain the Canadian Certified Administrative Professional (CCAP) designation. The CCAP program can be attempted through a variety of modalities, including online, face-to-face, and correspondence courses (Association of Administrative Professionals [AAP], 2018a). There are several branches of AAP throughout Canada (Toronto, Barrie/Simcoe County, Calgary, Edmonton, Hamilton, and Moncton) offering memberships, conferences, publications, and discounts for office supplies and shipping services. For professionals who do not live in branch cities, they offer a "member-at-large" category. Students enrolled in a variety of administrative programs receive discounted membership rates and may serve on AAP committees (AAP, 2018b).

International Association of Administrative Professionals (IAAP)

International Association of Administrative Professionals (IAAP) is a professional association for administrative assistants from all backgrounds, including health care. This international association began as the National Secretaries Association in Kansas in 1942 and opened its first Canadian branch in Niagara Falls, Ontario, in 1954. It now offers opportunities for administrative professionals in every province of Canada and around the world (see Fig. 2.6). The association offers annual conferences, helpful publications, job search options, leadership opportunities, and certifications. The association has also been the sponsor of the now-popular Administrative Professionals Week/Day since 1952. Its well-known Certified Administrative Professional (CAP) program provides many benefits for its recipients (see Box 2.8) and even provides information on how to get employers to realize the benefits of supporting administrative assistants through membership. For students, membership fees are greatly reduced, and some student members may be eligible to receive credit toward the CAP certification by transferring college credits (International Association of Administrative Professionals [IAAP], 2018).

ARMA Canada

ARMA Canada is a division of ARMA International, an information management association with a membership that includes health records specialists and managers. There are ARMA Canada branches in New Brunswick, Prince Edward Island, Nova Scotia, Newfoundland, Ontario, Alberta, Manitoba, Saskatchewan, British Columbia, and Québec. Together, the ARMA Canada membership works to create standards of record information management (RIM) based on and supported by Canadian laws and regulations. Members support their goals through annual conferences, publications, and professional development. Currently, their focus involves best practices for moving businesses, including health care institutions, from paper-based records to digital records.

For new graduates interested in the records management field, ARMA offers a mentorship program whereby they connect new members with experienced information managers that assist them while they navigate the information management aspects of their jobs. All medical administrative assistants manage records in some way, even if they do not have a "records management" title. ARMA Canada membership can provide valuable resources that will help you navigate the privacy, retention, and maintenance issues that are associated with health records.

Canadian Health Information Management Association (CHIMA)

Canadian Health Information Management Association (CHIMA) is "the certifying body and national association that represents leadership and excellence in health information management (HIM). CHIMA supports continuing education and professional practice of HIM professionals" (CHIMA, 2018, para 1). Students enrolled in a recognized HIM program can apply for a student membership at a discounted rate, and students who graduate from an accredited HIM program can apply to CHIMA to write a national certification examination. Passing the examination earns the candidate the use of the Certified Health Information Manager (CHIM) designation for a period of three years (e.g., Jane Smith, CHIM). To maintain the CHIM credential, continuing education courses must be taken during the three-year period. CHIMA offers continuing education courses and specialized HIM certificates in both face-to-face and online formats to their membership and anyone else who is eligible. CHIMA has chapters in all Canadian provinces and territories.

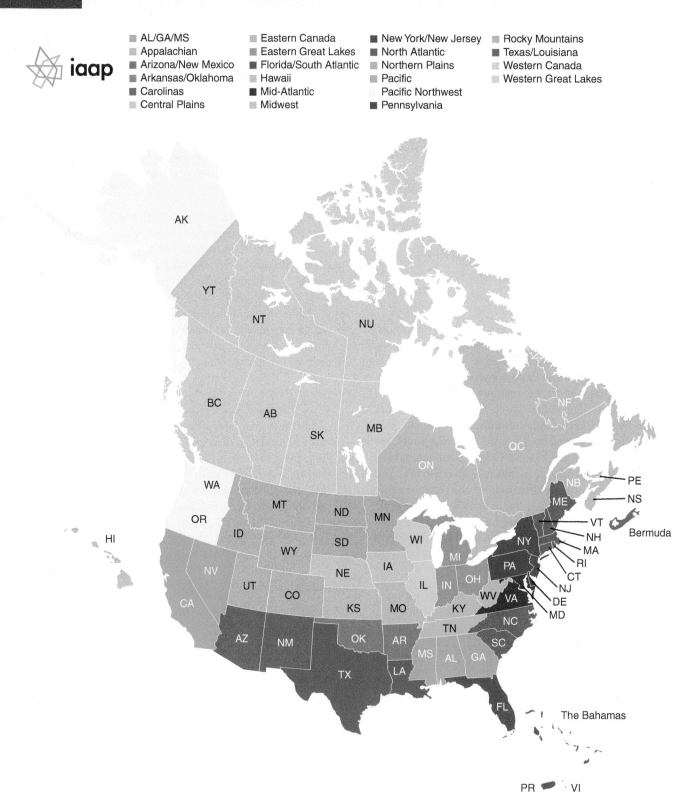

● **Fig. 2.6** International Association of Administrative Professionals membership map. (Source: Adapted from IAAP. (2018). *2018-2019 branch locations*. Retrieved from https://www.iaap-hq.org/page/ branch_map.)

Association for Healthcare Documentation Integrity (AHDI)

Association for Healthcare Documentation Integrity (AHDI) is a professional association for medical administrative assistants who perform medical transcription or speech recognition editing as a component of their job, or as their main area of employment. AHDI publishes *The Book of Style for Medical Transcription*; this publication is considered the gold-standard style manual for the health care documentation that you will encounter every day in your workplace.

AHDI provides many professional benefits of membership. The first benefit to students is that membership fees are waived, providing a great opportunity to get involved early in your career. AHDI also offers many opportunities for professional development through articles, webinars, conferences, online forums, and certifications. To prepare medical transcriptionists for certification, AHDI offers training, resources, and guidance on how to achieve success in the certification process. Certification is a two-level progression where candidates can first achieve their Registered Healthcare Documentation Specialist (RHDS) designation and then their Certified Healthcare Documentation Specialist (CHDS) designation. In May of each year, AHDI sponsors National Medical Transcriptionist Week to celebrate the achievements of medical transcription specialists and their contributions to patient safety through accurate, timely, and standardized documentation.

National Association for Health Unit Coordinators (NAHUC)

Many medical administrative assistants take courses in health unit coordinating in conjunction with, or in addition to, their medical administrative training so that they may work in hospitals as unit clerks, ward clerks, or unit secretaries. The National Association for Health Unit Coordinators (NAHUC) is an association focused on providing support, certification, and standards of practice for health unit coordinators. As with the other associations mentioned, the benefits of belonging to the association include opportunities for networking, leadership, and continuing education. The association is based in the United States but is recognized across Canada with many members, some of whom have become certified, allowing them to use the designation of Certified Health Unit Coordinator (CHUC; e.g., Jane Smith, CHUC). NAHUC certifies practising health unit coordinators through a national examination process created by practitioners, educators, and supervisors from the health care industry. Certification is valid for three years, at which point recertification is required and can be obtained by reexamination or by earning educational credits over the three-year period of certification. NAHUC offers discounted membership rates for students enrolled in an educational program related to health unit coordinating. The association also hosts annual conferences and celebrate Health Unit Coordinator Recognition Week in August of each year.

Medical Office Assistants Association of British Columbia

British Columbia has a provincial organization known as the Medical Office Assistants Association of British Columbia (MOAA of BC). The group is dedicated to the professional advancement of its members and also to providing networking that binds the groups together. Anyone who is employed in a medical office in an assisting capacity is eligible. Members include receptionists, secretaries, office managers, nurses, and technicians. MOAA of BC also provides student memberships at half the cost of regular membership.

Legal Considerations

Medical administrative assistants and other medical aides who are employees of doctors are usually considered to be doctors' agents. Doctors are likely to be held responsible for the acts of their agents. In its Medical-Legal Handbook for Physicians in Canada, CMPA calls this principle *respondeat superior*—let the principal answer (CMPA, 2016). Hence an awareness of medico-legal problems is of great importance to medical administrative assistants so that they do not cause negative consequences for their employers; they need to be knowledgeable about the rules and regulations that govern the practice of medicine and about the consequences when rules are not followed. It should be noted that medical administrative assistants and other related medical staff may also be held personally responsible for their own actions.

Rules and Regulations

Just as all other disciplines and human endeavours are subject to rules and regulations, so too is the practice of medicine. As you have already discovered, doctors practise their profession under a well-defined and time-honoured ethical code. Even though doctors have the same general responsibilities as all citizens do, they have special additional responsibilities specific to their profession.

To practise medicine in Canada, a doctor must be licensed by the provincial or territorial College of Physicians and Surgeons or its equivalent, such as the CMQ. The profession and the College must operate under clearly defined rules as set out in the relevant provincial or territorial legislation and the regulations made under the medical acts. For example, each province has a *Physicians' Administrative Manual,* or similarly named publication, which discusses statutes relevant to the practice of medicine in that province. A *Physicians' Legal Manual* or its equivalent should also be available. All doctors and medical administrative assistants should obtain and read a copy of the legislation and regulations that apply to them. Copies of regulations and pertinent statutes can be obtained by contacting the Queen's Printer for the province or territory, or the government bookstore.

Health care facilities have facility bylaws, medical staff bylaws, and medical staff rules. Any physician with privileges to practise within that facility must abide by these bylaws and rules.

DID YOU KNOW?

In 2018, there were 84,260 physicians licensed to practise medicine in Canada. Of these, 43,500 were family physicians, and 34% of these family physicians practised in Ontario.

Source: CMA. (2018). Physicians by Province/Territory and Specialty. Retrieved from https://www.cma.ca/Assets/assets-library/./01-physicians-by-specialty-province-e.pdf

Other Statutes

Doctors and their staff should also be acquainted with other statutes that touch on or affect the practice of medicine in their province. Some examples of these statutes are listed in Box 2.9.

Consideration should also be given to the fact that the practice of medicine may be controlled by certain federal statutes, most notably the *Food and Drugs Act, the Controlled Drugs and Substances Act, the Cannabis Act*, and others.

Reporting

Practising physicians should be particularly aware that the statutes mentioned previously require mandatory reporting in certain circumstances. For example, reports may have to be submitted to the children's aid society of your province or territory as outlined in the associated *Child and Family Services Act* (CFSA) for your region. Reports may also need to be submitted to the Registrar of Motor Vehicles under most Highway Traffic acts or Motor Vehicle acts, to your provincial or territorial Workers' Compensation Board under the *Workers Compensation Act*, and so on. If a doctor does not know how to go about reporting to these boards and agencies, a telephone call or letter to them will produce the desired procedures. A copy of *Determining Medical Fitness to Operate Motor Vehicles: CMA Driver's Guide* (9th ed.) can be obtained from the CMA. Information about reporting communicable diseases can be obtained by contacting the local, regional, provincial, or territorial health department. Not reporting something that is required by law to be reported can result in the imposition of fines or in charges of professional misconduct, or both.

Medico-Legal Problems

Doctors may be faced with a number of legal situations, such as partnership agreements, contracts with employees, estate planning, leases, and so on. In addition, doctors can encounter problems of a medico-legal nature. Rarely will a doctor face a criminal charge related to the practice of medicine. However, fraud, violations of the *Controlled Drugs and Substances Act*, and allegations of sexual assault are examples of possible instances in which a doctor could be charged. Most physicians will have a nurse or the medical administrative assistant present when a patient presents with a problem that requires a vaginal examination, or when the patient is booked for an annual physical examination. A doctor is seldom charged with criminal negligence as a result of the professional care of a patient. (The term *criminal negligence* refers to reckless or wanton disregard for a patient's welfare.)

It is more common for physicians to face civil medico-legal problems. Medical malpractice actions can be brought against doctors in small claims or provincial courts or in courts of superior jurisdiction, such as the supreme courts or Court of Queen's Bench in each province. There may be one or several claims asserted for any one action.

A contract exists between a doctor and the patient. Although this does not take the form of a written document, a "contract" is implied when the patient requests an examination and treatment from the doctor and the doctor makes a commitment, probably unspoken, to treat the patient. Either party could breach the contract: A claim by the doctor against the patient is likely to be related to the financial aspect of the relationship; the patient may feel that the doctor has not met the patient's expectations and may be tempted to start a legal action. The patient may claim that the contract was breached because the result of treatment was not what the patient thought was promised by the doctor.

More often, however, a medico-legal action is commenced against a physician from allegations of negligence. What is negligence? Negligence is a term used to describe the alleged failure of a person to exercise a reasonable and acceptable standard of care, thereby causing harm or injury to another.

Malpractice actions alleging negligence generally fall into one of two categories. The first category includes those cases in which a patient alleges that the treatment rendered by the doctor was negligent in a medical sense. For example, while the patient is undergoing surgery for removal of a gallbladder (cholecystectomy), his or her bowel is punctured by the surgeon. The second category, increasing in frequency, includes claims by the patient that the physician was negligent by failing to disclose sufficiently beforehand the risks of the treatment. Claims of this nature come under the expression "lack of informed consent" (see Box 2.10 for a definition of informed consent and Box 2.11 for criteria).

• BOX 2.9   Statutes

Child and Family Services Act
Coroners Act
Health Insurance Act
Health Protection and Promotion Act
Highway Traffic and Aeronautics Acts
Nursing Home Act
Pharmacy Act
Public Hospitals Act
Vital Statistics Act

• BOX 2.10   Informed Consent

The patient must be aware of the nature and risks of the treatment, of not having the treatment, and of any alternative treatment. The general rule is that, unless there is an emergency, before any medical treatment or medication can be undertaken, the patient must give his or her consent (verbal or written); without consent, there can be no treatment or medication (see Box 2.11 for the criteria for valid consent). The proposed treatment must be explained to the patient by the physician, never by the administrative assistant or the nurse. Consent can be witnessed by someone other than the physician after the proposed treatment has been explained to the patient.

• BOX 2.11   Criteria for Valid Consent

- The consent must be given voluntarily.
- There must exist in the patient the mental capacity to provide the consent.
- The patient must have the legal capacity to give the consent.
- The patient's consent must be directed or related to a specific treatment or set of treatments.
- The consent given by the patient must be an informed consent.
- The patient must consent to the person who will be treating him or her.

• BOX 2.12   CMA Code of Ethics on Diversity

"In providing medical service, do not discriminate against any patient on such grounds as age, gender, marital status, medical condition, national or ethnic origin, physical or mental disability, political affiliation, race, religion, sexual orientation, or socioeconomic status" (CMA Code of Ethics, 2004, para 5).

Special considerations and practices must be in place when seeking consent from patients with differing religious beliefs, practices, and attitudes. CMPA offers physicians and other health care providers advice and education on "cultural safety" that directly addresses physicians' responsibilities as outlined in CMA's Code of Ethics (see Box 2.12).

CMPA outlines how physicians can broaden their cultural knowledge to meet the expectations of patients from all cultures; it provides advice on how to avoid discrimination, deal with issues when duty clashes with cultural beliefs, and manage special requests based on culture and religion. In the case of informed consent, physicians may need to take extra time to make sure a patient whose first language is not English understands any procedures being explained; they may need the assistance of an interpreter to ensure that the patient fully understands the proposed procedure because some cultures have restrictions related to blood products and organ donations. As the physician's agent, the medical administrative assistant must also make efforts to become more culturally knowledgeable and communicative. It is important for the patient and, in some cases, the patient's family to feel welcome and respected. You should have resources in place for contacting interpreters; you should also be willing to adjust your communication style (use pictures, use simple language, and pay special attention to nonverbal cues) and be prepared to provide written material that the patient can take home.

If patients feel that they have received treatment for which consent was not given, they may allege assault and battery. Recent case law has established that for there to be a claim for assault and battery, the treatment carried out must be wholly unrelated to or different from that treatment

• BOX 2.13   Competent Adult

The person has the ability to understand the subject matter in respect of which considered requests are made and is able to appreciate the consequences of giving or withholding consent.

discussed earlier with the patient. Overriding the issue of consent is the "emergency rule," whereby in circumstances in which it is essential to treat someone to save the person's life or prevent serious permanent injury and it is impossible to ask the person's consent, a health professional can treat that person. If the patient in an emergency situation refuses treatment, the health professional cannot act, assuming the patient is competent. For a definition of what constitutes competency, see Box 2.13.

DID YOU KNOW?

"Medical tourism," or patients seeking medical care outside of Canada, is an emerging trend in health care. Patients may consent to treatments without being fully informed by the out-of-country physician. They may also receive substandard care due to inadequate regulations for medical tourism. If that patient seeks advice or advocacy from a Canadian physician before becoming coming a "tourist," the Canadian physician may be at risk of legal action.

Source: CMPA. (2016). Emerging trends and medical-legal risks in medical tourism. Retrieved from https://www.cmpa-acpm.ca/en/advice-publications/browse-articles/2016/emerging-trends-and-medical-legal-risks-in-medical-tourism

Other civil claims, in addition to medical negligence, lack of informed consent, or assault and battery, may be those that allege breach of medical confidentiality or defamation.

As well as, or perhaps instead of, suing a doctor, a patient may complain about the doctor's professional work. The complaint may be expressed directly to the doctor or to a member of the doctor's staff. It may be submitted to officials of the hospital that the doctor is affiliated with or to the College of Physicians and Surgeons or its equivalent.

Complaints or claims against doctors sometimes arise out of certain aspects of the practice of medicine with which medical administrative assistants have considerable involvement. The competent medical administrative assistant should pay heed to the following considerations.

Confidentiality

Every patient has the right to expect that the information the doctor has obtained about him or her, on the basis of what the patient or others have told the doctor or what the doctor has discovered by examination and other means, will be kept confidential by the doctor. This duty applies also to the doctor's staff.

Information about a patient must never be revealed to anyone (except, of course, the patient) unless required by law or unless authorized by the patient or by the person legally responsible for the patient (in the case, for example, of a minor or developmentally delayed patient). The physician can disclose patient information under the mandatory reporting requirements of certain statutes that require physicians to provide information that otherwise would be confidential. A physician who has questions about specific situations can contact the CMPA through his or her provincial or territorial College of Physicians and Surgeons (see Fig. 2.5). Unauthorized persons should not have access to appointment lists or other information, and certainly not to patients' records or to the information contained therein. Even the information that the patient was seen by the doctor should be considered confidential.

A doctor or medical administrative assistant should not release medical information to a third party unless properly authorized in writing to do so. An authorization should state clearly what is intended, and it should be dated. The authorization should be kept in the doctor's possession in case it is later alleged that a breach of medical confidentiality occurred.

If an inquirer, other than the patient, approaches a medical administrative assistant for information about a patient, it should be pointed out that the request for information should be put in writing and should be accompanied by an appropriate authorization, signed by the patient or the person responsible for the patient. Inquiries by the patient's lawyer, insurer, or employer must be in writing and must, as with all other requests for medical information, be accompanied by the patient's signed authorization.

CRITICAL THINKING

An official you know to be a member of the Royal Canadian Mounted Police (or your local police service) presents to your office and asks for the list of patients attending your office that day. What do you tell them? If you do not know what to tell them, who can you consult?

All patients have the right to know where their information is and what it is used for after being collected by your office. To protect these rights, the federal government developed the *Personal Information Protection and Electronic Documents Act* (PIPEDA), which governs all "commercial activities" and came into force in January 2004. Publicly funded hospitals, long-term care facilities, and home-care services are exempt from PIPEDA; however, their private counterparts are generally not. PIPEDA would apply to private physicians' offices, including family doctors, medical specialists, chiropractors, optometrists, and so on. However, federal law contains a provision stating that if a province can demonstrate to the federal government that it has legislation that is substantially similar in terms of the level of privacy protection it affords, the provincial or territorial law will prevail. Many provinces have created comparable legislation that has a specific focus on health care. Some of the new laws are applied in conjunction with PIPEDA (Saskatchewan, Manitoba, Yukon, and Northwest Territories), and some are substantial enough to replace it

(British Columbia, Alberta, Québec, Ontario, New Brunswick, Nova Scotia, Newfoundland, and Labrador) (Office of the Privacy Commissioner of Canada, 2018). In 2017, Prince Edward Island enacted its *Health Information Act*; however, it has yet to go through the process of being deemed "substantially similar." The Office of the Privacy Commissioner of Canada provides an up-to-date list of provincial and territorial privacy laws and oversight. It is good practice to have your provincial or territorial privacy statement displayed where patients can easily read it.

Medical Records

Proper medical records are considered an essential component of the physician–patient relationship. Whether your office uses an electronic medical record, a paper record, or some combination of the two, the main reason for making and keeping records is to assist the doctor and health care team in the continuing care of the patient.

The importance of complete and comprehensive records from a medico-legal point of view cannot be overemphasized. CMPA offers guidelines and advice on records management through many publications, including the *Electronic Records Handbook* that was previously noted in Box 2.5. This important handbook provides information on how to select an appropriate electronic records system, on regulations associated with electronic records, on security and privacy issues, and on transferring and destroying electronic records. In some provinces, the regulations or bylaws of the College of Physicians and Surgeons or its equivalent specify minimum standards for maintaining, organizing, and retaining medical records by physicians. For example, a section of the regulations under the *Regulated Health Professions Act* requires that a member shall do the following:

(1) Keep a legible written or printed record with respect to each patient of the member containing the following information:
   (a) the name, address, and date of birth of the patient
   (b) if the patient has health insurance, the health insurance number
   (c) for a consultation, the name and address of the primary care physician and of any health professional who referred the patient
   (d) every written report received respecting the patient from another member or health professional
   (e) the date of each professional encounter with the patient
   (f) a record of the assessment of the patient including
      i)   the history obtained by the member
      ii) the particulars of each medical examination by the member, and
      iii) a note of any investigations ordered by the member and the results of the investigations
   (g) a record of the disposition of the patient, including
      i)   an indication of each treatment prescribed or administered by the member
      ii) a record of professional advice given by the member, and
      iii) particulars of any referral made by the member

(h) a record of all fees charged that were not in respect of insured services under the *Health Insurance Act*, which may be kept separately from the clinical record

(i) any additional records required by regulation

(2) Keep a daybook, daily diary, or appointment record containing the name of each patient who is encountered professionally or treated or for whom a professional service is rendered by the member.

Generally speaking, entries in a patient's record—paper or electronic—should be accurately dated when written, typed, or entered into a software. All significant information should be entered into the record, including personal and family data, the past and present history obtained by the doctor, the doctor's findings, advice and recommendations concerning investigation and treatment, discussion of risks of treatment, alternative forms of therapy, and any other pertinent information about the patient's medical management. Events that may or may not involve the doctor should also be entered in the record—for example, vital signs taken by the nurse, changed or cancelled appointments, the issuance of printed instructions or pamphlets to the patient, referral arrangements, consents for disclosure of personal health information (see Fig. 2.7), and so on.

If a patient is thought to be allergic to certain medications, the office record should contain a clearly discernible warning to that effect, so that this important information is readily available whenever a prescription is given to the patient. Likewise, patient charts should be "flagged" when follow-up appointments, review examinations, and so forth are necessary.

Some doctors use "Problem Lists" in their records. These are a type of flow sheet on which diagnoses and other important clinical information are recorded. Such information is thereby readily available to the doctor for review at the time of each encounter with the patient.

Many doctors find it useful to keep a copy of each prescription given to the patient in the patient's record. An entry should be made in the record whenever a prescription is given or renewed by telephone.

Your access to the medical record may be different based on its format—whether paper or electronic. In an electronic system, medical administrative assistants may have access only to areas of the record that relate specifically to administrative tasks and may have no access or limited access to other areas. For instance, you will likely have full access to the appointment schedule, but you may be able only to view (and not to edit or enter) clinical information such as vital signs or medications. It is important in an electronic system that you do not share your password with co-workers because every entry, every deletion, and every page viewed can be tracked. If you share your access with someone who is "snooping" or making inappropriate changes to a record, you may get the blame for breaching privacy or worse.

Retention of Records

Although each province has its own regulatory act that states the appropriate retention schedules in the province or territory, you can easily obtain the information from the College of Physicians and Surgeons for your province or territory. Confirming retention times with the College of Physicians and Surgeons will avoid errors and allow you to adapt to any changes. In some cases, the College may recommend a retention schedule that is different from the provincial or territorial act. Hospitals and physicians' offices sometimes have different retention requirements, and different types of records within the same institution may need to be kept for different lengths of time. For instance, documents needed for continuing care, such as history and physicals or operative reports, may need to be kept longer than documents that are not required for the future care of the patient, such as dietary records or administrative checklists. Medical administrative assistants in private offices should be aware of the requirements and establish appropriate practices to ensure that the schedule is followed. If you are a member of ARMA or CHIMA, these associations may be able to assist in the establishment and maintenance of these important practices. Government-run facilities employ dedicated records information managers or health information managers.

Apart from the aforementioned statutory requirements, it is wise for doctors to keep their medical records for as long as there is an appreciable risk that the records may be required for the purpose of defence against a complaint or claim. Clinical records are often the most important single factor in the defence of a lawsuit arising out of a doctor's work. They are also often necessary when dealing with a complaint to the provincial or territorial licensing authority. A doctor should maintain control over records as long as possible.

When doctors leave a practice because of retirement or for any other reason, or when they relocate their practices, they should ensure that their records are kept intact, that they are accessible, and that the information contained in them is available to their patients' new doctors. When a doctor dies, the estate should make appropriate arrangements for the safekeeping of records until there is no likelihood that a claim will be made against the estate. It is prudent for physicians to include in estate planning provisions for the care of their medical records. When a physician in family medicine and primary care ceases to practise medicine, the physician can either transfer records to a member with the same address and telephone number or notify each patient that the records will be destroyed two years after the notification. The patient may obtain the records or have the member transfer the records to another physician within the two years.

Release of Records

Occasionally, patients or relatives of patients will ask for their records for one reason or another. It is generally considered that the record is the property of the doctor or clinic and not that of the patient. However, patients are entitled to have access to and receive copies of their entire medical record, including all notes made by the attending

**Standard Consent Form
to Disclose Personal Health Information to a Third Party**

I, _____ , authorize ___*Dr. Plunkett's Office*___ to disclose my personal health
  (Print your full name)   *(Name of health care practitioner)*

information listed below for the purpose of

_____
(Describe the purpose/use for the request)

_____

consisting of _____
    (List the personal health information to be disclosed)

_____

_____

to _____
  (Print name and address of third party requesting health information)

**I understand the purpose for disclosing this personal health information, and I understand how
the information will be used. I understand that I can refuse to sign this consent form.**

Name: _____

Address: _____

City: _____ **Province:** _____ **Postal Code:** _____

Telephone (home): _____ **Telephone (cell):** _____

Signature: _____ **Date:** _____

Witness Name: _____

Address: _____

City: _____ **Province:** _____ **Postal Code:** _____

Telephone (home): _____ **Telephone (cell):** _____

Signature: _____ **Date:** _____

• **Fig. 2.7** Consent to disclose personal health information. (Source: Ontario Ministry of Health and Long-Term Care. [2018]. *Authorization to disclose* personal health information [Sample form]. Retrieved from http://www.health.gov.on.ca/english/providers/project/priv_legislation/consent/consent_disclose_form.pdf.)

physician and all consultation reports that are part of the attending physician's records, even where these are marked as confidential. This applies to information compiled in the context of the physician–patient relationship. Physicians may charge a reasonable fee for preparing and copying records; the CMA or its local branch may provide guidelines on how much to charge for this uninsured service. Similar information can be found in most *Personal Health Information Acts.*

DID YOU KNOW?

General guidelines for copying medical records can include a *general fee* for locating and preparing the file (approximately $30), *direct fees* for mailing or couriering the file, and *specific fees* for photocopies, electronic transmissions, microfilm creation, audio recordings, review of record by the custodian, and so on.

A physician may refuse to give a patient access to his or her records if the doctor believes that such access would result in a substantial risk to the physical, mental, or emotional health of the patient or would result in harm to a third party. The physician must exercise this discretion reasonably and for very limited purposes. The patient may challenge the physician's decision in court. The onus is on the physician to justify the denial of access to records in such cases.

Medical administrative assistants should not give the doctor's office record (or a photocopy of it), or the information contained in the record (including consultants' reports, laboratory and x-ray reports, and so on), to a patient or a relative to read. Such records and reports frequently require interpretation for the patient, and the doctor's administrative assistant should arrange for the patient to have time with the doctor to discuss the information in the record.

Of course, if the doctor is presented with a court order to produce a patient's record, the doctor must comply, but steps should be taken to ensure that a duplicate copy of the record is kept by the doctor. The doctor should also retain a copy of the court order.

A second exception to releasing patients' records might arise when the doctor is served with a subpoena or a summons requiring submission of evidence in any legal action or other proceeding. The doctor may have to bring along a copy of the patient's office record. On occasion, a doctor may also be directed to forward a copy of a patient's record to the College of Physicians and Surgeons or its equivalent.

If a lawyer requests records, the physician can send only patient records that apply to the physician's direct patient care. Consultation notes, correspondence, and such from other physicians involved in the patient's care *must not* be released.

When organizing referrals and the supporting documentation to specialist physicians, medical administrative assistants should be careful to include only information that is relevant to the referral. For instance, if your doctor is sending a patient referral to an orthopedic surgeon, information about the patient's gynecological history is not relevant. Never release more information than is necessary for the proper treatment of the patient in each circumstance.

CRITICAL THINKING

At the patient's request, and with the doctor's permission, you have prepared a photocopy of her medical file. You present the patient with an invoice for the uninsured service, and she expresses that she cannot afford the charge. Unfortunately, you did not provide her with a quote prior to copying the file. What do you do? How could you have prevented the situation?

Transfer of Records

If a patient decides to transfer to another doctor's practice, the patient may ask the first doctor to forward the record to the second doctor, or the new doctor may ask for the record. A doctor should comply with such a request by sending a summary of the record or, if the first doctor prefers, a photocopy of pertinent portions of it. The first doctor should retain possession or control of the actual record. On occasion, a doctor may have custody of another provider's record. Before transmitting such records or photocopies, the doctor might like to obtain medico-legal advice. See Box 2.14 for a list of steps to follow when transferring patient records.

The doctor should obtain appropriate authorization from the patient, or the patient's legal guardian, even when transferring medical information or clinical record material to the patient's new doctor.

When a summary or photocopy of the record is sent to another doctor, a notation should be made in the record indicating when and to whom it was sent.

Medical Reports

The Code of Ethics of the CMA adopted in most provinces states, "An ethical physician will, on the patient's request, assist him by supplying the information required to enable the patient to receive any benefits to which the patient may be entitled." This ethical duty is also affected in the province of Ontario by the regulations under the

• BOX 2.14 Transfer of Records

- Obtain written authorization from the patient, the patient's Power of Attorney, or legal guardian.
- Obtain a prepared summary or copy the pertinent information.
- Send requested information, including a copy of the release of information.
- Make a notation in the chart stating when and where the information was sent.
- Retain the original chart for the first physician.

Regulated Health Professions Act, which requires the doctor to provide within a reasonable time "any report or certificate requested by a patient or his authorized agent in respect of an examination or treatment performed by the member." There is therefore a clear obligation, imposed ethically and by law, for a doctor to provide the patient or the patient's authorized agent with a report when requested to do so.

Unless reporting is required by legislation, as mentioned earlier, a doctor should obtain a signed authorization from the patient before releasing medical information (see Fig. 2.7). In other words, if a doctor is going to provide information about a patient to a third party, appropriate authorization must be obtained before doing so. When the information contained in the report is of a particularly sensitive nature, the patient should be alerted to the contents of the report. Whenever a doctor prepares a report, issues a certificate, or completes a form, a copy should be filed in the patient's chart. In some situations, the patient will not be entitled to receive a copy of the report from the physician and should be so advised.

A special kind of report is a medico-legal report, that is, one that is requested by a lawyer. The College of Physicians and Surgeons expects a doctor to provide a patient's lawyer with a report if requested to do so. The lawyer's request should be written, providing the doctor with an appropriate authorization signed by the patient or, if the patient is deceased, by the executor or administrator of the patient's estate. This authorization should outline specifically what information is required. If a proper authorization (sometimes called a "direction" or "release") does not accompany the lawyer's request, the doctor should ask the lawyer for one before submitting a medical report. The doctor's report should be forwarded to the lawyer within a reasonable period of time. The doctor should keep a copy of the report. Medico-legal reports are considered an uninsured service in many areas, so your doctor may charge the requesting lawyer for this report based on time spent to create the document.

If the doctor has reason to believe that the patient consulted a lawyer because of dissatisfaction with the doctor's care, the doctor may wish to seek the advice of a medical defence organization, such as CMPA, before responding to the lawyer.

Miscellaneous

Medical administrative assistants are active members of the health care team and may encounter problems that could have legal implications for their employers. A knowledgeable, engaged, and caring medical administrative assistant can play a significant role in the prevention of some of these problems. Alternatively, a medical administrative assistant who is not actively engaged in the patient care experience may unintentionally overlook or contribute to unprofessional, or even negligent, actions while dealing with the day-to-day events in doctors' offices and clinics. The paragraphs below highlight some common situations and offer advice on how to avoid problems.

Each medical administrative assistant should discuss with the doctor in advance the type of advice he or she may give by telephone and should confirm the doctor's instructions about dealing with requests for appointments, referrals, reports, and so on.

Problems may be averted by an efficient system for handling incoming telephone calls and for noting the nature of the call in the patient's record. Chapter 5 offers a more detailed discussion about handling calls.

Medical administrative assistants who witness patients signing consent for treatment forms should assure themselves that the forms correctly describe the proposed treatment. Information should be cross-checked with patients' charts, or the doctor should be consulted if there is any question about the treatment noted on the consent. Medical administrative assistants should recognize the characteristics of informed consent and understand their contributions to the process. For instance, medical administrative assistants should satisfy themselves with the identity and competence of the patients who sign such forms. Should a patient have questions about the proposed procedure, the doctor should be notified specifically that the patient has unanswered questions and concerns.

The physician will assess whether the patient is competent. If there is any doubt, he will notify the patient's family, the legal guardian, or the person holding the Power of Attorney (POA) before obtaining consent.

A child of any age can give or refuse consent. The physician will assess the child's competency to understand the information presented to obtain informed consent. The child's consent must meet the criteria of the adult's consent.

Bookings for operative and investigative procedures should be exact and clear. Copies of booking slips should be retained. Notations should be made in patients' records about the arrangements that have been made.

Injuries sustained by a patient in a doctor's office can lead to a claim for damages. Those who work in medical offices should always be alert to situations that could put patients' safety in jeopardy.

Historically, the medical profession has been very aware of the confidentiality of patient information. The enactment of federal and provincial freedom of information legislation reinforces the importance of confidentiality. Before releasing any information concerning a patient, it is imperative that you secure in writing the permission of the patient. It is also important to remember that freedom of information and access legislation may allow patient access to records upon application to the appropriate provincial or territorial privacy and access department. Medical administrative assistants should make themselves familiar with this process by consulting with the appropriate government department.

Summary

Medical administrative assistants need to develop a holistic view of Canadian health care to become competent, valuable members of health care teams. An understanding of the associations that affect the decisions and drive the actions of health care employers is essential for forming this outlook. This chapter has provided valuable insight into potential medico-legal problems and the rules and regulations that guide the medical profession. You have discovered practical information related to confidentiality, medical records, and consent. Insight into the connection between the responsibilities of a medical administrative assistant and health care laws, ethical codes, and the associations that address them has been provided.

Assignments

Assignment 2.1

Go to the IAAP website (https://www.iaap-hq.org/). Find the IAAP Code of Conduct and review its contents, including the ethical standards section. Find the similarities between the ethical standards section of the IAAP's Code of Conduct and the CMA's Code of Ethics. Outline your comparisons.

Assignment 2.2

Go to the AHDI website (https://www.ahdionline.org/) and navigate to the *Certification* tab on the *Home* page. Create a report on eligibility for each of the certifications offered by AHDI. Include a reflection on how a membership in this association could advance your career.

Assignment 2.3

Using the contact information provided in the chapter, compare the goals and responsibilities of your provincial or territorial College of Physicians and Surgeons with those of your provincial or territorial branch of CMA. Note the main differences between the two organizations. Describe why it is important for you as a medical administrative assistant to be familiar with each.

Assignment 2.4

Navigate to your local College of Physicians and Surgeons or equivalent and find information on records retention for your province or territory.

Topics for Discussion

1. Read the Oath of Hippocrates and try to find information within it that relates to everyday ethical and legal issues in modern medicine. Do you think the Oath still applies to medicine in modern times?
2. In 2015 the government of Canada amended its position on medical assistance in dying. Visit the Canadian government website at https://www.canada.ca/en.html and navigate to the Health/Health System and Services/Health Service/End-of-Life Care/Medical Assistance for Dying. Read the information on the page and consider your opinions about this issue. How will you separate your feelings about the topic from your role as a medical administrative assistant?
3. A patient has disclosed to you that the physician has done something inappropriate. The patient wants to report the doctor and is asking you for guidance on how to do this. How would you handle this situation?
4. Discuss some ways in which you can become more culturally competent, communicate with non-English-speaking patients, and be more sensitive to the needs of minority groups in your community.
5. Medical administrative assistants and other medical aides act on behalf of the doctor. Discuss some scenarios in which the doctor may be held responsible for his or her staff's actions. How can you avoid unprofessional, negligent, or illegal behaviours that your employer may be responsible for?

References

Association of Administrative Professionals. (2018a). *CCAP designation*. Retrieved from https://canadianadmin.ca/qaa-designation/overview/.

Association of Administrative Professionals. (2018b). *Members*. Retrieved from https://canadianadmin.ca/members/member-benefits/.

Canadian Health Information Management Association. (2018). *About CHIMA*. Retrieved from https://www.echima.ca/chima/about.

Canadian Medical Association and Joule Inc. (2000). *About CMA and CMA companies*. Retrieved from https://www.cma.ca/En/Pages/about-cma.aspx.

Canadian Medical Protective Association. (2016). *Medical-legal handbook for Canadian physicians* (2 ed). Retrieved from. https://www.cmpa-acpm.ca/en/advice-publications/handbooks.

Canadian Medical Protective Association. (n.d.). *About CMPA*. Retrieved from https://www.cmpa-acpm.ca/en/about

International Association of Administrative Professionals. (2018). *Certified administrative professional*. Retrieved from https://www.iaap-hq.org/page/Certification.

Office of the Privacy Commissioner of Canada. (2018). *Provincial legislation deemed substantially similar to PIPEDA*. Retrieved from https://www.priv.gc.ca/en/privacy-topics/privacy-laws-in-canada/the-personal-information-protection-and-electronic-documents-act-pipeda/r_o_p/provincial-legislation-deemed-substantially-similar-to-pipeda/.

Rodgers, T. L. (2017). *The battle of the snakes-staff of Aesculapius vs. Caduceus* [Web log post]. Retrieved from http://www.premiumcaremd.com/blog/the-battle-of-the-snakes-staff-of-aesculapius-vs-caduceus.

Royal College of Physicians and Surgeons. (2018). *What we do*. Retrieved from http://www.royalcollege.ca/rcsite/about/what-we-do-e.

World Health Organization. (2018). *ICD purposes and uses*. Retrieved from http://www.who.int/classifications/icd/en/.

World Medical Association, Inc. (2018). *Declaration of Geneva: The "Modern Hippocratic Oath"*. Retrieved from https://www.wma.net/what-we-do/medical-ethics/declaration-of-geneva/.

3

Reception, Booking Appointments, and Clinical Responsibilities

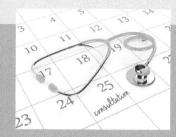

Source: © CanStock Photo Inc./compuinfoto

The reception area is a location of paramount importance in a medical facility because it sets the tone for each patient visit while delivering an overall message about the practice priorities and competency. Scheduling appointments is a foundational reception task performed and has a significant impact on operational success. This chapter explores frontline reception and clinical responsibilities, along with effective and efficient booking methodologies.

CHAPTER OUTLINE

Introduction
Elements of the Reception Area
Booking Appointments

Summary
Assignments
Topics for Discussion

LEARNING OBJECTIVES

After reading this chapter, you should be able to:

1. Explain the responsibilities of the medical administrative assistant regarding patient reception
2. Understand and explore methods for patient appointment scheduling

3. Recognize components of scheduling diagnostic appointments
4. Demonstrate the procedure for booking surgery
5. Explain and practise basic clinical skills

KEY TERMS

E-health: A general term used to describe communication technologies connecting to the electronic patient record.

Electronic Medical Record (EMR): Electronic collection of patient health information. These data move across health platforms and networks to support quality of care. Each patient health record stored in the EMR consists of the patient demographic, medical history, test results, and billing information.

Encounter: When a patient sees the physician for one symptom or problem, for example, a sore throat, this is considered one encounter. If the same patient wants another symptom or problem (e.g., a mole) looked at by the doctor within the same appointment time, this would be a second encounter. Many doctors will see a patient for one encounter per visit. If the patient needs to see the doctor for a second encounter, he or she will need to book another appointment.

Matrix: Identifies a pattern of working and nonworking hours for the medical office by blocking out times on the calendar.

Medical asepsis: The state of being free from disease-causing microorganisms; it is concerned with eliminating the spread of disease-producing microorganisms.

Ministry of Health (MoH): A government ministry responsible for administration of public health services.

Most responsible physician (MRP): The MRP is the physician who assumes primary care for a patient admitted to the hospital. The MRP may change during the patient's hospital stay, depending on the patient's medical needs. For example, a patient may be admitted for a cholecystectomy (surgical removal of the gallbladder). The patient recovers from the surgery only to develop a secondary condition (not related to the surgery) before being discharged. The MRP responsibility may then be transferred to a physician who treats the patient for the secondary condition.

Noninvasive: A procedure defined as when no break in the skin is created and there is no contact with a skin break, or introduction to an internal body cavity beyond a natural opening.

Open-hours scheduling: Scheduling that involves a set time period available for patients to come into the office and be seen on a first-come, first-served basis. Often utilized in urgent care or walk-in types of environments.

Patient self-scheduling: This involves a patient accessing the web page of the health care practice to book his or her own appointment.

Stream scheduling: With stream scheduling, patients are booked at fixed times depending on the nature of their appointment. This system makes it easier to ensure a steady flow or stream of patients during the day.

Triage: To assess the sense of medical urgency.

Venipuncture: To puncture a vein, typically to obtain a specimen of blood (*Taber's Cyclopedic Medical Dictionary* [20th ed.]).

Version code: A version code consists of one or two letters assigned to a health card number depending on province or territory. This additional code is issued on a replacement card with the same original health card number. Circumstances requiring a replacement card include damage, theft, expiration, or loss of original card.

Wave scheduling: Wave scheduling is based on the average time spent with each patient within a half hour or an hour. If a physician spends 10 minutes with each patient, then three patients can be seen within a half hour. Three patients would be given the same time at the beginning of the hour, for example 10:00. Another three patients would be given the same time on the half hour, for example 10:30.

Introduction

Patient wait times have been a long-standing matter of focus in health care. Waits occur throughout the continuum of care, and the current status quo is evolving with the development and implementation of various booking tools, such as web-based patient self-scheduling.

A medical facility may book several appointments every day, and a systematic approach is essential to ensure the smooth management of workflow. An effective medical administrative assistant understands how appointments are the primary resource for patients to utilize the facility services. Poor management of the schedule increases stress for both staff and patients.

When you assume your professional role, your responsibilities likely will include appointment scheduling, reception duties, and a variety of clinical tasks (see Box 3.1). As you explore this chapter, you will cultivate an understanding and an opportunity to develop these primary skills for your professional growth and employability.

Elements of the Reception Area

Waiting Area

The reception waiting room typically is the first and last place a patient will connect with a medical facility. Ideally, a peaceful, comfortable area for patients to be received and await their appointment is essential (see Fig. 3.1). No matter the type of medical facility, an attractive decor, comfortable chairs, reading materials, soft music, and various other items such as a TV with various DVDs to pass the wait time create an impression. Many offices have Wi-Fi available in the reception area as well. Periodically, throughout office

---

• BOX 3.1 Common Responsibilities

- Office reception
- Booking appointments
- Managing an electronic medical records (EMR) system
- Collecting patient information for data entry into the health record
- Arranging referrals to specialists/practitioners and diagnostic procedures
- Booking outpatient procedures and surgery, or both
- Maintaining charts in the appropriate format
- Filing patient information
- Billing provincial health care plans and workers' compensation claims
- Billing patients for services not covered by their health care plans
- Billing third-party insurances
- Managing pharmacy inquiries
- Ordering and maintaining supplies
- Noninvasive clinical skills
- Maintaining examination rooms
- Sterilizing instruments
- Assisting the physician when required
- Medical transcription and speech recognition editing

---

hours, the waiting area will need to be surveyed and tidied as appropriate. Many patients will be handling reading materials, chairs, and doorknobs, of course; cleanliness and tidiness are the two most important features. Some offices have toys for young children and a designated children's play area. These toys should be washed or sprayed with disinfectant during and at the end of the day (depending on usage); therefore soft plush toys are not suitable. Books for small children that can be washed with disinfectant are encouraged. Some facilities also offer a selection of coffee, tea, and water for patients to enjoy.

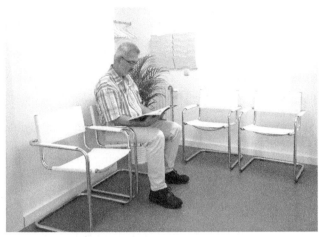

• **Fig. 3.1** The waiting area should be peaceful and comfortable for your patients. (© CanStock Photo Inc./compuinfoto.)

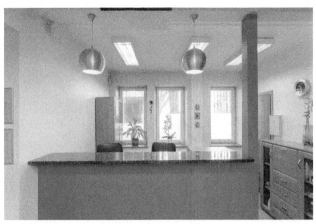

• **Fig. 3.2** Reception desk. (Source: istockphoto.com/Katarzyna Bialasiewicz.)

Reception Desk

The reception desk in a medical facility is often the focus of concentrated activity. The reception area is the first point of contact for patients and provides an impression about the facility based on its layout and front office support staff. From greeting patients to managing phone calls, scheduling appointments, preparing communication, and carrying out billing procedures, the reception activities are pivotal. The reception desk should be a central point of the reception area and should be viewable from each facility entrance point.

Ensure that the reception desk is spacious enough for computers, phone systems, and printers. The importance of maintaining confidentiality is a key consideration of the reception desk area; therefore the height and layout of the desk should allow for patient communication while protecting sensitive data from view. For infection control, consider having sanitizer available at the front desk; avoid shaking hands because this is also a transmitter of infection in the medical office. Most people who visit a medical office are ill, so be mindful of infection control practices.

Fig. 3.2 shows a standard reception desk.

The Receptionist

The role of receptionist is often a career entry point for the medical administrative assistant, also referred to as *a patient services representative*. An effective receptionist focuses on a customer service approach, often interacting with patients who have a compromised health status requiring a higher level of empathy and understanding. Recent patient satisfaction surveys report that the attitudes of health care workers experienced during patient visits at medical facilities balance at a level of importance similar to that of treatment processes. Consider the following four customer service steps for exceptional patient service.

Prioritize Patients

Acknowledge patients upon arrival and when they have questions or complaints. Go beyond expectations. Seek out answers to patient questions even when you do not initially know the answer; follow up and provide a response. Timely follow-up is essential to a positive patient experience.

Recognize Errors

If you forget to call back a patient or you have double-booked two patients in error, apologize and acknowledge the mistake.

Respect

Remember to show respect for your patients with a customer service approach, and also remember to display the same qualities of respect toward your health care team members. It will help to set a harmonious positive tone with patients and with others in the facility.

Patient Information

It is the responsibility of the front office staff to establish and maintain an accurate file, also known as *the health record,* containing information for each new, current, and inactive patient. An inactive patient is a patient who has had no contact with an office for 2 to 3 years. To obtain the required information from a new patient, you may ask the patient to complete a patient information form, as shown in Fig. 3.3. If questions are answered orally, move to a private place to protect confidentiality. If a private place is not available, have patients fill out the information on their own. Provide them with a clipboard and pen and be available if they are in need of assistance. Ask them to print so you are able to read their information. This is the information you will depend on for accurate data management and billing processes. Strive to ensure that *all* information is current, including the mailing address and telephone number. On repeated visits, ask whether there are any changes in the patient information.

Greeting Patients

A warm, friendly smile and immediate attention are two things to remember when greeting patients. If you are

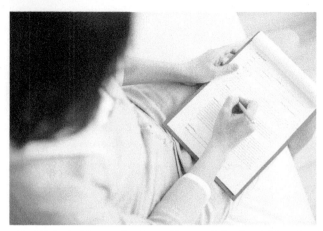

• **Fig. 3.3** Patient information form. (Source: © CanStock Photo Inc./ pressmaster.)

transcribing a letter or preparing a chart, these activities can wait; the most important duty is patient relationship management. If you are busy with a patient and someone else comes into the office, look directly at the new arrival and acknowledge his or her presence ("I will be with you in just a moment"). If you are on the telephone, look at the person and smile or raise your hand to show you are aware that someone has entered the office. Do not simply ignore the person. Attend to the person as soon as you are finished. Do not start on something else first.

Whenever possible, greet the patient by name. Initially, it is best to use the formal greeting (Mr., Mrs., Ms.) when receiving patients. Recent studies have shown that the majority of people under the age of 65 prefer to be addressed by their first name. Some patients will request that you refer to them by their first name after you have become acquainted. This practice is acceptable, but only after you have been instructed to take that liberty. The patient information form or the patient information in the health record will assist you in establishing the marital status of the patient, for example, single, married, separated, divorced, or widowed. Checking this information for an unfamiliar patient can help avoid some uncomfortable situations.

As mentioned in previous chapters, the majority of patients visiting the doctor are under stress. It is important for the medical administrative assistant to be considerate and caring. The following guidelines assist with greeting patients:

- Acknowledge the arrival of a patient by greeting them by name and introducing yourself as you maintain eye contact.
- Verify and/or record their information.
- Note the time of their arrival compared with the scheduled time of the visit. If there is a delay, inform the patient accordingly.
- Invite the patient to take a seat in the waiting area.
- Keep small talk to a minimum around the reception desk area.

Health Card Verification

All provinces and territories in Canada provide eligible residents with a health card (see Chapter 7). Patients must present their health card when accessing services covered by the provincial and territorial health care system. When a patient arrives for an appointment, you must ask for the health card and verify that the card is current and belongs to the patient. In some cases, depending on the province or territory, a version code is issued along with the health card number. It is important to *ask* whether the patient's card has been replaced for any reason. Some health cards have an expiry date. The majority of patients do not pay attention to this detail; therefore if the expiry date is coming up, you can remind them when you check their card.

Some provinces offer health card number validation availability to a service provider through an **eHealth** system with authorization from the patient. The general term *e-health* is used to describe communication technologies connecting to the electronic patient record. If the patient does not have their health card with them when requesting a health service covered under their provincial or territory plan, they may be billed for services because the responsibility for presenting a valid card is the patient's. In the physician's office, electronically swiping the card or keying the number into the electronic medical records system will bring up the patient's information. The medical administrative assistant can then confirm that the health card belongs to that patient. If there is a question about the authenticity of the health card, it is your responsibility to report this information to the provincial or territorial ministry. If a patient possesses two health cards, it is your responsibility to confiscate the outdated card. The patient must voluntarily submit this card to you.

As mentioned, verification procedures may vary between offices. In most hospital settings, a direct e-link is made to the Ministry of Health (MoH) once the health card is swiped or the number is keyed into the computer. The system can then validate the number immediately. It is flagged if the number is invalid.

Booking Appointments

The scheduling system is an important component in the smooth operation of the health office. A successful system depends on collaborative decision making by the medical administrative assistant and health care provider(s). Scheduling systems vary and consist primarily of computerized systems; in some instances paper-based appointment scheduling is used. The booking system maintains a record of each day's functions in the office, but it is also an official record that can be used for billing purposes or for legal documentation in case of legal action. When initiating

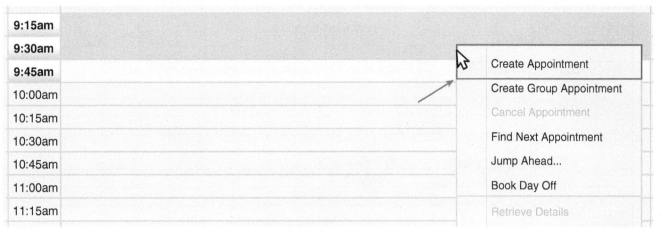

• **Fig. 3.4** Computerized schedule.

a daily booking schedule, you must also be aware of the health care provider's schedule outside of the office. This includes meetings, hospital rounds, luncheon dates, speaking engagements, surgery schedule, and on-call responsibilities. It is a critical operational responsibility to record such information as well as a full schedule for patient visits. Everyone involved in the practice will refer frequently to this daily activity record to keep on schedule. Many physicians have adopted mobile technology enabling smartphones and tablets to view, record, and update their schedules both in and out of the office. Research has shown that at least 25% of physicians use mobile technology tools daily in their practice management. It is therefore imperative that you as the administrative assistant be exact when making entries in the appointment scheduling system. Accuracy is essential.

There are several variations of appointment booking systems, but most have the capability to segment time periods according to the doctor's practice and preference. Most offices today use an electronic scheduling system; Fig. 3.4 shows an example.

Many specialists book half-hour and one-hour appointments. General practitioners have 10- or 15-minute segments in their appointment schedule. Complementary therapy clinics will also book half-hour and hour-long appointments, depending on the type of treatment required. Some chiropractic offices will book patients every 5 to 10 minutes.

Walk-in and urgent care clinics and some private practices do not schedule appointments. Patients are seen on a first-come, first-served basis. This, of course, could lead to long waiting periods for some patients because the most urgent cases are seen first. In this type of practice, the office does not run at a steady pace. There is also no time to prepare for a patient's needs ahead of their visits.

Determining the Appointment Schedule

Several considerations are navigated in developing an appointment schedule. The physician and the scheduling team are consultative and based on variables the parameter of the schedule is often formed. These scheduling variables can include several factors such as age demographic of the patient base, the specialty of the physicians practice, and the preferences of the provider(s).

Scheduling Guidelines

In a medical practice, patients schedule visits for a variety of reasons. Depending on the nature of the reason, the appointment length and resources needed are impacted. As a best practice, many facilities will formulate a category system for appointment scheduling to assist the scheduling team to determine the appropriate length of time for a visit. For instance, a complete physical would require a longer time than a follow-up on a skin infection. The facility can determine the guideline for the types of visits requiring 15-, 30-, and 45-minute increments. This will ensure enhanced patient and provider satisfaction because neither the patient nor the provider will feel rushed when the appropriate length of time is recognized in the daily schedule.

The majority of medical offices use an Electronic Medical Record (EMR) system for practice management, and scheduling is a key component of facility management. An EMR is the electronic collection of patient health information comprising an e-health record. This data can be shared across health platforms and networks to support quality of care. Each patient health record stored in the EMR consists of the patient demographic, medical history, test results, and billing information. Across Canada, several EMR systems offering many clinical tools have revolutionized the way a health office functions. The selection of clinical tools available through an EMR system typically consists of automated patient appointment reminder, online appointment booking, waiting room check-in kiosk, virtual care, patient questionnaires, and data analytics.

Types of Scheduling

With the scheduling parameters and appointment categories established, a scheduling matrix is constructed. This involves noting times in the schedule where the provider is unavailable for patient visits and indicating times when

APPOINTMENT SCHEDULE

DOCTOR _Plunkett_

Day_____ Month_____ Year_____

TIME	PATIENT	PHONE	REASON FOR APPOINTMENT
0930			
1000	Eliz. Green	427-3774	
	Erik Shultz	427-9977	
	Heather Smith	576-3225	
1030			
1100			
1130			
1200			
1230			
1300			
1330			

REMARKS: _____

• **Fig. 3.5** Wave scheduling.

appointment selection is available. This matrix process is essential to ensure that nobody on the scheduling team mistakenly books the wrong time.

The most common type of scheduling consists of a patient securing a specific time for an appointment. This enables the scheduling team to organize the day so that the patients arrive in a steady flow. This type of scheduling is also known as _stream_ scheduling.

Wave scheduling is another method for booking appointments (see Fig. 3.5). This method can help alleviate problems created by late arrivals. Assume that you use a schedule that books a patient every 10 minutes, allowing three patients scheduled each half hour and at the time scheduled. If you changed to wave scheduling, three patients would be scheduled at the beginning of each half-hour interval and seen in order of arrival. Your initial schedule would be

1000	Mrs. Green
1010	Mr. Shultz
1020	Ms. Smith

Your revised schedule would be

1000	Mrs. Green
	Mr. Shultz
	Ms. Smith

TABLE 3.1	Comparison of Wave Scheduling	
Advantages	**Disadvantages**
Provides ample time for unexpected visits	Excessive downtime when no-shows occur
Permits time for staff to keep up with charting, filing, and other tasks	A lag in scheduling may affect the flow of work in the office
Allows more patients to be seen in the allotted time period	Irritated patients when they discover other people with the same appointment time
May allow for work-in appointments	Can create a significant backup when patients arrive late

If one patient were late for the appointment, it would not affect the other two, and the longest waiting interval would be 20 minutes.

Modified wave scheduling would have two patients booked at 1000 and one patient booked at 1020.

Double-booking is not recommended, except for appointments such as allergy shots, blood pressure checks, or flu shots. These appointments should take less than 5 minutes per patient. See Table 3.1 for a comparison of the advantages and disadvantages of wave scheduling.

Patient self-scheduling is another method that is continuing to gain in popularity. This involves a patient accessing the web page of the health care practice to book his or her own appointment. Studies show that it takes upward of 8 minutes to book an appointment when a patient calls in. It can save significant time and offer convenience for patients to select their appointment time online. It typically is available to patients 24 hours a day.

CRITICAL THINKING

You are assigned the responsibility of researching the viability of an online patient self-scheduling platform and delivering a recommendation to the management team. What information would you need to know in advance of your research, and what information do you think is critical to making a recommendation?

Open-hours scheduling involves a set time period that is available for patients to come into the office and be seen on a first-come, first-served basis. This type of scheduling is often utilized in urgent care or walk-in types of environments.

DID YOU KNOW?

Missed appointments or no-shows are problematic in the medical environment for a number of reasons. For starters, a missed medical appointment could present health risks for patients in terms of early-stage disease detection and timely treatment. Additionally, missed appointments can wreak havoc for the office scheduling systems.

Appointment Time Allotment

When a patient requests an appointment, ask the reason for the visit to assess the time allotment required; for example, a minor sore throat or cold may need a 10-minute appointment, whereas counselling or a complete physical could require a half-hour appointment.

Always allow for travel time, from hospital to office, for example, when required. It is wise to leave a 15-minute open appointment each morning and afternoon, if possible. This allows for catch-up time if the doctor is behind schedule. If the doctor is on schedule, the time is used to discuss telephone messages or even to take a quick break. However, not every doctor may want you to follow this procedure. Discuss with the physician to determine booking preferences before implementing such a practice in the appointment schedule. When arranging your appointment schedule, it is important to anticipate that Mondays and Fridays tend to be very busy days.

An earache, chest pain, and high temperature are considered urgent, and patients *must* be seen. On the other hand, someone with cold-like symptoms may be seen the next day. When your daily schedule is completely filled and a patient insists on seeing the doctor, check with the doctor and call back with instructions. Refusing a critically ill patient could result in legal action against the doctor. *Never* make such a decision on your own. The health care provider is responsible for patient triage. Triage means to assess the sense of medical urgency. Remember—your responsibility is to book appointments, not to make a diagnosis.

Never put off an emergency patient. If the doctor should become involved in an emergency and cancellations prove necessary, always make arrangements to have urgent patients seen by another physician or referred elsewhere to obtain care. If another physician is not available to see your patients, it is then necessary to send them to a walk-in clinic or the nearest emergency department. Many jurisdictions have family health care teams that include on-call physicians; physician preference may be discussed in advance. Routine appointments can be booked for a later date. If time allows, contact the patient before he or she leaves for the doctor's office.

If you need to contact a patient to cancel, ensure that you can access their contact information through the EMR; for a new patient, secure their contact information at the time of the appointment booking.

Additional Recommendations Concerning Appointments

1. Consider giving preprinted reminder cards to patients who book appointments in the office (see Fig. 3.6). Any special instructions to the patient can be recorded on the back of the card; for instance, "Bring Medication." This eliminates misunderstandings and errors. If time allows, missed appointments can be virtually eliminated by setting up an electronic generating reminder system that will contact the patient the day before the scheduled visit. If a patient needs a follow-up appointment, arrange the time before the patient leaves the office.

APPOINTMENT REMINDER

An appointment is scheduled with

DR. J.E. PLUNKETT

Date _____

Time _____

• **Fig. 3.6** Appointment reminder card.

• **BOX 3.2** **Common Abbreviations Used in Scheduling**

F/U	Follow-Up
Pap	Pap Smear
WB	Well Baby
BP	Blood Pressure
N/S	No-Show
Inj	Injection
NP	New Patient

2. Make appointments for homemakers, preschoolers, and retirees early in the day. This leaves time open for school-age children after 4 p.m. and for working patients after 5 p.m.

3. If a patient cancels an appointment and does not request a rebooking, follow these steps:
   - Make a comment/note in the EMR and push out to the doctor.
   - If the missed appointment will jeopardize the patient's well-being, suggest making another appointment.
   - If you are employed in a specialist's office and a patient cancels or misses an appointment, advise the referring/family physician.

4. Do not book several long appointments together (unless your doctor/employer does all annual health examinations on a specific day).

5. When the doctor is called away from the office for an emergency and a patient arrives for an appointment,
   - Apologize for the inconvenience.
   - Explain the doctor's absence (without going into too much detail).
   - Tell the patient approximately how long the doctor will be detained.
   - If the doctor is not going to be away too long,
     i. Suggest that the patient might like to wait, and offer a magazine.
     ii. Suggest that the patient might have some errands to run and would like to come back later.
     iii. Suggest rebooking for a future date.

6. If a patient may be infectious to other patients, try to book him or her as the first appointment of the morning or as the first appointment of the afternoon. Take the patient into an examination room upon arrival so he or she will not be seated in the waiting room with other patients. Refer to Box 3.2 for common scheduling abbreviations.

CRITICAL THINKING

You notice that your office is experiencing a significant number of missed appointments, also known as *no-shows*. The physicians are concerned and addressed the situation at a recent team meeting. What strategies do you suggest to help manage this more effectively? Consider the pros and cons of each strategy.

Patients Without Appointments

If a patient arrives and wishes to see the doctor without having first made an appointment, you would point out that the doctor sees patients by appointment only and that, in the future, arrangements should be made before coming to the office. If you can arrange to have the doctor see the patient without inconveniencing anyone, you would then explain that there will be a waiting period (state time, for example, approximately one hour) before the patient can be seen by the doctor.

Of course, you may be faced with an emergency situation in which a patient arrives at the office and needs to be seen immediately. In such an instance, you would usher the patient into the first available examining room, secure the patient's health record, and inform the doctor.

No-Shows

Inevitably you will have patients who do not arrive for their scheduled appointments. When this occurs, you will need to call the patient and rebook if necessary. If you need to leave a message, be as confidential as possible. One way of leaving your message may be, "Please have Mr. Baxter call this number when he arrives" versus "This is Dr. Plunkett's office. Please have Mr. Baxter call this number when he arrives." Some health facilities and doctors' offices will choose to have "Private Name, Private Number" as opposed to the office number or facility name shown on a phone's call display.

Be sure to document in the patient health record that the patient did not arrive for the appointment and the date of the new appointment, if applicable. Inform the physician, who can then adjust his or her daily schedule.

House Calls

The delivery of health care has changed radically over the years. If we compare health care in the early 1900s with health care delivery today, we see that early in the last century the doctor came to the patient's home, whereas today the patient usually sees the doctor in the office or in a hospital. There are occasions, however, when it may be necessary for the doctor to visit the patient at home. If you are responsible for making arrangements for a house call, you must get explicit instructions regarding the location of the house or apartment as well as the name, telephone number, and complaint. You must also advise the patient about the approximate time of the doctor's arrival. If a doctor is making a house call, it will usually be after office hours, or before or after hospital rounds. It is important to have the patient's health record available. Remember—house calls are expensive and time-consuming. Always urge patients to come to the office if at all possible.

New Patients/Patient Education

It is good practice to have a new patient arrive earlier than his or her appointment time so any required paperwork can be completed.

When a new patient arrives in your office, you should supply a brochure or outline of your office policies, including the following information:

- Office phone number
- Hours of operation
- Any additional costs not covered by the provincial health care plan
- What to do in the case of an emergency outside of office hours
- Office policy with regard to visits (i.e., if the physician will see only one **encounter** per visit)

Arranging for Diagnostic Testing and Appointments With Specialists

At the end of the doctor's consultation with the patient, you may be required to complete requisition forms for specific tests. (A more thorough outline of completion of requisition forms will be covered in Chapter 12.) It may be necessary to arrange appointments for such tests—for example, an ultrasound or blood work. It may also be necessary to arrange an appointment with a specialist. These appointments in some instances are self-arranged by the patient. This will depend on regional preferences and test requirements.

Some points to consider when making arrangements for special tests follow:

1. Some patients who are very ill can tolerate only so much in one day. Be sure you do not overtax someone with too many tests at one time.
2. Ask about any required special preparations for the test. Ensure that instructions are clearly communicated to and understood by the patient. It is good practice to provide instructions both verbally and in written form.
3. If more than one test is required, determine whether the patient can be booked consecutively, or whether the appointments must be booked on separate days. See Box 3.3 depicting best practices for diagnostic testing requisitions.
4. If a series of weekly appointments must be booked, try to arrange them for the same day and time each week. This will make it easier for the patient to remember.

• BOX 3.3 Diagnostic Test Best Practices

Diagnostic tests typically require a requisition. If the facility does not receive the requisition, the appointment may be cancelled. Provide the patient a copy of the requisition, or send electronically through the EMR platform when possible. A copy of the requisition should also be saved in the patient health record; make note of when you provided or sent the requisition.

---

5. Inform the patient of the approximate amount of time required to complete the test.
6. Try to be aware of your patients' comfort level with pending tests. Allay their fears, or encourage them to ask questions.
7. Discuss time availability with the patient before arranging for the testing.
8. Inform the receptionist at the testing location of any special needs of the patient.

When arranging a referral to a specialist, you will also be required to do the following:

1. Provide the patient's sociological information (name, address, date of birth, telephone number, and health card number).
2. Supply the reason for the referral.
3. Electronically send the referral letter and relevant diagnostic test results.

Scheduling Surgery

In most areas, hospital operating rooms are booked to capacity many weeks in advance. Procedure requirements for booking surgery will differ according to hospital and area, but the following information will be required by any operating room scheduling officer or admitting department:

1. The patient's sociological information (name, address, phone or cellular phone number as well as the medical care plan number)
2. Whether the surgery is elective or urgent
3. Type of surgery that will be performed
4. The admitting diagnosis
5. Surgeon performing surgery (most responsible physician [MRP])
6. The name of the patient's family physician

Many hospitals now have a presurgical information package to be completed prior to surgery. Either the hospital's presurgery clinic or the surgeon's office staff may supply the package. Components of the required information may vary among institutions.

It is important to inform your patient that if he or she experiences fever, diarrhea, sore throat, or any other flu-like symptoms, he or she must contact your office immediately. If your office is closed, the patient must contact the hospital admitting department. There is a chance that surgery will need to be postponed if any of these symptoms occur. See Box 3.4 identifying common forms completed in relation to a surgical patient preoperatively.

• BOX 3.4 Preoperative Forms

Form	Completed by
Letter of instruction to patient	Surgeon
Preanaesthetic questionnaire	Patient
Preregistration questionnaire	Patient
History and physical examination form	Surgeon/family physician
Consent form	Surgeon must ensure completion by patient
Order sheet (including preoperative testing requirements)	Surgeon

---

Many hospitals will run a presurgery clinic in which the patient meets with the anaesthetist and relevant instructions for the surgery are given. This provides the patient with education and information as well as an opportunity to ask any questions.

Emergency surgery usually results after a patient has been examined in the emergency department at the hospital. The arrangements for emergency surgery would then be made within the hospital by the emergency department and the operating room scheduling officer.

Booking for Two or More Physicians/ Practitioners

Many offices have multiple physicians or practitioners working out of a shared area. It is very important to be aware of equipment, facilities, and staff that need to be available for appointments. For example, at 1300 Robert Baxter is having a benign mole removed by Dr. Plunkett. This would be done in the minor treatment room. This room is also used for venipuncture, baby weights, and blood pressures. Dr. Park shares office space with Dr. Plunkett, and you book the appointments for both physicians. Amelia Jackson is being seen by Dr. Park for a blood test on the same day that Robert Baxter is being seen. You will need to make sure that the minor treatment room will be available for Amelia's appointment.

Pharmaceutical Representatives, Supply Salespersons, and Nonpatient Visitors

Pharmaceutical representatives and supply salespersons often have innovative medicines and supplies in which the doctor may be interested. They are usually aware of doctors' preferences for booking time to see them, and they arrange their appointment times well in advance of their visits. Always ask for the pharmaceutical representative's or salesperson's business card because you may have a follow-up inquiry.

The appearance of someone without an appointment on a very busy day may present you with a problem. Most doctors/ employers will have a preference for scheduling appointments for nonpatient visitors, so you will have clear-cut guidelines on how to deal with them. If, however, there are no set rules, an efficient medical administrative assistant will tactfully but firmly advise all nonpatient callers that the doctor will see them only by appointment. Remember, the patients are the doctor's

first priority, and their appointment times should not be interrupted by those who have failed to make an appointment.

Daily Schedule

Many doctors prefer to have their administrative assistants print up a daily appointment schedule to have on their desks. In this way they know which patients are scheduled to be seen that day. The schedule might be formatted as follows:

DR. PLUNKETT
APPOINTMENTS FOR JANUARY 23, 20___

Morning
0900–1130   Assist Dr. Jones in surgery—Gary Green—bypass
1200–1300   Speaking engagement—Kinsmen Lunch Bunch—Holiday Inn, Green Room

Afternoon
1300–1315   Hazel Davis, O.B. checkup

Some physicians will opt to view their daily schedule from their office computer or digital device. If your physician is able to do this, make sure that the computer monitor is at an angle that cannot be viewed by someone who may be sitting in the physician's office.

24-Hour Clock

You will notice in the previous appointment example that times are written in a style that is different from the norm. In the medical environment, many areas use a 24-hour schedule to identify time.

Rather than dividing the day into two sections (morning and afternoon), the schedule begins at one minute after midnight and proceeds cumulatively through to midnight. At one minute after midnight, the time is written 0001 and referred to as 0-0-0-1 (pronouncing O rather than saying zero). One o'clock in the morning is written 0100 and spoken as "O one hundred hours" rather than 1 a.m. Twelve o'clock noon is written 1200 and spoken as "twelve hundred hours." After noon hour, the time does not begin at one again but continues to be cumulative. Therefore 1 p.m. would be written as 1300 and spoken as "thirteen hundred hours," 5 p.m. would be written as 1700 and spoken as "seventeen hundred hours," and so on (see Fig. 3.7).

Clinical Responsibilities

Along with clerical duties, many medical administrative assistants have clinical responsibilities as a component of the role. Clinical responsibilities may include:

- Prepare and maintain examination rooms
- Prepare patients for examination and treatment
- Obtaining a health history and interviewing the patient
- Taking and recording vital signs
- Specimen handling and collection

- Adhering to standard precautions related to infection control, handwashing, disposal of biohazardous materials, sterilization, and quality assurance practices

Preparing and Maintaining Examining Rooms

The examining rooms should be prepared for the patients; instruments to be used should be readily available for the doctor; sufficient paper should be available to ensure a clean

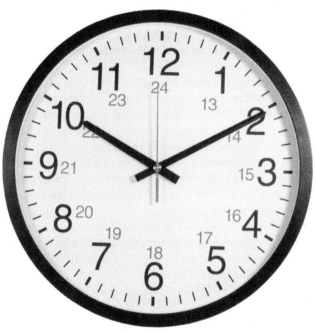

• **Fig. 3.7** 24-Hour clock. (Source: © CanStock Photo Inc./ dcwcreations.)

examination table at all times; light bulbs in examining lamps must be working; and all medical supplies required for the patient should be placed in an easily accessible area (see Fig. 3.8). Of course, all areas of the medical office must be kept clean, and medical instruments must be sterile. To secure the examination rooms, ensure that drugs and supplies are kept locked away from patient access.

The layout of the room generally revolves around three key considerations: efficiency, patient comfort, and physician convenience (see Fig. 3.9). For general setup suggestions, see Box 3.5.

All confidential, patient-sensitive materials *must* be kept where only the physician(s) or the medical administrative assistant can access them. They should never be left in view of nonmedical personnel or patients. Never leave them in the examination rooms.

Now that you are ready, the patients can be allocated to the examination rooms. If working from paper-based records, the patient's file should be readily available to the doctor, but not to the patient. If there is a holder outside the examination room door, the file is placed inside it. If such a holder is not available, the file can be placed somewhere on your desk so the physician knows who is to be seen next.

After each patient, you should change the paper on the examination table if necessary and ensure that all is in order in the examining room.

Preparing the Patient for Examinations and Treatments

Consider your responsibilities in preparing the patient for the physician. Try to put the patient at ease before you begin by speaking softly and explaining how they will prepare for the physician's examination. Does the patient need to disrobe? If so, most offices provide a gown or sheet. Is a specimen required, such as a urine sample? You would collect this first before having the patient disrobe. Additional particulars may be required, for instance, if the patient is having a Pap smear. The best approach is to determine the expectations of patient

Blood Pressure Cuff	Bandages	Lancets
Syringes	Telfa	Peak Flow Meter
Needles	Ear Syringe	Slides (glass)
Alcohol	Otoscope	Fixative (cytology)
Sutures	Vaginal Speculum	Forceps
Needle Driver	Tongue Depressors	Curette
Scissors	Cotton Swabs	Height and Weight Chart
Mosquito Forceps	Reflex Hammer	Weight Scales
Skin Hooks	Eye Chart	Biological Supplies
Scalpel (and blade)	Gown	Ophthalmoscope
Cotton	Examining Table Paper	Silver Nitrate Sticks
Gauze	Stethoscope	Sample Bottles
Tensors	Hemoglobinometer	

• **Fig. 3.8** Common instruments and supplies used in a general practitioner's office.

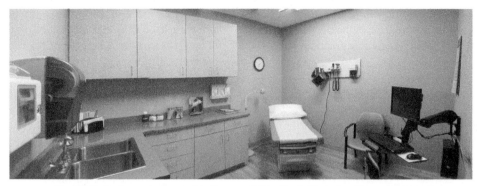

• **Fig. 3.9** Patient examination room. (Source: © CanStock Photo Inc./jfergusonphotos.)

• BOX 3.5   General Examination Room Setup

- One or more chairs, a rolling stool. Adjustable examination table, wall brackets for equipment. High-intensity lamps or lighting. Computer stand or cart. Sink or counter and storage cabinetry, completes the examination room set up.

---

preparation in advance with the physician prior to welcoming the patient into the examination room. Each physician will have their preparation preferences depending on the type of examination, along with common expectations for you to become familiar with and practise in a safe manner. Medical administrative assistants can provide assistance with specific clinical skills considered noninvasive. A noninvasive procedure is defined as when no break in the skin is created, there is no contact with a skin break, and there is no introduction to an internal body cavity beyond a natural opening.

According to the Canadian Medical Protective Association (CMPA), invasive procedures such as giving injections, treatments such as suturing injured tissue, and similar clinical procedures are beyond the terms of reference of a medical administrative assistant. Several guides are available on the website, including "Patient Safety and Professionalism." You can find more information at the CMPA website located at www.cmpa-acpm.ca. Refer to Chapter 2. Many health practices and functions fall under the scope of practice for a nurse or a doctor. Never engage in a health care practice outside of your scope.

You may be required to weigh and measure the patient. In addition, you may be required to perform tasks such as taking blood pressure, temperature, checking pulse and respiration, and so on. These statistics are entered in the patient's health record. The physician will instruct you whether these responsibilities are required of you, and as a matter of preference, some physicians will choose to do their own vital sign readings.

Obtaining a Health History and Interviewing the Patient

The purpose of obtaining a health history is to gather subjective data from the patient and/or the patient's family to enable the health care team to promote health and effectively manage health problems. Subjective data is information the patient provides to the health care team. Asking

questions collects the subjective data; an appropriate questioning pattern will help source the pertinent information (see Fig. 3.10). Consider the following sample questions for subjective information gathering:
- "What brings you here today?"
- "How has your health been lately?"
- "How long have you been experiencing these symptoms?"
- "Do you have other concerns?"

Conducting the interview helps capture key information for the physician's examination process. Chief complaint, also known as *the history of the present illness,* is the statement made by the patient indicating the subjective reason for the health care visit. The medical history forms a basis for medical treatment; the documenting of this history should be accurate. To ensure success of the interview, prepare in advance by noting the reason listed for the visit in the appointment schedule and by reviewing the last patient chart note. Approach the patient and conduct the interview in private with the door closed in the examination room or treatment room. Manage information with sensitivity. Additional guidelines include:
- Record exact patient words.
- Record all dates in chronological order.
- Follow the SOAP method of information data recording. SOAP is an acronym representing Subjective = patient tells, Objective = you observe, Assessment = assessment by examination of physician, and Plan = plan of action for treatment by health care provider.

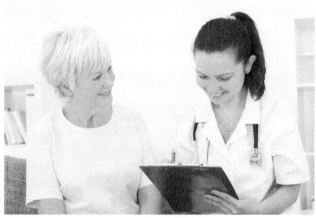

• **Fig. 3.10** Patient interview. (Source: © CanStock Photo Inc./ AndreyPopov.)

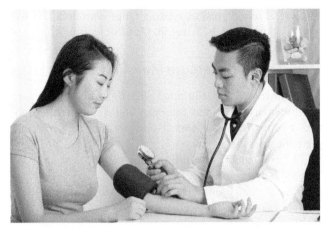

• **Fig. 3.11** Assistant measuring blood pressure. (Source: © CanStock Photo Inc./Bialasiewicz.)

Measuring and Recording Vital Signs

Vital signs are measurements of the body's basic functions. There are four main vital signs routinely assessed by health care providers, including the following:
• Body temperature
• Pulse rate
• Respiration rate
• Blood pressure – not considered a vital sign but often is measured in collaboration with the signs listed (see Fig. 3.11)
Variations in vital signs assist in monitoring medical problems.

Temperature

Several factors affect a normal body temperature reading. Some of these variations include activity, food and drink consumption, time of day, and gender. Generally, the body temperature ranges from 36.5°C to 37.2°C. When taking a body temperature, several routes are possible, and they include:
1. **Oral.** Temperature taken by mouth using digital thermometers that use an electronic probe to measure body temperature. This tends to be a convenient and accurate methodology.
2. **Rectal.** Temperatures taken rectally tend to be almost 1°C higher than when taken by mouth.
3. **Axillary.** Temperatures taken under the arm using a glass or digital thermometer. Temperatures taken by this route tend to be 1°C lower than those taken orally.
4. **Ear.** An ear thermometer quickly measures a temperature, often in seconds. Ear temperatures can be 0.3°C to 0.6°C higher than those taken orally.
5. **Temporal.** A special thermometer can quickly measure the temperature of the skin on the forehead. As with the ear temperature, the same variation in reading applies.

Steps for Taking a Temperature (Oral)

• Wash your hands.
• Ask the patient or spokesperson for consent to take a temperature.

• Obtain a digital or glass thermometer.
• Use a disposable thermometer probe cover.
• Landmark close to the sublingual artery (under the tongue) for the insertion of the probe and for accuracy.
• If you are using a digital thermometer, activate the systems and wait for the audio sound indicating that a reading has been obtained. If you are using a glass thermometer, insert it for one minute before removing the thermometer and reading the temperature.

Indications for Measurement

There can be many clinical reasons for measuring a body temperature, including:
• Obtaining a baseline to compare all future readings
• Monitoring a patient with variations indicating an infection
• Monitoring response to treatment for an infection

Measurement of Pulse Rate

The pulse rate is a measurement of the rate of the heartbeat. You can say your pulse rate is your heart rate; it is measured in beats per minute (bpm). A heart rate can be measured at various pulse points throughout the human body. The wrist, where the radial artery is found, is often a common point because it is easily accessible and accurate. Other locations for pulse measurement points include the brachial artery located in the fold of the arm, the carotid artery located in the neck region, and the apical pulse point located in the chest region near the heart.

Steps for Pulse Measurement

• As with all procedures, wash your hands and obtain consent from the patient.
• Place the tips of your index and middle fingers on the palm side of the wrist, below the base of the thumb. You will need an instrument to measure the seconds of time.
• Press lightly with your fingers until you feel the blood pulsing beneath them. You may need to move your fingers around until you feel the pulsing.
• Count the beats you feel for one minute. Some health care professionals will use a shorter timeline for a reading, but it may not establish a pattern for an accurate reading.
• Normal adult pulse rate range is 60 to 100 beats per minute; it will vary by age and gender.
• Children under 10 can range from 70 to 110. Infants can be as high as 140 beats per minute.

Indications for Measuring a Pulse

• Respiratory complaints
• Complete physical
• Asthma, chronic respiratory conditions
• Cardiac arrest
• Sedation monitoring

Measurement of Respiration Rate

The respiration rate is the number of breaths a person takes per minute.

- The rate is usually assessed when a person is at rest and simply involves calculating the number of breaths for one minute by counting how many times the chest rises and falls.
- Each rise and fall of the chest equals one respiration. Inspiration is breathing in, and expiration is breathing out. Some patients will experience greater challenges with inspiration than with expiration depending on their health issues.
- Conduct the reading over 30 seconds, and double it. Normally, take the pulse and respirations over one minute with 30 seconds dedicated for each measurement. It is best not to inform the patient that you are checking their respiration rate because they will alter their breathing.
- Normal adult respiration rate is 12 to 20 breaths per minute. In children, the range is 20 to 30, and infants can be as high as 60 respirations per minute.

Indications for Measuring Respiration Rate

Respiration rates may increase with fever, illness, and other medical conditions. When checking respiration, it is important to note whether a person has any difficulty breathing. Note these results in the health record.

Measurement of Blood Pressure Digitally

Blood pressure is the pressure exerted by circulating blood upon the walls of blood vessels. Systolic pressure is the blood pressure when the heart contracts. Diastolic pressure is the pressure when the heart relaxes.

- Have the patient sit comfortably.
- Place the cuff on the exposed arm 2 cm (approximately two fingerbreadths) above the elbow.
- Make sure the tubing is placed at the centre of the arm toward the front and that the sensor is correctly placed.
- Pull the end of the cuff so that it is wrapped evenly and firmly around the arm.
- Check that the tightness of the cuff is appropriate.
- When the cuff inflates, it should not cause any painful sensation.
- Press the start button. During measurement, keep the arm relaxed.
- The cuff will inflate and then slowly deflate. When the measurement is complete, readings of the systolic and diastolic blood pressure will display.

- Normal blood pressure reading range is around 120 over 80 and less than 140 over 90 (120/80 to 140/90).

Manual Blood Pressure Measurement

Some offices are not equipped with digital blood pressure instrumentation. In this case you will need a stethoscope and a sphygmomanometer (blood pressure cuff) to complete the following steps:

- To begin blood pressure measurement, use a properly sized blood pressure cuff.
- Wrap the cuff around the upper arm with the cuff's lower edge 1 inch above the elbow.
- Palpate for the brachial artery pulse point with your fingertips. Once it is located, lightly press the stethoscope's diaphragm over the brachial artery, just below the cuff's edge.
- Quickly inflate the cuff to approximately 160 to 180 mm Hg. Release air from the cuff at a slow rate.
- Listen with the stethoscope, and simultaneously observe the sphygmomanometer. The first Korotkoff sounds heard are the knocking sounds of the patient's systolic pressure. Korotkoff sounds are the sounds produced when blood flows through the artery while blood pressure is being measured. When the knocking sound disappears, that is the diastolic pressure.

Indications for Blood Pressure

Usually patients will have no symptoms and feel fine when experiencing high blood pressure or hypertension. Hypertension is indicative of stroke and cardiac disease.

Additional Clinical Responsibilities

Many reasons for visits result in shifting and differing responsibilities. For instance, during a complete physical, often the patient's weight and height are measured. Alterations in either of these could indicate health concerns. The physician may require you to conduct these assessments prior to the examination. Weight is usually measured in kilograms. Each kilogram is equal to 2.2 pounds. Height is measured in centimetres.

A well-baby check is an examination that assesses the status of a baby's health and development. This is another visit whereby the medical administrative assistant may participate in some of the assessment by weighing the baby and measuring the infant's head circumference.

For the comfort and protection of a patient during a gynecological examination, the physician will require the assistant to be present.

Routine collection of urine is another common clinical duty. See Box 3.6 outlining the forms of urine collection.

• BOX 3.6 Collection of Urine Specimens

Medical office personnel often collect urine specimens for a variety of tests that are performed at a hospital or outside laboratory.

Some are collected at the office, but some are to be collected by the patient at home, so it is important that you are familiar with proper instructions. In either case, proper labelling is essential. Place the label on the container, not the lid, and use indelible markers.

Many specimens are kept under refrigeration because bacteria will grow as early as within one hour if the specimen is kept at room temperature.

Routine Urinalysis Specimen

The preferred specimen for routine urinalysis is the first morning sample. Urine concentration varies considerably throughout the day from very dilute to very concentrated. Because it is not practical to collect the first morning specimen at the medical office, the patient would collect this sample at home and bring it into the office or drop it off at the designated laboratory (with a requisition).

24-Hour Urine Specimen

This specimen must be a full 24 hours. The patient would void on arising, but this sample is not collected. The patient needs only to note the time of voiding. The test now begins with an empty bladder. The patient collects all urine voided in a small cup and pours it into the large 24-hour container (which can be picked up at a laboratory). The container is returned to the laboratory by the patient.

Midstream Specimen

The patient collects the specimen *after* approximately one-third of the specimen is passed into the toilet. This acts to "flush" the lower urinary structures of normal contaminants; it is not saved. The patient then collects the second one-third portion (approximately 20 mL); after collection, the patient completes urination into the toilet.

To evaluate the patient's understanding of the proper procedures for a urine specimen collection, have him or her repeat the steps of the procedure to you.

Aseptic Health Practices and Infection Control

In any clinical practice, routine infection control practices are essential to reducing the spread and transmission of infection. Medical asepsis is the state of being free from disease-causing microorganisms; it is concerned with eliminating the spread of disease-producing microorganisms. Infections are the invasion of the body by disease-producing pathogens; many infections are communicable in nature, meaning that they are spread from

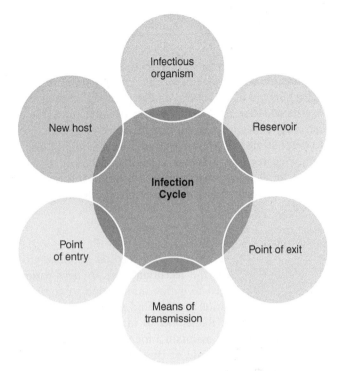

• **Fig. 3.12** Infection cycle.

contact, such as person-to-person. Consider the infection cycle (see Fig. 3.12).

Routine infection control practices are used with all patients to prevent the transmission of diseases. These can typically include:

- Handwashing, the single most effective method to reduce disease transmission
- Gloves, not required when contact is with intact skin; required for invasive procedures, when contact is with membranes
- Facial protection, used when splash of fluids is a possibility
- Gowns, again to protect clothing if any backsplash is a possibility
- Droplet and airborne precautions
- Proper equipment care, use disposable equipment when possible
- Sterilization and disinfection of instruments

For more information and detailed guidelines, contact the Centre for Communicable Diseases and Infection Control, Public Health Agency of Canada (ccdic-clmti@phac-aspc.gc.ca).

Summary

Interactions between receptionists and patients are shaped by the administrative tasks completed jointly by them. Receptionists typically follow established patterns, even when faced with unusual situations. Adopting an approach that balances a task-based focus with a polite, relationship-building demeanor will foster an efficient, welcoming environment in the medical facility. Staff will rely on your competency as a frontline receptionist and will trust you to ensure that the patient experience is positive from the first point of contact. Be mindful that the patient experience often begins and ends with effective appointment scheduling management.

Assignments

Assignment 3.1

As a receptionist, you will be required to secure patient information for the health record. The importance of this collection and of the security of this information cannot be overstated. Research online in your location (province or territory) concerning health care privacy legislation related to the collection, disclosure, and security of health information. Prepare a brief overview in a written document to your instructor detailing what you have learned in your research.

Your instructor may choose to evaluate your performance of this assignment.

Assignment 3.2

Role play—Assume the role of a medical administrative assistant working at the reception desk. A new patient arrives, and you need to gather information to complete the patient information record. Find a partner in the class to be your patient. Remember to introduce yourself and to explain your role; maintain a friendly and relaxed manner. Explain the purpose of data collection and address the issue of privacy regarding the information provided. A blank form to complete the assignment can be found on the Evolve site.

Assignment 3.3

Assume that you are the medical administrative assistant and that a patient has arrived for an appointment. Dr. Plunkett has been called to the hospital to deliver a baby; he expects to return in approximately one hour. You were unable to contact the patient. Think about how you would handle the situation and then write a scenario.

Assignment 3.4

Dr. Plunkett's office is very busy today. Due to an emergency, he is running behind schedule. An aggressive sales representative insists on seeing Dr. Plunkett that day because he is from out of town. He assures you that he will take only five minutes of the doctor's time.

From experience, you know that five minutes is not realistic. Dr. Plunkett has told you not to accept additional appointments today. The sales representative is very insistent.

Jot down some suggestions on how you would handle the situation.

Assignment 3.5

For this assignment, you will create an appointment schedule matrix using today's date.

a. The following appointments have been scheduled and entered in your book. Use an electronic format created in your class to schedule appointments. This scheduling can be completed in manual format as your instructor determines.

Dr. Plunkett and his wife have a dinner engagement at 1700.

The president of the Downtown Kinsmen Club has asked Dr. Plunkett to speak to the Kinsmen Lunch Bunch at 1200. (Dr. Plunkett agreed.)

Dr. Jones, a vascular surgeon, is performing a bypass and graft for hemodialysis (synthetic) on Gary Green and has asked Dr. Plunkett to assist. Surgery will take approximately 2.5 hours beginning at 0900 in O.R. 6 at St. Joseph's Hospital. (Note: When a physician is asked to assist in surgery, the surgeon's office administrator will call the physician's office administrator and advise the time, date, place, type of surgery, patient's name, and approximate length of time for surgery.)

Erik Shultz is "at the end of his rope" with his wife's drinking and needs to talk to the doctor immediately. (Note: Erik works from 0900 to 1900 and finds it difficult to arrange time off work. You feel there is some urgency in this situation. Because Dr. Plunkett usually comes into the office early in the morning, you book Erik in before Dr. Plunkett's scheduled surgery time. You discuss this with the doctor, and he agrees.)

Elizabeth Green has requested an appointment for her annual health examination.

Tim Peters has a large boil on his forearm.

b. Complete the appointment schedule by entering the following appointments, allowing appropriate time periods. If you feel that some appointments do not need to be seen on this schedule, document when you would book them and your reasons for doing so.

Thomas Bell (427-5327) and Heather Smith (576-3225) have requested appointments for complete physicals.

Jean Belliveau and Mary Jane Brown have requested a premarital consultation and physicals. Mary Jane is a regular patient (427-3333), and her fiancé has requested that Dr. Plunkett consider him as a patient.

Hazel Davis (427-7006) is coming in for her monthly O.B. checkup.

There is a flu epidemic, and the following patients are coming in with temperatures, sore throats, and congestion: Peter John Scott (427-2245), Mel Thompson (427-5432), Amelia Jackson (748-3192), Bob Baxter (652-3179), and Lisa Basciano (742-2717).

Lois Elliott (748-3355) is coming in to have a dressing changed.

At 1 p.m. you receive a call from Mrs. Harris, whose 4-month-old baby, William, has been crying and upset all morning. He is screaming in obvious pain, and Mrs. Harris is very upset. What will you do?

Assignment 3.6

Choose an appropriate scheduling system as determined by your instructor. Use today's date. The doctor will see patients from 9 a.m. to 6 p.m. with lunch from 12 to 1:30.

Rosie Smythe (236-7712) has a boil on her arm.

Sara Downs (471-3327) is becoming drug dependent and requests some counselling.

Gary Groves (236-8717) has been experiencing severe dizziness when he stands up and lies down.

Annabell Ford (236-3131) has an excruciating pain in her left thigh.

George Arthur (471-3728) has large sores in his mouth.

Ryan Elder (471-3515) has oozing sores on both ankles. He thinks it might be poison ivy.

Deanna Duggan (236-4131) has had intermittent chest pains over the past few days. The pain radiates into her neck and right shoulder blade.

Brad Nichols (471-3112) is experiencing tightness in his chest, and his heartbeat races periodically.

James Noris (236-3449) has a bunion on his left toe; it is causing severe discomfort.

Walter Page (471-9952) is very uncomfortable because of constipation.

Janie Packer (471-8987) has several warts on her fingers.

Chuck Leahy (236-3577) has just been fired from his job and is very depressed.

Bunni Rill (471-8338) has had a cold; she now has a fever and is having trouble getting her breath.

Kendra Hall (236-1122) is experiencing severe pain in her lower back that radiates into her left leg.

Mohamed Nasir (471-8772) is booked to have stitches removed from a laceration on his right hand.

Sue Jessup (471-5567) has a broken wrist, and her cast is getting loose. She is booked for a new cast.

Cheryl Page (236-3396) has had diarrhea for almost two weeks.

Diane Stevens (236-4747) is having hot flashes and experiences occasional periods of depression.

Jack Porter (236-3991) has a cloudy film over his left eye.

John Bard (471-9988) needs to have his blood pressure checked.

Harry Duffell (236-9991) has had pains in his stomach and some blood in his stool.

Ted Lang (236-6667) needs an allergy shot.

Harold Topper (236-1112) has severe laryngitis.

Assignment 3.7

Clinical skills practice role-play. Find a partner in the classroom. This person will be your patient for today, and they have arrived for a complete physical examination. Conduct the following:

a. Patient interview and record patient's subjective statements

b. Practise taking and recording the vital signs and blood pressure

c. Instruct the patient on how to prepare for the physician's examination

Your instructor will observe your performance.

Topics for Discussion

1. What amenities add to the atmosphere of the waiting room? Discuss pros and cons of clocks and televisions in the waiting room.

2. Discuss with your classmates the importance of the reception role in a health care practice. Share a positive experience you have encountered. Share a negative experience you have encountered. What made it positive, and what made it negative?

3. If a patient arrives in your office before you have had a chance to call them to rebook a cancelled appointment, how would you handle the situation?

4. Rate the following medical situations in terms of how urgently an office appointment is needed by circling a number on the scale provided; 1 is most urgent, and 5 is least urgent.

	Most			Least	
Annual checkup	1	2	3	4	5
Infected toenail × 1 week	1	2	3	4	5
Worried about moles (read about melanoma)	1	2	3	4	5
Painful urination × 3 days	1	2	3	4	5
Missed period—pregnancy test?	1	2	3	4	5
Baby coughing at night	1	2	3	4	5
Sore on leg won't heal	1	2	3	4	5
Camp medical (must be within 30 days)	1	2	3	4	5

5. As discussed in Chapter 1, it is necessary to prioritize your work to maintain an organized and efficient office. You are working alone in a physician's office. Number the following scenarios in the order you would deal with them, and discuss the reasons for your chosen order.

a. The mail has just arrived.

b. The doctor is looking for test results on a patient he is currently seeing.

c. The phone is ringing.

d. The next two patients have arrived.

e. Mrs. Jackson is leaving and requires an urgent referral for a diagnostic test.

f. The examination room needs to be made ready for the next patient.

g. Mr. Baxter would like you to call him a taxi.

4

Patient Records Management

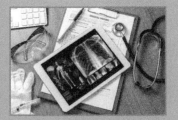

Source: istockphoto.com/metamorworks

The chapter provides practical information related to the creation, maintenance, and storage of medical records. The contents of the typical medical file are introduced, and the concepts and associations related to keeping medical records safe are reinforced. Standardized rules for alphabetic, numeric, and subject filing are presented, along with how to use charge-out cards, tickler files, and Soundex files. The chapter offers best practices related to efficient and accurate filing.

CHAPTER OUTLINE

Introduction

Patient Chart Basics

Folders

Cabinets

Filing

LEARNING OBJECTIVES

After reading this chapter, you will be able to:

1. Describe the status of technological advancements with respect to patient files
2. Describe the procedures for preparing patient file folders (e.g., charts)
3. Understand the rules for alphabetical filing
4. Understand general correspondence filing, subject and tickler filing, preparing correspondence for filing, charge-out systems, and updating files
5. Describe the purpose of colour-coding files
6. Recognize the points to follow for efficient filing procedures

KEY TERMS

Canada Health Infoway: Canada Health Infoway works with the federal government, provinces, and territories to bring digital health solutions to Canadians.

Charge-out card: The charge-out card is made of heavy cardboard and is inserted where a file has been removed. The patient's name, the date the file was removed, who removed it, and the current location are documented on the card.

Cross-reference: Cross-referencing is used when charts are filed numerically. A system is required that will match the name of the patient or individual with the number that has been assigned. Cross-referencing can also be used when two names sound the same but are spelled differently, for example, "Thompson" and "Thomson." A cross-reference page would be filed with these charts. This page would be coloured (for easy identification) and lightweight (to conserve space).

Electronic Health Record: "An electronic health record (EHR) refers to the systems that make up the secure and private lifetime record of a person's health and health care history. These systems store and share such information as laboratory results, medication profiles, key clinical reports (e.g., hospital discharge summaries), diagnostic images (e.g., x-rays), and immunization history. The information is

available electronically to authorized health care providers" (Canada Health Infoway: Solutions, 2018, para 1).

Guides: Visual markers that lead the filer to a specific location in either open cabinets or file drawers. They may be primary subject guides (accounting), letter guides (highlighting the start of new section of the alphabet), or number guides (highlighting the start of new number or series of numbers). They may be used in conjunction with colour coding to increase the efficiency of the filing process.

Out-folder: The out-folder is similar to the charge-out card in that it is also inserted where a file has been removed. Information that is to be filed in the missing chart is placed in the folder and can be easily filed when the chart is returned to the filing system.

Purging: The removal of inactive files from active files. These files would include patients who have moved out of town, transferred to another physician, or are deceased. The files on these patients are moved to a secure separate storage area, either onsite or offsite.

Tickler file: The tickler file is a reminder system. Its purpose is to "tickle" your memory.

Introduction

The use of electronic medical records (EMRs) in medical offices has increased substantially since the early 2000s. Canada Health Infoway measured a 69% increase from 2004 to 2017 (Leaver, 2017). Some provinces, including Alberta, Ontario, and Nova Scotia, have offered health service providers assistance with EMR funding, allowing them to be more progressive than other provinces; however, all Canadian provinces have substantially increased their use of EMRs and electronic health records (EHRs). The solutions provided by these computer information systems have decreased the need for numerous file cabinets and the process of manual filing; however, many medical environments dealing with patient information (e.g., private practices, hospitals) are still using manual filing systems or a combination of manual and electronic files. No matter which type of system your place of employment chooses, you must understand the rules and concepts of manual filing to be an effective medical administrative assistant. The concepts, rules, regulations, and expectations that apply to the management of manual records also apply to or complement those related to electronic records management.

Patient Chart Basics

Because patient charts are the backbone of the physician's practice, the administrative assistant must be precise when handling them. Any office personnel responsible for filing charts and charting information must have accurate spelling skills and knowledge of record keeping policies as outlined by the College of Physicians and Surgeons. They should also keep up to date on health information management practices through association with the Canadian Health Information Management Association or ARMA (discussed in Chapter 2).

Doctors' offices generally maintain a personal file folder (chart) for each patient. The chart provides a chronological history of the patient's care. This includes diagnostic tests, hospital visits, admissions, and consultative visits with other providers. Information is filed in reverse chronological order, which means that the most recent visit or test is on the top. The folders are usually filed in alphabetical order and colour-coded, or both, for easy reference.

Here are a few important things to keep in mind when you are handling files:

- A lost file could cause a disaster and negatively affect patient care. When paper files have been removed from the stacks or drawers, be sure you use a charge-out card (discussed in more detail later in this chapter), and promptly return the files to their proper place when they are no longer needed.
- Do not leave files (electronic or paper) in open view of nonmedical personnel in the office—remember the importance of maintaining confidentiality. If you leave your desk, even for a moment, cover the files, turn them face down, minimize your computer screen, or log out of your EMR screen.
- When colour-coding is used, a periodic scan for misplaced files can be accomplished quickly and ensures that each chart is in the correct location.
- Be sure to put all relevant material in the correct patient's manual or electronic chart. Do not simply check for a patient's name; also look at a unique identifier, such as a personal health number. Documents misfiled in electronic systems can be just as difficult to find as those misplaced in a manual system.
- All paper charts should be filed by the end of the day. If this is not possible, it is good practice to put them in the order in which they are to be filed, either alphabetically or numerically, and then to place them in a storage area (a drawer or empty file area) where they can be locked up.

DID YOU KNOW?

When personal health information is inappropriately accessed, lost, or stolen, it is necessary to consider whether patients should be notified. In some cases, it is mandatory to contact the affected patient(s), the College of Physicians and Surgeons, the Office of the Privacy Commissionaire, and/or the ministry of health. Because the regulations are different in each province and territory, the Canadian Medical Protective Association (CMPA) recommends that it be contacted directly for advice and clarification (Canadian Medical Protective Association [CMPA], 2018).

Each doctor has preferences for the setup of individual patient files. For paper charts, the outside and inside cover of the file folder, or both, can be utilized to provide patient information, thereby saving time when looking up patient details. (A rubber stamp can be designed and ordered to suit the physician's requirements, or a computerized label maker may be used—see Fig. 4.1.)

NAME _____ D.O.B. _____

HEALTH CARD # _____ VERSION CODE _____

PHONE # (HOME) _____ WORK _____

ALLERGIES _____

EMERGENCY CONTACT _____

• **Fig. 4.1** Rubber stamp/label format.

Special notations regarding allergies, medications, or serious illnesses may be noted on a form and attached to the left inside cover of the folder, so that they will be immediately noticeable. Some paper charts have preprinted inside covers that include an area for medications and allergies. Patient allergies may be written in red pen, or a coloured sticker (preferably red) may be placed beside the word *allergies* to alert the doctor that a patient has allergies. What the patient is allergic to should be easily visible on the chart. Each page that is added to the patient's history should also include an allergy notation. In an EMR, medication allergies are noted by navigating to the allergy or adverse reaction screen and choosing the medication or substance from a drop-down list. Caution must be used when choosing the correct medication or substance, and often the system will require a physician to verify the allergy, its severity, and its reaction.

A typical paper patient chart may include the following:
1. A family medicine form (also referred to as a *progress note* or a *patient history note*) (see Fig. 4.2). This will provide all the details about the patient's past history up to and including the most recent illness. This sheet should have the patient's name and medical billing number displayed at the top. Each entry must include the visit date, and medical administrative assistants should always ensure that there is sufficient space for physician notes; new sheets should be readily available and added to the chart if space is limited or previous sheets are full.
2. Other relevant forms that the doctor requires. These may include infant and child progress record forms (see Figs. 4.3 and 4.4), prenatal or antenatal records, and results of routine and diagnostic tests, including blood work, x-rays, and so on. These forms should be filed behind the family medicine sheet.
3. Correspondence is filed behind all pertinent medical information. This would include consultative notes from other providers, operative notes, and hospital notes.

Items (1), (2), and (3) would be filed on the right side of the folder with the history sheet on top, followed by reports in date order, and then correspondence in date order, with the most recent on the top. In an EMR, these items can be grouped into their respective folders for easy retrieval.

Small forms and notes should be taped or stapled to a full-size (8.5 inch × 11 inch) sheet of paper to avoid misplacement in a paper file. Most laboratory results and other diagnostic reports are now printed on 8.5 × 11 paper. Some physicians prefer that all records concerning a specific illness be organized or stapled together; this is called a problem-oriented medical record (POMR). Paper clips are not recommended because papers can pull away from the clip and become mixed with unrelated documents, or the clip may catch onto other documents.

The patient's chart is a legal document, and maintenance of this record is extremely important. In the event that it is necessary to add, modify, or correct an entry in a patient's medical chart, CMPA recommends that the changes be dated and signed (or initialed) or, in the case of electronic records, authenticated. When amending a clinical record, the original entry must not be destroyed (CMPA, 2009).

Information concerning transfer of files, the release of information from files, and the length of time files must be retained was discussed in Chapter 2. Not only must these regulations be complied with, but CMPA also recommends that after the required retention period has been met, records should be destroyed in a manner such that they cannot be reconstructed. This means that records must be shredded, pulverized, or incinerated. A list of any destroyed records must also be kept. For electronic records, permanent deletion is required (CMPA, 2016). Medical records management in a hospital setting, including the use of EHRs, will be discussed also in Chapter 12.

Folders

Heavy-duty, letter-size manila file folders are generally used in medical offices. The tab is the projection at the top or side (end) of the folder. Top-side, 1/5 or 1/2, tabs are used in file drawers as shown in Figs. 4.5 and 4.6. Bar-style end tabs are used in open-shelf cabinets.

Some physicians prefer file folders that have inside fasteners embedded into the chart. When using this chart type, all diagnostic tests are filed on the left side of the chart, with all visits and correspondence on the right side (see Fig. 4.7). A special hole-punch is needed to prepare your information for filing in this type of chart. The benefit of this type of file is that it reduces the risk of information falling out of the chart. The downside is that it takes longer to file the information.

Cabinets

The most popular types of file cabinets used in medical offices are open-shelf file cabinets and four- or five-drawer upright steel cabinets. Open-shelf cabinets save floor space and provide quicker access than drawer-type cabinets. They are available with covers that pull down to close and lock for security purposes, and they are available in a double-sided rotary format that revolves to hide and secure files. The drawer-style cabinets use "Hang-a-file" systems for easy access. The five-drawer cabinet unit will hold approximately 720 files, and the open-shelf unit with seven 90-cm (36-inch) shelves will hold approximately 1000 files. A lock is essential on any type of medical record holder to maintain confidentiality.

If ordering new filing cabinets, keep in mind how many people will be accessing the cabinets at the same time. Some cabinets have a safety feature built in that will not allow another drawer to be opened if one is in use.

Filing

Filing is the process of uniformly arranging information so that it can be easily accessed and efficiently used. In a

FAMILY MEDICINE						
Name			Insurance #			S M W D
Address			Phones (H)	(O)		
Occupation			Date of Birth			Age
Medical Data	HT	WT	BP	PULSE	RESP	TEMP
Allergies			Drug Allergies			
DATE	HISTORY & PHYSICAL					

• **Fig. 4.2** Family medicine chart.

INFANT PROGRESS RECORD
0 – 24 Months

Name _____

Date of Birth _____ Sex M/F

B.Wt. _____ Kg _____ lb. Length _____ cm. Head _____ cm. Chest _____ cm. D.Wt _____ Kg _____ lb.

Maturity _____ wks. Apgar _____ / _____ Blood Gp. _____ Rh _____ P.K.U. _____ Thyroid _____

Problems: Prenatal _____ Labour _____ Neonatal _____

Defects: _____ Marks _____ Circ. _____

Breast until _____ Bottle until _____ Started juice _____ Started solids _____

Landmarks — 25th Percentile – 90th Percentile in months

Motor	Date	Mo
Prone lifts head 1.3 – 3.2		
Follows light 1.8 – 4.0		
Rolls over 2.3 – 4.7		
Grasps 2.5 – 4.2		
Reaches out 2.9 – 5.0		
Sits unsupported 4.8 – 7.8		
First tooth		
Stands holding 5.0 – 10.0		
Stands alone 9.8 – 13.9		
Walks 11.3 – 13.3		
Kicks ball 15.0 – 24.0		

Social	Date	Mo
Blinks to clap		
Smiles back – 1.9		
Laughs 1.4 – 3.3		
Sleeps through night 6 + hours		
Turns to voice 3.8 – 8.3		
Things to mouth		
Feeds self 4.7 – 8.0		
Says Dada or Mama 5.6 – 10.0		
Drinks from cup 10.0 – 14.3		
Uses spoon 13.3 – 23.5		
Combine 2 words 14 – 23		

DPTp: 1 _____ 2 _____ 3 _____ 4 _____

O.T.T. _____ M.M.R. _____ Reactions _____ Allergies _____

Months	1	2	3	4	6	9	12	15	18	24
Date										
Wt. kg.										
Length/cm.										
Head circ.										
Heart sounds										
Breath sounds										
Abdomen										
Skin										
Legs										
Other	Hips	Hearing	PKU	Hips	Babbling	Hb				

• **Fig. 4.3** Infant progress report.

CHILD PROGRESS RECORD
2 – 15 Years

Name _____

Date of Birth _____ Sex M/F

INFANT & HEREDITARY PROBLEMS _____

_____

LANDMARKS 25-90%ile in Yrs.	Date	Age
Testes Descended		
Clean at night		
Dry at night		
Throws ball 1.4 – 2.6		
Gives own name 2.0 – 3.8		
Does up buttons 2.6 – 4.2		
Recognizes 3 colours 2.7 – 4.9		
Hops on one foot 3.0 – 4.9		
Catches ball 3.5 – 5.5		
Ties shoelaces		
First menstruation		
Voice breaks		
Axillary hair		

ILLNESSES	Date	Age
Eczema		
Croup		
Bronchitis		
Allergies		
Tonsillitis		
Ear infections		
Pyrexia over 40°C		
Convulsions		
Chicken Pox		

IMMUNIZATIONS:

Pre School
DPTp x 3 + 1 _____
M.M.R. _____
DPTp _____
O.T.T. _____

10 Years
DPT _____
O.T.T. _____
Hb _____
Rubella Titre _____

15 Years
DPT _____
O.T.T. _____
Hb _____
ASOT _____

Years/Months	2	3	4	5	6	7	8	9	10	11	12	13	14	15
Height cm.														
Height %ile														
Wt. kg.														
Wt. %ile														
Vision Right														
Left														
Near														
Urine Albumin														
Glucose														
Blood Pressure														
Ears														
Eyes														
Nose														
Throat														
Teeth														
Neck														
Lungs														
Heart sounds														
Abdomen														
Legs														
Back														
Posture														
Other														

PUBERTY STATUS

Female
1. Flat
2. Breast buds
3. Enlargement – Slight raising
4. Separate breast contour

Male
1. Infantile
2. Testes enlarging, scrotum & coarse
3. Penis lengthening
4. Penis enlarging, scrotal skin pigmented

Pubic Hair
1. None
2. Sparse, downy
3. Pigmented, coarse, curling
4. Adult

• **Fig. 4.4** Child progress record.

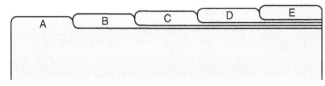

• **Fig. 4.5** 1/5 cut folders.

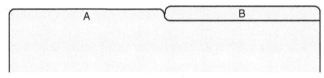

• **Fig. 4.6** 1/2 cut folders.

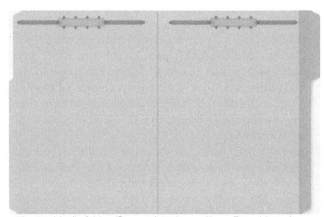

• **Fig. 4.7** Manila folder. (Source: istock.com/Anna Pogrebkova.)

TABLE 4.1	**Indexing Patient Names**		
Patient Name	**Unit 1**	**Unit 2**	**Unit 3**
Mary Jane Brown	BROWN	Mary	Jane
Lisa Basciano	BASCIANO	Lisa	
Thomas William Bell	BELL	Thomas	William
Robert T. Baxter	BAXTER	Robert	T
Jean Etienne Belliveau	BELLIVEAU	Jean	Etienne

TABLE 4.2	**Patient Names Alphabetized by Indexing Unit 1**		
Patient Name	**Unit 1**	**Unit 2**	**Unit 3**
Lisa Basciano	BASCIANO	Lisa	
Robert T. Baxter	BAXTER	Robert	T
Thomas William Bell	BELL	Thomas	William
Jean Etienne Belliveau	BELLIVEAU	Jean	Etienne
Mary Jane Brown	BROWN	Mary	Jane

medical office, it is the alphabetical or numerical arrangement of patient charts and patient information that you will be most concerned with. Before patient information can be filed alphabetically, you need to know how to arrange the units of patients' names into the correct filing order. This is called *indexing*. Patient names are indexed into units (each part of the name is a unit) in the order of last name, first name, and middle name (or initial) if one is available. When file labels are used on chart tabs, the patient names should also be arranged in this order to assist in the filing process. Punctuation is not considered during indexing. See Table 4.1 for how to index an average patient name.

Rules for Alphabetical Filing

To alphabetically file indexed names, you first compare the first units (last names), letter by letter. For example, the first letter of all last names in Table 4.1 is the same. Because of this, you need to move on to the second letter of the last names for comparison. There are two names that begin with "BA," two that begin with "BE," and one that begins with "BR." You know the "BAs" will come before

the "BEs," but you still need to determine which "BA" comes first and which "BE" comes first. To do this, you need to look at the next letter in each pair. In this scenario, the third letters are different in the "BA" pair, so you can now put the names in correct alphabetical order. In the "BE" pair, you have to look to the fifth place to determine which goes first. Because there is no fifth letter in "Bell," it will come before "Belliveau" because of the "nothing before something" rule (discussed below). See Table 4.2 for the correct alphabetization of the indexed names from Table 4.1.

If all the letters of the first unit are identical, the second unit is then considered, letter by letter (see Table 4.3).

If all the letters in the second unit are the same, the third unit is then considered (see Table 4.4).

Three units will be sufficient for filing purposes in most medical offices. The following rules should also be applied to the process and will provide explanations for what to do in some special circumstances.

1. When identical names occur (all indexing units are the same), the next consideration may be town or city, province, followed by street address. For example, Thomas Bell, 175 Park Street, Ottawa, Ontario; Thomas Bell, 134 King Street, Ottawa, Ontario; and Thomas Bell, 283 King Street, Ottawa, Ontario would be indexed as seen in Table 4.5.

   Other options for when identical names occur are the patients' dates of birth or health numbers. All options are acceptable; however, unique numbers such as health num-

TABLE 4.3 Patient Names Alphabetized by Indexing Unit 2

Patient Name	Unit 1	Unit 2	Unit 3
Andrea T. Brown	BROWN	Andrea	T
Andrew Brown	BROWN	Andrew	
Bethany A. Brown	BROWN	Bethany A	
Marie Anne Brown	BROWN	Marie	Anne
Mary Jane Brown	BROWN	Mary	Jane

TABLE 4.4 Patient Names Alphabetized by Indexing Unit 3

Patient Name	Unit 1	Unit 2	Unit 3
Robert A. Baxter	BAXTER	Robert	A
Robert Andrew Baxter	BAXTER	Robert	Andrew
Robert Brian Baxter	BAXTER	Robert	Brian
Robert T. Baxter	BAXTER	Robert	T
Robert Zane Baxter	BAXTER	Robert	Zane

TABLE 4.5 Indexing Units for Identical Names

Unit 1	Unit 2	Unit 3	Unit 4	Unit 5	Unit 6
BELL	Thomas	Ottawa	Ontario	King Street	134
BELL	Thomas	Ottawa	Ontario	King Street	283
BELL	Thomas	Ottawa	Ontario	Park Street	175

bers may be the most fail-safe. This is because people with the same name can also have the same date of birth, and, although less common, people with the same name can live at the same address. Whichever option is used at your office, it must be applied consistently.

2. Always use the patient's proper name and not a nickname. For example, use Robert even though the patient is known as *Bob* or *Rob*. You can add the patient's nickname to the file label (in parentheses) to remind yourself to use it when speaking with them, but do not use it for filing purposes. It is also important to ask the patient what his or her legal name is; Betty or Bette is not always a short form for Elizabeth. Do not guess the meaning of a nickname. If you do encounter abbreviated names on correspondence, you should consider them in full when filing; for example, Jas. is James, Chas. is Charles, and Wm. is William.

3. Always remember the rule "nothing before something" when considering all alphabetizing. See Table 4.4 for an example. Notice Robert A comes before Robert Andrew in the alphabetical order. This is because there is "nothing" to consider after the "A" in Robert A, and there is "something" to consider after the "A" in Robert Andrew.

4. Hyphenated names (first, last, or middle) are considered to be one indexing unit; for example, MacKenzie-King, Betty-Jean, and Knockwood-Redsky would all be indexed as one unit. No punctuation is considered. For example, MacKenzie-King would appear as MACKENZIEKING. See Table 4.6 for more examples.

5. Last names that begin with prefixes are considered one unit, even if there is a space between the prefix and the name. If you are not sure whether a name includes a prefix, ask the patient for clarification. Examples of common prefixes are Del, Du, El, Fitz, Las, Los, Mac, Mc, O', Saint, San, St. (do not write out as Saint), Van, Van de, Van der, and others. NOTE: Names that begin with "Mac" and "Mc" are not indexed or filed the same, despite sounding the same. However, some offices may treat them similarly for simplicity. Some commercial colour-coded tabs include a "Mc" tab and not a "Mac" tab. Be sure that you understand how your office deals with these and other similar names with prefixes and remain consistent with office procedures. Table 4.7 provides an alphabetized example.

6. Degrees (M.D., Ph.D.), professional titles (Dr., Senator), military titles (General, Major, Private), and personal titles (Mr., Mrs., Ms.) are not considered in filing. If patients wish to be addressed with any of these titles, you can add the preference to their file label in parentheses as a reminder.

7. Seniority designations are considered as the last indexing unit and used only with identical names. They are filed in numerical and alphabetical order, depending on their origin. For instance, 1st, 2nd, 3rd are examples of Arabic numbers; I, II, and III are Roman numbers; and Jr. and Sr. are generational terms expressed as abbreviated suffixes (or written out in full). Within these designations, the order of alphabetizing is Arabic numbers first, Roman numbers second, and generational suffixes last. No punctuation is considered. See Table 4.8 for an alphabetized example.

8. When a name consists of a title (such as religious or royal titles) and either a given name or a surname, do not transpose the name; you can make the title an indexing unit. However, this can cause some confusion when filing in a medical office, so it is always good to ask the patient for his or her other name for filing purposes. You can add their title to their file label in parentheses to indicate how to address them during conversation (see Table 4.9).

General Correspondence

A doctor's private practice is classified as a small business. As a result, you will be dealing with records other than patient charts. Some general correspondence files would be kept separate from patient charts. The following are examples of general correspondence types you may encounter:

- Drug suppliers
- Travel agents
- Building and equipment maintenance
- Insurance companies
- Utilities, heat, and telephone

TABLE 4.6 Indexed and Alphabetized List Including Hyphenated Names

Patient Name	Unit 1	Unit 2	Unit 3
Lisa Basciano	BASCIANO	Lisa	
Lisa Jane Basciano	BASCIANO	Lisa	Jane
Lisa-Jane Basciano	BASCIANO	LisaJane	
Lisa-Jane J. Basciano	BASCIANO	LisaJane	J
Lisa D. Basciano-Lee	BASCIANOLEE	Lisa	D

TABLE 4.7 Last Names With Prefixes

Patient Name	Unit 1	Unit 2
Ashley Del Rio	DELRIO	Ashley
Paul MacDonald	MACDONALD	Paul
John McDonald	MCDONALD	John
Rick Van der Veen	VANDERVEEN	Rick
Erin Van Duzee	VANDUZEE	Erin

TABLE 4.8 Alphabetized Seniority Designations

Patient Name	Unit 1	Unit 2	Unit 3	Unit 4
Todd A. Bernard, 3rd	BERNARD	Todd	A	3rd
Todd. A. Bernard, II	BERNARD	Todd	A	II
Todd A. Bernard, Jr.	BERNARD	Todd	A	Jr
Todd A. Bernard, Sr.	BERNARD	Todd	A	Sr

- Office supplies
- Medical supply companies

You may choose to file your general correspondence alphabetically, or you may use a subject filing system that combines alphabetizing with primary subject guides. When filing correspondence for medical facilities and other businesses alphabetically, names are filed as they are written (introductory and connecting words such as *the, and,* and *A* are not considered when indexing). Symbols, except for ampersands (&), are filed as spelled out and used as indexing units (see Table 4.10). If a business name consists of a person's given name and surname, treat it as you would any other personal name (last name, first name, middle name).

If you wish to file by subject instead of company, follow the guidelines in the Subject Filing section below.

TABLE 4.9 Religious or Royal Titles

Patient Name	Unit 1	Unit 2
Princess Victoria	DUPONT	Victoria (Princess)
Reverend Mulhaney	MULHANEY	Robert (Rev.)
Sister Veronica	O'NEILL	Veronica (Sister)

TABLE 4.10 Alphabetical Filing by Company Name

Company Name	Unit 1	Unit 2	Unit 3
Diagnostics + Incorporated	Diagnostics (+)	Plus	Incorporated
The Drug Shoppe	Drug	Shoppe	
Ottawa General Hospital	Ottawa	General	Hospital
Park & Davis	Parke (&)	Davis	
Parker James Limited	Parker	James	Limited
Stevens and MacDonald	Stevens	MacDonald	
Stevens Medical Supplies	Stevens	Medical	Supplies

Subject Filing

In a subject filing system, the main subject (for example, drug suppliers) is identified on the divider tab, and all drug suppliers' files are placed in alphabetical order in the drug suppliers' section. The main sections are also filed in alphabetical order. In the example below, the main subjects are illustrated with all uppercase letters, and the subsidiary files are beneath them with each word in each entry having an initial capital.

The order of your general correspondence file system would appear as follows:

BUILDING AND EQUIPMENT MAINTENANCE
    Adams Carpentry Service
    Brintnell General Maintenance
    Dynamic Maid Service
DRUG SUPPLIERS
    Best Buy Drugs
    Medicare Drug Company
    Zanzibar Clinical Supplies
INSURANCE COMPANIES
    Component Property Insurance
    Friendly Automobile Insurance
    Jackson Life Insurance

TRAVEL AGENCIES
Fly Safe Travellers
Plan-a-Trip Agencies
Quiet Vacations Limited
UTILITIES, HEAT, AND TELEPHONE
Bell Canada
Public Utilities Ltd.
Research Gas Company

Numerical Filing

Hospitals and large group practices generally use numerical filing systems. Doctors may choose to file by number for reasons of confidentiality. Each patient chart is assigned a special number and filed in numerical order. This number can be generated by the EMR when patient information is registered to the system. It can also be a personal health number (as it is read left to right), a terminal-digit version of a health number (as it is read right to left), or some combination of these. For instance, a clinic may choose to flip the last four digits and the first four digits of an eight-digit health number (01234567 becomes 45670123). Regardless of which arrangement is chosen, a cross-reference file is required in which the patients' names are listed with their assigned numbers and filed in alphabetical order. Most EMRs will have built-in cross-referencing systems. When the patient information is accessed, the patient's assigned number also appears on the screen. If your files are numerical, you will need to look up each patient every time you need his or her chart or to file patient reports. If you are not using an EMR, you can create cross-referencing lists in your word-processing or database software rather than using a manual file (see Fig. 4.8). A paper copy should be kept in a safe and confidential space for use during power outages or other computer downtimes. Most doctors' offices file alphabetically, which removes the need to look up every patient in the computer each time the chart is needed.

Soundex Filing

Soundex filing is generally used to overcome the problem of names that sound similar but are spelled many different ways, for example, Bare, Bear, Baher, and Bayer. The Soundex system incorporates six basic phonetic sounds with coded numbers. Some computer systems have this built in as an additional patient search. Although not widely used, it is efficient and allows for rapid filing. Because it is fairly complex, it will not be discussed further in this text.

Tickler File

Every efficient medical administrative assistant has some type of reminder system. In a busy medical office, it is impossible to remember all the details for efficient patient health care. A

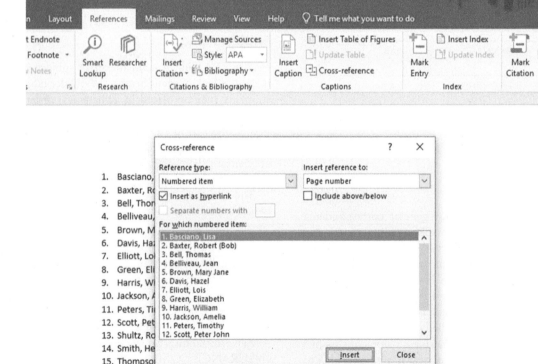

• **Fig. 4.8** Cross-reference in word processor.

reminder system is often referred to as a "tickler file" because the system is designed to "tickle" your memory. There are several ways to implement a tickler system. You may choose simply to record reminder notes on your daily calendar and asterisk them with a red pen. A more complex system is to have a small file box with 12 divisions for each month of the year. A subdivider for each day of the month is placed behind the month divider. Reminders are recorded on cards and placed behind the appropriate month/day division.

Most eCommunication tools have built-in or downloadable reminder systems. They may be accessed through calendar apps, e-mail reminders, scheduling apps, or some combination of these. Be sure the tools you choose are mandated by your employer and do not cause you to breach any policies—such as cell phone or mobile device restrictions. Regardless of the system you choose, it is important to refer to your tickler system each day, as soon after your arrival in the office as possible. If you are using electronic reminders, make sure they are set for when you arrive in the office. This system will only work if you use it faithfully.

Filing Preparation

Offices use various methods to prepare documents for filing. Some routines include the following:

- All documents need a visible indicator of what action is to be taken. Once the doctor has seen a document (report, letter, or request), he or she needs to code it according to an agreed-upon system. A code number, checkmark, doctor's initials, or other consistent symbol(s) can be used to tell you whether a document is ready for filing or whether it needs further action. For example, when the physician has viewed the information, he or she writes a "C" on it, which means that you will need to pull the chart. If an "F" is written on it, it can then be filed. Charts that are returned for filing can be placed in a designated area that is identified as "To Be Filed."
- Prepare a cross-reference page to be filed with material that may be under a different heading. Cross-reference sheets should be coloured (for easy identification) and lightweight (to conserve space). Here are some situations that would require cross-referencing:
  a. When names sound the same but are spelled differently (e.g., "Thompson" and "Thomson").
  b. When it is difficult to distinguish between a given name and surname (e.g., Lloyd George, when George is the surname). It is a good idea to capitalize or underline the last name.
  c. When a woman retains her maiden name after marriage and you want to have a cross-reference to her husband's name.
- Sort all materials in preparation for filing. If you have a large stack of filing, you can start with a "rough sort." This is when you split a large stack into smaller stacks by letters of the alphabet (or by number series for numerical filing). Make one pile for each letter, or a small range of letters, and alphabetize these small groups first. Then, you can combine all the smaller piles together into one

large alphabetized stack. This process reduces the chance for errors and makes what may seem like an overwhelming task much more manageable. This procedure generally takes place on a desk or by means of a collating rack. The sorted documents are then taken to the file area for quick and easy insertion into the appropriate file folders.

It is important that your filing take priority, even though it is the one responsibility that seems to get postponed. Inefficient filing will result in an inefficient office and may cause delays or errors in patient care. If you have incomplete filing at the beginning of your day, you need to check it for reports or other essential information about the patients being seen in the office that day.

Charge-Out Systems

If a file is removed, a charge-out card (sometimes referred to as an "out" card) may be inserted in its place (see Fig. 4.9). The card is generally made of heavy, coloured cardboard and has lines on which to write the date of removal, the name of the person who removed the file, and the file's current location. It would be very time-consuming for a medical administrative assistant to "charge-out" the files of patients visiting the office each day, so for regular patient visits you should not insert an "out" card in place of the patient's file, because it should be either on your desk or with the doctor. Removal of a patient's chart from the files for any other reason, however, requires a "charge-out."

Some offices may use a computerized chart location system to eliminate the need for a manual charge-out system. This is usually utilized by large facilities that share a central records department or a hospital records department.

Out-Folders

An out-folder is used for temporary filing of data. It is used in the same way as a charge-out card. The folder is placed where the chart should be, and test results or correspondence for the patient are placed in the folder. When the chart is returned, it is easy to file the information.

CRITICAL THINKING

A patient chart is missing from your cabinet; it is not on the doctor's desk, and you do not have it. The patient was recently at the office for a visit, and you remember he requested a letter for his employer. You suspect that the physician may have taken the chart home, but you don't know for sure. What can you do to ensure that other staff members are aware of the missing file and that any papers you have to file do not get misplaced in its absence?

FILE LOCATION

Date Removed	By	Can Be Found	Date Returned	Initial When Ret.
Dec. 20/18	Jane Smith	In Business Office	Dec. 23/18	J. S.
Jan 1/19	Dr. Plunkett	My Desk	Jan 15/19	JEP
Mar. 18/19	Dr. Pelham	at my home	Mar. 22/19	E.J.P.

• **Fig. 4.9** Charge-out card.

Purging Files

To maintain an efficient filing system, it is necessary to perform periodic purging of your records. This task may be done when the physician is absent from the office and your workload is not as heavy as usual. Files of patients who have moved out of town, have transferred to another physician, or are deceased would be removed from your active files and stored as inactive files in a storage area. You may also have patients who require that their files be "thinned" because of their large size. This means that older material should be removed from the file and placed in a separate file that can be stored. This process requires you to give each chart a version or volume code, usually a number. For instance, the first time you thin a file, the material you remove and store is volume 1, and the active file becomes volume 2. (Note: An accurate and current list of stored files and their location must be maintained.) Some offices store their purged files in a secure off-site location, due to lack of space. The services of a document-scanning and archiving company may also be sought, provided the proper security, retention, and access can be ensured.

Colour-Coded Files

The use of colour-coded files is a very efficient system for identifying file folders and is used extensively in the medical environment. It is easy to find misplaced files in a colour-coded system: If a purple label is mixed in with the red labels, it is easily spotted. Colour-coding also makes filing records faster and easier.

There are many colour-coding systems (Oxford; Smead) produced by office supply companies. They consist of adhesive coloured tabs with each colour stamped with a letter of the alphabet or set of numbers (usually 0 to 9). The tabs can be purchased in kits with all of the letters or numbers present in one box (see Fig. 4.10), or each letter and number can be purchased separately on a roll. Offices have different ways of coding their files, and all are acceptable as long as the system is agreed upon and consistently applied. In some offices, the first three letters of a patient's last name may be identified with colours. For example, if your colour-coding system stipulated that the letter "A" would be pink, the letter "G" would be green, the letter "U" would be purple, and the letter "T" would be light blue, then the folder for "Agar" would have a pink tab, a green tab, and another pink tab. The folder for "Autum" would have a pink tab, a purple tab, and a light blue tab. The folder end-tab (also called "bar-style" because the tab runs the entire length of the chart—it is not 1/2 cut or 1/5 cut like a top-tab) would still have a label with the patient's full name typed on it, last name first. In other offices, there may be a combination of letters from the patient's last name and first name; fewer or more tabs may be used. In specialists' offices, the coding often includes a number tab that indicates

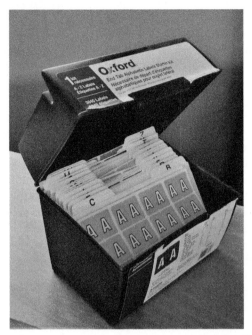

• **Fig. 4.10** Colour-coded tab kit. (Source: Courtesy of Heather Ramsay.)

the year of consultation, and in hospitals the number tab may indicate the last date of admission. Be sure that you understand the colour-coding requirements of your office before you create any new charts or purge any old charts.

In Fig. 4.11 the numeric coloured tabs on the end-tab folders are facing out on the open-shelf cabinet. When colour-coding your alphabetic charts, the first letter of the patient's last name should be on the outer edge of the chart, and the second and subsequent letters should be placed beneath it; a label with the patient's name can be added either below or above the coloured tabs. File folders provide indicators for where to add tabs and labels. When using this type of system, you can see at a glance where the charts are for patients with the last name beginning with an "A" because they all have pink tabs facing out. If you are looking for Elizabeth Autum's chart, for example, you simply go to where the charts show a pink, purple, and light blue tab combination and begin your search from there.

It is important that you inspect your cabinets or stacks regularly to detect any charts or folders that have been misfiled. It is often necessary to secure patient information on a moment's notice; misfiled charts may result in serious problems. Colour-coded charts make this task quite easy.

Suggestions for Efficient Filing

- File behind the guides. This is common practice because it is more efficient.
- Place the miscellaneous folder behind its matching primary guide so that it is the last folder before the next primary

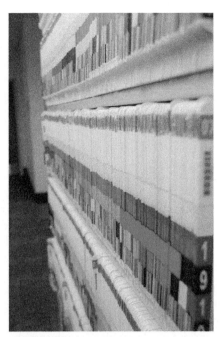

• **Fig. 4.11** Colour-coding patient charts makes it easy to see a file that is misplaced. (Source: © CanStock Photo Inc./makimg.)

guide. For example, the miscellaneous folder for accounting documents would be filed as the last folder in the "accounting" section. That section's primary guide is the divider at the beginning of the section labelled "accounting."

- Collect a maximum of five items for one firm or customer in a miscellaneous file. Miscellaneous files are not usually used in a patient file system. However, the doctor would have miscellaneous files in his or her business files.
- Arrange letters and other material in individual folders by date, with the most recent appearing at the front. Generally, you are dealing with current information, and using this system allows easier access.
- Allow 10 to 15 cm of working space in drawers to prevent jamming and tearing material.
- When removing folders from the shelf or drawer, always grasp them by the side or centre, never by the tab. When filing or removing papers, lift up the folders partway and rest them on the side of the drawer to avoid inserting papers between folders.
- Ensure that all headings of papers appear to the left as you face the file to facilitate correct placement and easy finding.
- To prevent injuries to staff, close all file drawers when not in use.
- To locate misplaced files, charts, or documents, do the following:
  a. Look immediately in front of and behind the place of the file folder—materials may not have been put in the folder.
  b. Look under names that have a similar spelling or that sound alike.

Summary

In this chapter, you have discovered how to become an efficient, safe, and accurate organizer of medical records and documents. You have learned how to index patient names for proper alphabetical filing and chart label creation. You are now aware of the common documents found in a typical chart and understand the order of these documents. You have been introduced to a variety of chart creation methods, cabinet types, and folder types that are typical in medical offices. With this knowledge and keen attention to the tips provided throughout this chapter, you are well prepared to encounter and work with patient files in a medical office.

Assignments

Assignment 4.1

For this assignment, you will apply all the rules presented in the chapter by alphabetizing the sample patient names from the chapter. The first step is to index all the patient names—try not to refer back to the chapter examples. Begin by writing unit numbers 1 to 5 at the top of a piece of paper (do not use a word processor for this assignment). Then index all the names according to the rules. The next step is to begin alphabetizing. Because the list is longer, you can consider starting with a "rough sort" by clumping together all the names that begin with the same letters. Finally you can put all the names together to form the complete list. Print out your final list on a new piece of paper in order (leave the units in their indexed positions) and double-check your work by using the letter-by-letter, unit-by-unit process. Make sure you are spelling names correctly when you transfer them over to your paper—attention-to-detail errors are the most common errors related to filing.

Andrea T. Brown
Andrew Brown
Ashley Del Rio
Todd. A. Bernard, II
Bethany A. Brown
Erin Van Duzee
John McDonald
Lisa Basciano
Todd A. Bernard, 3rd
Lisa D. Basciano-Lee
Lisa-Jane J. Basciano
Todd A. Bernard, Sr.
Marie Anne Brown
Mary Jane Brown
Paul MacDonald
Rick Van der Veen
Robert A. Baxter
Robert Andrew Baxter
Robert Brian Baxter
Mary-Jane Brown
Thomas Bell (421 King Avenue, Ottawa)
Thomas William Bell
Lisa Jane Basciano
Todd A. Bernard, Jr.
Thomas Bell (420 King Street, Ottawa)

Assignment 4.2

Use the same steps as in Assignment 4.1 to place these new patient names in alphabetical order.

Indexing may be keyed or handwritten. Submit both the indexing exercise and the alphabetized list. For the purposes of this assignment only, consider all shortened names to be abbreviations of the full name; for example, Nick would be Nicholas.

Mary Shier-Sorrie
Don Bruce, 156 Park St., Ottawa
Dr. Rob T. Durin
Mrs. John L. Kingston (Rena)
Masie Shierman
Nicholas Maziotti, 223 George St., Virgil, BC
Delbert J. McCall
Robbin Durin
Nick Mazzioti, 107 George St., Virgil, NS
Jamie Dickens
Connato DiCarlo
Michael Terry Masters
Wm. Ainsworth
John Kingston
Mike T. Masterson
Nicholas Mazziotti, 372 George St., Virgil, AB
Wilma Ainsworth
Nick Mazziotti, 315 George St., Virgil, ON
Donald Bruce, 101 Park St., Ottawa
D.J. MacCall
Mrs. Donalda Bruce, 96 Park St., Ottawa, ON

Assignment 4.3

For this assignment, 15 file folders are required. Your instructor will decide between end-tab and top-tab files.

Prepare file folders using the information found on the patient information forms (see Fig. 4.12). Use age, birthday, and current year to calculate each patient's year of birth. If colour-coding tabs are available, use a three-letter colour code to create your folders. If no tabs are available, colour-code the folders using coloured pencils or markers—use the following colour key.

A = pink
B = red
C = light orange
D = dark orange
E = yellow

G = dark green
H = light blue
I = purple
J = lilac
L = light brown
M = pink
O = light orange
P = dark orange
R = light green
S = dark green
T = light blue
U = purple
V = lilac
X= light brown

Blank stamp forms (as shown in Fig. 4.1) are on the Evolve site and can be pasted on the front of each file folder. Alternatively, you can print off a computer label, or your instructor may have an ink stamp prepared for this assignment.

Print the patient's name (or place a file folder label with the name) on the tab of the folder, last name first in capitals, for example, BASCIANO, Lisa. Insert a family medicine chart and a record form for allergies and medications in the appropriate place in each file. These and any other forms your instructor wishes inserted in the file will be provided. Forms are available on the Evolve site. Samples of these forms include a patient information form (see Fig. 4.12), a prescription record (see Fig. 4.13), a family medicine chart (see Fig. 4.2), and an infant and child progress record (see Figs. 4.3 and 4.4). It is your responsibility to file all information pertaining to each patient in the appropriate folder and in the order indicated in this chapter.

Topics for Discussion

1. What may be the consequences of a misplaced file in the following environments:
   a. In an office setting?
   b. In a hospital setting?

Assignment 4.4

a. Index and alphabetize the following names:
James Park
Sister Rosemary McManus
I.B.A. Drug Stores
Lois Armstrong, D.C.
Bob MacCarrell, Jr.
Dr. David Sniddon
Sister Veronica
Josie Iammancini

b. In the space provided below, or on a piece of paper, write a three-letter colour code for the units determined to be the first indexing unit of the names above. Use the following colour guide:
A = pink
B = red
C = light orange
I = purple
M = pink
N = red
P = dark orange
R = light green
S = dark green

1. _____
2. _____
3. _____
4. _____
5. _____
6. _____
7. _____
8. _____

2. Discuss the pros and cons of both an alphabetical and a numerical filing system.
3. What type of tickler file system would help you remember most easily, and why?

PATIENT INFORMATION

(Please Print Clearly)   Date _July 30 –_

NAME _Robert (Bob) Baxter_ AGE _27_ SEX _M_

ADDRESS _24 Stapleton Road_

CITY _Manotick_ PROV. _Ont_ CODE _K6Y 3T7_

Oct 7 ☑ Mar. ☐ Sing. ☐ Wid. ☐ Div.
Date of Birth

PHONE: Home _652-3179_ Work _652-6643_

EMPLOYED BY _Town of Manotick_

CITY _Manotick_ PROV. _Ont_

OCCUPATION _Township Clerk_

SPOUSE'S NAME _Sylvia_

EMPLOYED BY _Self_

CITY _Ottawa_ PROV. _Ont_

PHONE _652-6643_ OCCUPATION _Boutique Owner_

REFERRED BY _____

HEALTH CARD NO. _4892608532_ VERSION CODE _____

ALLERGIES _____

SERIOUS ILLNESS _____

EMERGENCY CONTACT _Sylvia_   _Wife_   _652-6643_
                    Name   Relation   Phone

• **Fig. 4.12** Patient Information Forms

PATIENT INFORMATION

(Please Print Clearly)   Date _Aug. 31, 20 -_

NAME _Lisa Basciano_   AGE _42_ SEX _F_

ADDRESS _2796 Waycross Cres._

CITY _Ottawa_   PROV. _Ont._ CODE _J7X 2X9_

Nov. 19   ☑ Mar. ☐ Sing. ☐ Wid. ☐ Div.

Date of Birth

PHONE: Home _742-2717_   Work _743-7776_

EMPLOYED BY _GOVERNMENT OF CANADA_

CITY _OTTAWA_   PROV. _ONT._

OCCUPATION _ACCOUNTANT_

SPOUSE'S NAME _DINO_

EMPLOYED BY _GOVERNMENT OF CANADA_

CITY _OTTAWA_   PROV. _ONT._

PHONE _743-7776_   OCCUPATION _M.P._

REFERRED BY _____

HEALTH CARD NO. _2719278836_   VERSION CODE _____

ALLERGIES _____

SERIOUS ILLNESS _Rheumatoid Arthritis_

EMERGENCY CONTACT _Dino_   _Husband_   _243-7776_
          Name   Relation   Phone

• **Fig. 4.12, cont'd**

PATIENT INFORMATION

(Please Print Clearly)   Date _June 23, 20-_

NAME _Melville Thompson_   AGE _75_ SEX _M_

ADDRESS _22 Edward Road_

CITY _Ottawa_   PROV. _Ont_ CODE _J7X 2X6_

Nov. 8   ☑ Mar. ☐ Sing. ☐ Wid. ☐ Div.
Date of Birth

PHONE: Home _427-5432_   Work _____

EMPLOYED BY _Retired_

CITY _____   PROV. _____

OCCUPATION _____

SPOUSE'S NAME _Laura_

EMPLOYED BY _____

CITY _____   PROV. _____

PHONE _____ OCCUPATION _____

REFERRED BY _____

HEALTH CARD NO. _6448417672_   VERSION CODE _____

ALLERGIES _____

SERIOUS ILLNESS _Emphysema_

EMERGENCY CONTACT _Laura_   _Wife_   _427-5432_
                    Name   Relation   Phone

• Fig. 4.12, cont'd

PATIENT INFORMATION

(Please Print Clearly)   Date _JULY 12, 20-_

NAME _AMELIA JACKSON_   AGE _57_ SEX _F_

ADDRESS _13 CROSS ST._

CITY _KEMPTVILLE_   PROV. _ONT_   CODE _KON 2LO_

APR. 29   ☐ Mar. ☐ Sing. ☐ Wid. ☑ Div.
Date of Birth

PHONE: Home _748 - 3192_   Work _748·5532_

EMPLOYED BY _KEMP HOSPITAL_

CITY _KEMPTVILLE_   PROV. _ONT_

OCCUPATION _NURSE_

SPOUSE'S NAME _____

EMPLOYED BY _____

CITY _____ PROV. _____

PHONE _____ OCCUPATION _____

REFERRED BY _DR. JAMES_

HEALTH CARD NO. _8806773712_ VERSION CODE _____

ALLERGIES _____

SERIOUS ILLNESS _____

EMERGENCY CONTACT _STEVEN_   _SON_   _427-0098_
                   Name   Relation   Phone

• **Fig. 4.12, cont'd**

PATIENT INFORMATION

(Please Print Clearly)   Date _March 12, 20-_

NAME _MARY JANE BROWN_   AGE _21_   SEX _F_

ADDRESS _731 HAMPOLE ST._

CITY _OTTAWA_   PROV. _ONT._   CODE _J8X 4X9_

JAN. 1   ☐ Mar. ☐ Sing. ☑ Wid. ☐ Div.
Date of Birth

PHONE: Home _427-3333_   ~~Work~~ SCHOOL _427-5566_

EMPLOYED BY _____

CITY _____   PROV. _____

OCCUPATION _STUDENT_

SPOUSE'S NAME _____

EMPLOYED BY _____

CITY _____   PROV. _____

PHONE _____ OCCUPATION _____

REFERRED BY _____

_____

HEALTH CARD NO. _3820703795_   VERSION CODE _____

ALLERGIES _SULPHA, ASPIRIN_

SERIOUS ILLNESS _____

EMERGENCY CONTACT _BERT_   _FATHER_   WORK _456-9321_
                  Name   Relation   Phone

• Fig. 4.12, cont'd

PATIENT INFORMATION

(Please Print Clearly)　　　　　　　Date __April 12, 20—__

NAME __HAZEL DAVIS__　　　AGE __30__ SEX __F__

ADDRESS __539 CHERRYHILL LANE__

CITY __OTTAWA__　　　PROV. __ONT__　CODE __KOW 3SS__

__FEB 2.__　　☑ Mar. ☐ Sing. ☐ Wid. ☐ Div.
Date of Birth

PHONE: Home __427-7006__　　Work __—__

EMPLOYED BY _____

CITY _____　　PROV. _____

OCCUPATION __—__

SPOUSE'S NAME __BRENT__

EMPLOYED BY __OTTAWA COLLEGE__

CITY __OTTAWA__　　PROV. __ONT__

PHONE __426-0001__　OCCUPATION __MAINT. MECH.__

REFERRED BY _____

HEALTH CARD NO. __178 105 0552__ VERSION CODE _____

ALLERGIES __—__

SERIOUS ILLNESS __—__

EMERGENCY CONTACT __BRENT__　__HUSBAND__　__426-0001__
　　　　　　　　　Name　　　　Relation　　　Phone

• **Fig. 4.12,** cont'd

PATIENT INFORMATION

(Please Print Clearly)   Date _Feb 13, 20—_

NAME _HEATHER SMITH_ AGE _18_ SEX _F_

ADDRESS _BEAVER CRES._

CITY _MANOTICK_ PROV. _ONT_ CODE _K6Y 3T7_

APRIL 4 ☐ Mar. ☑ Sing. ☐ Wid. ☐ Div.
Date of Birth

PHONE: Home _576-3225_ Work _____

EMPLOYED BY _GOVERNMENT OF CANADA_

CITY _OTTAWA_ PROV. _ONT_

OCCUPATION _FILE CLERK_

SPOUSE'S NAME _____

EMPLOYED BY _____

CITY _____ PROV. _____

PHONE _____ OCCUPATION _____

REFERRED BY _DR. JOHNSTON_

HEALTH CARD NO. _9086182038_ VERSION CODE _____

ALLERGIES _—_

SERIOUS ILLNESS _—_

EMERGENCY CONTACT _CHRISTINE_ _MOTHER_ _576-3225_
                        Name   Relation   Phone

• Fig. 4.12, cont'd

PATIENT INFORMATION

(Please Print Clearly)   Date   MARCH 11, 20—

NAME   BELLIVEAU, JEAN   AGE 22   SEX M

ADDRESS   729   UPPERHILL   DRIVE

CITY   OTTAWA   PROV. ONT.   CODE J8Z 4X7

DECEMBER   26   ☐ Mar. ☑ Sing. ☐ Wid. ☐ Div.
Date of Birth

                                    SCHOOL
PHONE: Home 427-3899   ~~Work~~   427-9987

EMPLOYED BY

CITY   PROV.

OCCUPATION   STUDENT

SPOUSE'S NAME

EMPLOYED BY

CITY   PROV.

PHONE   OCCUPATION

REFERRED BY

HEALTH CARD NO.   69 10 0 4 7635   VERSION CODE

ALLERGIES

SERIOUS ILLNESS

EMERGENCY CONTACT   BARB   MOTHER   427-3665
                    Name   Relation   Phone

• **Fig. 4.12, cont'd**

PATIENT INFORMATION

(Please Print Clearly)

Date __MAY 3, 20-__

NAME __ROBERT ERIK SHULTZ__ AGE __55__ SEX __M__

ADDRESS __17 BOND STREET.__

CITY __OTTAWA__ PROV. __ONT.__ CODE __J8Z 4H3__

__MAY 26__ ☑ Mar. ☐ Sing. ☐ Wid. ☐ Div.
Date of Birth

PHONE: Home __427-9977__ Work __427-3456__

EMPLOYED BY __TEXTILES LIMITED__

CITY __PERTH__ PROV. __ONT.__

OCCUPATION __PERSONNEL DIRECTOR__

SPOUSE'S NAME __MARY.__

EMPLOYED BY _____

CITY _____ PROV. _____

PHONE _____ OCCUPATION __HOMEMAKER__

REFERRED BY _____

_____

HEALTH CARD NO. __7819 749 313__ VERSION CODE _____

ALLERGIES _____

SERIOUS ILLNESS __CANCER, RIGHT THIGH - ON CHEM.__

EMERGENCY CONTACT __MARY__ __WIFE__ __427-9977__
                    Name   Relation   Phone

• Fig. 4.12, cont'd

PATIENT INFORMATION

(Please Print Clearly)   Date _June 18, 20—_

NAME _Peter John Scott_   AGE _14_ SEX _M_

ADDRESS _16 Binn St._

CITY _Ottawa_   PROV. _Ont._ CODE _J7X 2X6_

Aug. 18   ☐ Mar. ☑ Sing. ☐ Wid. ☐ Div.
Date of Birth

PHONE: Home _427-2245_   Work _____

EMPLOYED BY _____

CITY _____   PROV. _____

OCCUPATION _____

SPOUSE'S NAME _____

EMPLOYED BY _____

CITY _____   PROV. _____

PHONE _____ OCCUPATION _____

REFERRED BY _____

_____

HEALTH CARD NO. _9191807099_   VERSION CODE _____

ALLERGIES _Morphine_

SERIOUS ILLNESS _Epilepsy_

EMERGENCY CONTACT _Glen_   _Father_   _work 372-7687_
                    Name   Relation   Phone

• **Fig. 4.12, cont'd**

PATIENT INFORMATION

(Please Print Clearly)   Date _____ *Sept. 26, 20—*

NAME ___ LOIS ELLIOTT ___ AGE __ 51 __ SEX __ F __

ADDRESS ___ RR3 ___

CITY ___ Kars ___ PROV. ___ ONT. ___ CODE ___ W9U4W9

___ MARCH 19 ___ ☐ Mar. ☐ Sing. ☑ Wid. ☐ Div.
Date of Birth

PHONE: Home ___ 748-3355 ___ Work ___ 427-3478

EMPLOYED BY ___ GLOUCESTER CLOCK WORS

CITY ___ OTTAWA ___ PROV. ___ ONT.

OCCUPATION ___ EXECUTIVE SECRETARY

SPOUSE'S NAME ___

EMPLOYED BY ___

CITY ___ PROV. ___

PHONE ___ OCCUPATION ___

REFERRED BY ___ Dr. CARL ROLLINGS

HEALTH CARD NO. ___ L9541545092 ___ VERSION CODE ___

ALLERGIES ___

SERIOUS ILLNESS ___

EMERGENCY CONTACT ___ LORRAINE ___ DAUGHTER ___ 799-5473
                          Name   Relation   Phone

• Fig. 4.12, cont'd

PATIENT INFORMATION

(Please Print Clearly)   Date __UCT 3, 20—__

NAME __TIMOTHY PETERS__   AGE __36__   SEX __M__

ADDRESS __10 LORD ST.__

CITY __KEMPTVILLE__   PROV. __ONT.__   CODE __KOW 2LO__

__JAN 1__   ☑ Mar. ☐ Sing. ☐ Wid. ☐ Div.
Date of Birth

PHONE: Home __743-2525__   Work __743-5550__

EMPLOYED BY __SMITH AND SMITH LIMITED__

CITY __OTTAWA__   PROV. __ONT.__

OCCUPATION __LABOURER__

SPOUSE'S NAME __KRISTA__

EMPLOYED BY __KEMPTVILLE COLLEGE__

CITY __KEMPTVILLE__   PROV. __ONT.__

PHONE __743-7557__   OCCUPATION __TEACHER__

REFERRED BY ____

HEALTH CARD NO. __7031381135__   VERSION CODE ____

ALLERGIES ____

SERIOUS ILLNESS ____

EMERGENCY CONTACT   __KRISTA__   __WIFE__   __WORK OR HOME ABOVE__
                      Name   Relation   Phone

• Fig. 4.12, cont'd

PATIENT INFORMATION

(Please Print Clearly)   Date _JAN. 16, 20-_

NAME _ELIZABETH GREEN_ AGE _36_ SEX _F_

ADDRESS _72 HILLCREST ST._

CITY _OTTAWA_ PROV. _ONT._ CODE _J3Z 5X4_

AUG. 12   ☑ Mar. ☐ Sing. ☐ Wid. ☐ Div.
Date of Birth

PHONE: Home _427-3774_ Work _____

EMPLOYED BY _____

CITY _____ PROV. _____

OCCUPATION _____

SPOUSE'S NAME _GARY_

EMPLOYED BY _ABC DELIVERIES_

CITY _OTTAWA_ PROV. _ONT._

PHONE _427-4545_ OCCUPATION _MANAGER_

REFERRED BY _____

HEALTH CARD NO. _3777220777_ VERSION CODE _____

ALLERGIES _NIL_

SERIOUS ILLNESS _HYPERTENSION_

EMERGENCY CONTACT _GARY_ _HUSBAND_ _427-4545_
                          Name   Relation   Phone

• **Fig. 4.12,** cont'd

PATIENT INFORMATION

(Please Print Clearly)   Date __Jan. 20, 20-__

NAME __Thomas Bell__   AGE __82__ SEX __M__

ADDRESS __321 Adelaide St.__

CITY __Ottawa__   PROV. __Ont.__ CODE __J3Z-5X3__

__Sept. 25__   ☑ Mar. ☐ Sing. ☐ Wid. ☐ Div.
Date of Birth

PHONE: Home __427-5327__   Work __427-3227__

EMPLOYED BY __Self__

CITY __Ottawa__   PROV. __Ont.__

OCCUPATION __Freelance Writer (Retired)__

SPOUSE'S NAME __Janet__

EMPLOYED BY _____

CITY _____   PROV. _____

PHONE _____   OCCUPATION __Housewife__

REFERRED BY _____

HEALTH CARD NO. __6875231059__   VERSION CODE _____

ALLERGIES __Penicillin__

SERIOUS ILLNESS _____

EMERGENCY CONTACT __Janet__   __Wife__   __427-5327__
                        Name   Relation   Phone

• Fig. 4.12, cont'd

PATIENT INFORMATION

(Please Print Clearly)   Date _Nov 1, 20-_

NAME _William Harris_   AGE _2 month_ SEX _M_

ADDRESS _362 Blue Jay Cres._

CITY _Ottawa_   PROV. _Ont_   CODE _J7K 2X9_

Sept. 5   ☐ Mar.   ☑ Sing.   ☐ Wid.   ☐ Div.
Date of Birth

PHONE: Home _778 -2367_   Work _____

EMPLOYED BY _____

CITY _____ PROV. _____

OCCUPATION _____

SPOUSE'S NAME _____

EMPLOYED BY _____

CITY _____ PROV. _____

PHONE _____ OCCUPATION _____

REFERRED BY _____

_____

HEALTH CARD NO. _2722575673_   VERSION CODE _____

ALLERGIES _Sulpha, milk, Penicillin_

SERIOUS ILLNESS _____

EMERGENCY CONTACT _Brad_   _father_   _427-0009_
                Name   Relation   Phone

• Fig. 4.12, cont'd

NAME

# OF PRESCRIPTION	LONG TERM MEDICATION AND TREATMENT	DATE FILLED

• **Fig. 4.13** Prescription Record

References

Canada Health Infoway. (2018). *Understanding EMRs, EHRs, and PHRs*. Retrieved from https://www.infoway-inforoute.ca/en/solutions/digital-health-foundation/understanding-ehrs-emrs-and-phrs.

Canadian Medical Protective Association. (2018). *The new reality of reporting a privacy breach*. Retrieved from https://www.cmpa-acpm.ca/en/advice-publications/browse-articles/2018/the-new-reality-of-reporting-a-privacy-breach.

Canadian Medical Protective Association. (2016). *A matter of records: Retention and transfer of clinic records*. Retrieved from https://www.cmpa-acpm.ca/en/advice-publications/browse-articles/2003/a-matter-of-records-retention-and-transfer-of-clinical-records.

Canadian Medical Protective Association. (2009). *The medical record: A legal document—can it be corrected?*. Retrieved from https://www.cmpa-acpm.ca/en/advice-publications/browse-articles/2009/the-medical-record-a-legal-document-can-it-be-corrected.

Leaver, C. (2017). *Canada health infoway: Use of electronic medical records among canadian physicians*. Retrieved from https://www.infoway-inforoute.ca/en/component/edocman/resources/reports/benefits-evaluation/3362-2017-cma-workforce-survey-digital-health-results?Itemid=101.

5

The Telephone and eCommunication Tools

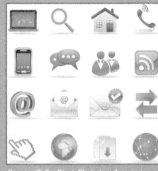

This chapter provides information about general telephone procedures and etiquette, the types of calls you will receive, and the types of outgoing calls you will generate. Some common requests you will experience as a medical administrative assistant are revealed. Telephone systems and their modern eCommunication counterparts are discussed. You will learn best practices and explore the special considerations required for using cell phones, e-mail, social media, and other modern communication modalities in the health care atmosphere.

CHAPTER OUTLINE

Introduction

General Telephone Procedures

Incoming Calls

Outgoing Calls

Answering Services

Voice-Messaging Systems

The Telephone Directory

Equipment

eCommunications

LEARNING OBJECTIVES

After reading this chapter, you will be able to:

1. Describe effective telephone usage including answering, screening, holding, and making outgoing calls
2. Describe how to handle calls regarding appointments, prescription requests, and emergencies
3. Describe how to use the telephone directory as a reference source
4. Identify the types of telephone equipment
5. Describe the eCommunication tools and usage guidelines
6. Describe the methods of dealing with callers other than patients
7. Recognize and practice good telephone etiquette

KEY TERMS

Allied health professionals: Groups of trained professionals working in health care to provide services outside of the nursing, dentistry, and medical professions. Examples of allied health professionals are physiotherapists, occupational therapists, dietitians, speech language pathologists, podiatrists, and others.

eCommunications: Communication that happens with the assistance of an electronic source, such as a computer or mobile device, and includes videoconferencing, e-mail messaging, social media posting, and texting.

Primary care physician (PCP): The medical professional who is a patient's first point of contact with the health care system. Usually the PCP is a general practitioner (family physician) who accepts responsibility for the care of routine, nonemergency, and chronic illnesses. PCPs refer patients to specialists for any secondary care that is required.

Provisional diagnosis What the physician suspects is wrong with the patient, based on presenting symptoms.

Telemedicine: The use of eCommunication tools and associated procedures to deliver health care services.

Introduction

As a medical administrative assistant, you will spend a great deal of your day answering calls, returning messages, delivering messages, and sending outgoing communications. You are the first person most patients will interact with, and it will be your responsibility to manage all calls efficiently, professionally, and accurately. Because it is difficult to imagine the types of requests you will receive, these responsibilities may seem intimidating at first. The information provided in this chapter will help you understand what to expect and how to deal with a number of common situations. With this information, a bit of practice, and some on-the-job experience, you will feel confident in your telephone and eCommunication skills.

General Telephone Procedures

The telephone is the main link between patients and the physician's office. It is also important for connecting with other doctors' offices, hospitals, suppliers, pharmaceutical companies, allied health professionals, and other institutions your office must do business with regularly. Medical administrative assistants spend a great deal of time on the telephone, and practicing some general telephone procedures creates a professional impression while using this important communication tool.

Equipment Basics

When you begin employment in an office, clinic, or hospital, you should familiarize yourself with the telephone system. Many clinics have multiline systems that may take a bit of practice before "going live" on the telephones. Taking the time to review simple processes with your co-workers may prevent some embarrassment when dealing with patients, physicians, and other callers. You should practice how to forward calls, how to pick up your voicemail, how to transfer a call, and how to record, delete, and change your greeting. If you do not have a co-worker who can assist you, locate the phone's user manual—if you cannot find the manual in the office, you can likely locate it online by searching the telephone manufacturer's website.

Medical administrative assistants are often required to listen as well as write or find information from a chart. A headset (as shown in Fig. 5.1) is recommended because it leaves both hands free and does not require you to hold your head and neck in an uncomfortable position for extended periods of time. A headset provides mobility throughout the office, but you need to remain aware of those around you. You must maintain confidentiality and practice discretion while you are away from your desk; be mindful of patients waiting in examination rooms as you make your way through the office. Patients may not intend to overhear private information but may do so accidentally; it is not their responsibility to ensure the privacy of patients—it is yours. Do not answer calls while assisting a physician with an examination and, just as you would with your desk-style equipment, ensure that you know how to use all the functions of the headset so that you do not accidentally hang up or misdirect callers.

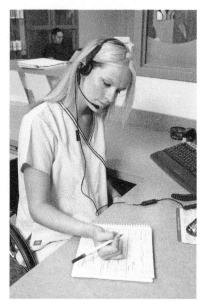

• **Fig. 5.1** A good telephone headset leaves the hands free and facilitates good body posture. (Source: Procter, D., Niedzwiecki, B., Pepper, J. et al. (2017). Kinn's the administrative medical assistant [13th ed]. St. Louis, MO: Elsevier.)

If a headset is not available to you, be sure to have your desk set up with correct ergonomics so that you can maintain good posture (as seen in Fig. 5.2). If you regularly need to cradle the phone between your shoulder and ear to have your hands free, ask your employer to invest in a proper telephone shoulder rest so that you can avoid injury to your neck.

Answering Calls

You should not let the phone ring while you finish with less pressing tasks. For instance, if you are informally chatting with another patient or staff member, or updating a spreadsheet, you should leave those tasks and make answering the telephone your priority. A good rule of thumb is to answer within three rings. This allows you to get to the caller before he or she receive your office voice mail and before they become impatient or feel frustrated. Remember, people calling your office often are not feeling well; they may be under great stress or may be highly anxious about their physical or mental health. A simple unanswered phone call can increase the stress of a vulnerable patient. In turn, the patient's reaction, when you finally do speak, may be unpleasant.

"Holding" Callers

Do not answer the phone and say, "Dr. Plunkett's office; will you hold, please?" and then immediately leave the line. In today's busy office, it is not uncommon to have two or three lines engaged at one time (see Box 5.1). If another line rings, make certain before you place the caller on hold that it is not an emergency. It is common courtesy to wait for an answer to the "Will you hold?" question. If the call is not an emergency and you cannot handle the call immediately, inform the caller that you are on the other line and give the caller a choice of holding or being called back. Some telephone systems have music playing or an intermittent sound such as a beep that lets callers know that they are still on

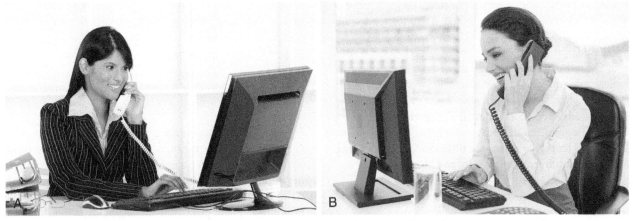

• **Fig. 5.2 A,** Good posture when answering the telephone improves voice quality and prevents muscle strain. **B,** Leaning back in the chair and using the shoulder to hold the telephone results in poor voice quality and muscle strain. (Source: A: © CanStock Photo Inc./michaeljung; B: © CanStock Photo Inc./ lightwavemedia.)

• BOX 5.1   Interrupting a Call to Answer Another Line

- Ask the person if he or she can hold while you answer the other line. Inform the person that you will be right back.
- When you answer the other line, ask the second caller if he or she can hold because you are on another call. If it is not an emergency, ask whether the caller wants to hold or have you call back.
- Return to the first caller as soon as possible and thank him or her for holding.

• BOX 5.2   Telephone Etiquette

- Answer the call within three rings.
- Clearly identify the doctor's office and then yourself.
- Answer your call with a smile.
- Speak clearly and slowly.
- Do not have candy, gum, or food in your mouth.
- Concentrate on the call—do not let your mind wander.
- Listen actively—ask questions to clarify.

---

hold and have not mistakenly been cut off. If the caller is waiting to speak with the physician and the physician is on another call, check back frequently to assure the caller that he or she has not been forgotten. Inform the caller that the doctor is still on the other line and ask whether he or she would like to continue holding or leave a message and have the doctor call back. If the caller is another physician, you can ask whether there is a chart that your physician will need for the call. If so, pull the chart and have it ready.

Personal Demeanor

When you answer the telephone, your voice should sound pleasant and friendly, calm and professional. If you put a smile on your face when you answer the phone, you will also put a smile in your voice. You cannot sound pleasant or friendly if you are distracted. Clear your mind and concentrate on the caller. Identify the doctor's office and then yourself: "Good morning. Dr. Plunkett's office, Ann speaking." This simple introduction tells the patient that he or she has reached the person intended, and it makes the encounter more personal and welcoming.

Be patient and courteous at all times. As mentioned, the people you are dealing with usually have medical problems. They are not like customers coming to buy a product. You must be sympathetic and empathetic; let them know you are listening to what they are saying and that you will do whatever is necessary to help. Your voice should be natural, interested, and expressive. Try to speak in a normal tone, and speak clearly and slowly. You need to present yourself as confident,

knowledgeable, and professional. If the patient is in distress, be sympathetic. Most important, be reassuring, but be careful not to offer medical or other advice that is beyond your normal scope of practice. See Box 5.2 for telephone etiquette tips.

Active Listening

How you listen is very important. A medical administrative assistant must practice active listening to provide the best service to patients. This means that you are fully concentrating on what the caller is saying and anticipating their needs. Do not allow your mind to wander or perform unrelated tasks while a patient talks to you. Be sure to get the caller's name, and use it during the conversation to show that you are attentive. Listen carefully to the patient's request or inquiry and ask for clarification when needed. Asking questions will encourage patients to be specific about their needs, making the call efficient without seeming rushed. It will also make you certain of your next task, which will ultimately bring a better result to the patient.

Responding to the Telephone Request

Once you have the information you need, determine whether you can accommodate the patient yourself or whether you need to refer the call or question to the doctor or other health care provider. If you need to pass along the message or consult with other team members, tell the patient, and try to give an approximate time when their call will be returned. This may help alleviate some anxiety or frustration during the patient's day. If the call cannot be returned in the approximate time frame you provided, you may want to update the caller on the status of their request to ease their mind.

Recording Requests and Inquiries

One of the most important aspects of telephone usage in a medical practice is to *record all incoming patient requests and inquiries (not appointment bookings)*. You should have a notebook and pencil, or alternative electronic solution, beside the telephone at all times.

When a patient calls, record the time, date, patient's name and telephone number, the message, and your initials or signature. After you have noted details of the call, it is good practice to repeat the message to the caller. This ensures that the information is correct. Most offices use message pads similar to the one shown in Fig. 5.3 (Note: If you receive an urgent message, highlighting the word *urgent* will indicate to the doctor that the message requires immediate attention). There are message books available with NCR (no carbon required) paper that transfers the information written on the top sheet to the underlying sheets. These are available in duplicate and triplicate options. This way, you can give a copy of the message to your physician and still have one available for your own records (see Fig. 5.4). Once you are sure that a task has been completed or a call has been returned, you can indicate this on your copy with a check mark. If there is more than one person working in your office, make sure that you write your initials on the message pad.

DID YOU KNOW?

You should record everything. Do not depend on memory.

Computer networks are a part of today's modern offices. If you work in an office where you have the responsibility of answering the telephone, and you have a computer network system in your office, you may no longer need to write telephone messages on paper. Your system will likely be equipped with electronic messaging capabilities. You will call up a preprogrammed message form (see Fig. 5.5) on your screen, key in the details of the call, and forward the message using the computer. The terminal of the message recipient will display the message for perusal. Computers enable you also to send your messages by e-mail. This system is dependent on the receiver frequently checking for messages. You will have to ensure also that your network is properly backed up on a regular schedule—electronic records, including e-mail messages, are considered a part of

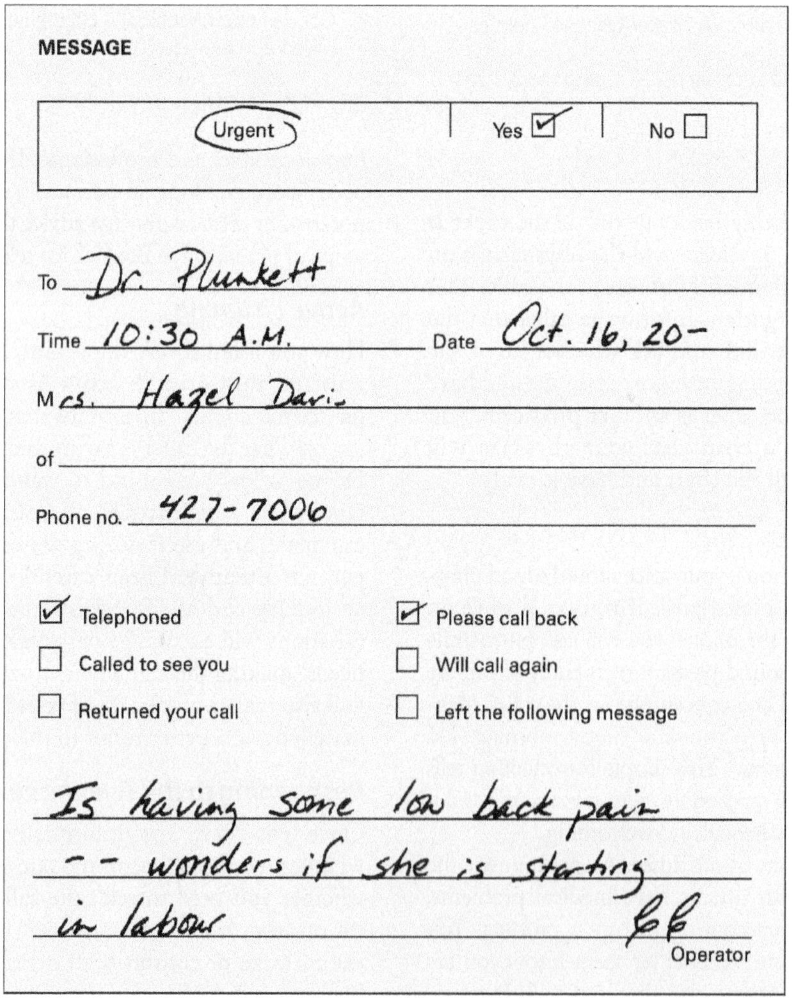
MESSAGE

Urgent | Yes ☑ | No ☐

To Dr. Plunkett

Time 10:30 A.M. Date Oct. 16, 20–

Mrs. Hazel Davis

of

Phone no. 427-7006

☑ Telephoned ☑ Please call back
☐ Called to see you ☐ Will call again
☐ Returned your call ☐ Left the following message

Is having some low back pain -- wonders if she is starting in labour

Operator

• **Fig. 5.3** Telephone Message.

PHONE MESSAGE

To		Date		Time	A.M. P.M.
From					**URGENT**
Company					PHONED
Telephone		Extension			PLEASE CALL
Cellular	Fax				RETURNED YOUR CALL
E-mail					WILL CALL AGAIN
Message					CAME TO SEE YOU
					WANTS TO SEE YOU
		Signature			

A1630-T

🔷 **Blueline**

• **Fig. 5.4** Telephone message pad with NCR (no carbon required) paper.

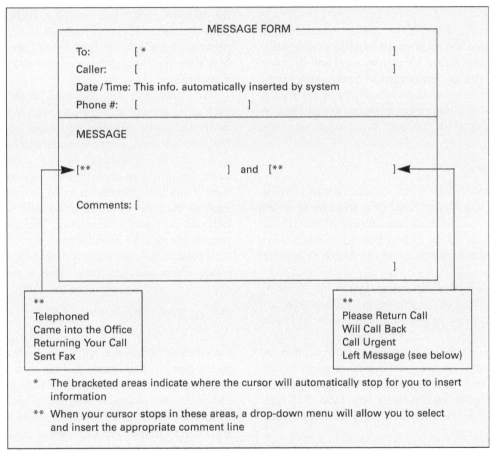

• **Fig. 5.5** Preprogrammed message form.

the medical record and subject to similar retention and privacy rules.

Incoming Calls

The medical administrative assistant is the barrier between the doctor and interruptive calls. Do not interrupt the doctor unless absolutely necessary. Some patients may insist on speaking with the physician; your job as "gatekeeper" is to offer solutions to the patient without interrupting the flow of the office. Once you determine the urgency of a request, you can suggest the patient book an appointment, you can offer to deliver a message, or you can explain how you can address their request yourself.

Although you must screen all incoming calls, be careful not to give the impression that the doctor is never available. If the doctor is with a patient, relay that to the caller. Don't say, "The doctor is busy." Saying the doctor is busy gives the unwanted and unintended impression that the doctor simply does not want to speak with the caller. Saying "The doctor is with a patient. May I give him a message?" helps the caller understand the reason the doctor is not available. And the statement still highlights the importance of the call by offering to provide a message—the caller is less likely to feel pushed aside. Discuss callback preferences with your doctor to determine what calls will be accepted during the day.

Although most calls will be from patients, you will also receive calls from hospital departments, other physicians, family members, and others. The following paragraphs will provide insight into what types of calls you will receive and how to deal these calls.

Patient Callers

As suggested above, many of the patient-related phone calls that come into the office can be handled by you without referring to the doctor. Of course, there will be some exceptions, and you are encouraged to communicate with the physician about these exceptions. Some of the typical patient call types you can expect to receive are outlined in the following paragraphs. Solutions and possible responses are included.

Telephone Advice

Patients often explain their symptoms and then ask, "What do you think I should do?" Your only response is to ask the patient to come in for an appointment or arrange for the patient to speak to the doctor. Box 5.3 provides a list of tasks you should perform to save the doctor time when returning a call.

The Canadian Medical Protective Association (CMPA) recommends that you *do not give any medical advice at any time*. Phone advice *can* be given through provincial health advice services, whereby patients can speak directly with a registered nurse or a nurse practitioner. Patients in most Canadian provinces can call 8-1-1 for nonurgent medical advice; however, make sure you have any alternate telephone numbers available for your patients (see Table 5.1). You may want to include this information on patient brochures,

---

> • **BOX 5.3** **Time-Saving Tasks**
>
> - Make complete and accurate notes concerning the patient's call.
> - Pull the patient's chart and attach the message to it.
> - Check the chart to see that any related test results have arrived *before* giving the chart to the doctor.
> - If the results have not arrived, call the referral facility and request a fax of the results or get a verbal report.

---

information sheets, and appointment cards. You may also want to have the numbers displayed in the waiting room. Encourage your patients to access this service when your office is closed.

Appointments

Booking appointments takes good judgement and accurate information. Physicians will wish to have specific amounts of time for different appointment types. For instance, an annual health examination takes much more time than the assessment of a sore throat. Until you are very familiar with the physician's preferences, keep a list of the most common appointments and the appropriate appointment lengths beside your phone. You should also keep some notes about the proper procedure for booking appointments with offices and departments you call often. This will make the call efficient for both parties and display your commitment to efficiency and professionalism.

Regardless of the appointment type, be sure to collect all the necessary patient information to book the appointment properly: name, reason for appointment, phone number, personal health number, time frame (how soon, if urgent), best time for the patient, and provisional diagnosis if necessary.

After booking a date and time, repeat the information back to the patient and give any further instructions, such as whether a urine sample is required or whether diet restrictions are necessary prior to laboratory tests. You may wish to have the patient repeat back any instructions to ensure that he or she heard you correctly and understand the information. If you have permission to do so, you may sometimes need to confirm the information with a caregiver, other responsible person, or translator. You could also offer to provide instructions in writing.

If patients are continuously calling for directions to hospitals, laboratories, etc., have copies of maps available and attach them to their referral or requisition when needed.

Prescriptions (Rx)

Patients will often call to request prescription renewals. If a prescription renewal is requested, ask the patient's name, phone number, and health card number. Record the name and drug identification number, or both, of the medication and ask at what pharmacy the prescription is required. If the medication information is not available from the patient, you can refer to the electronic medical record or paper chart.

At a convenient time, prescriptions should be transferred to a separate record. A steno pad is ideal if using a manual system, or you may utilize a computerized database. This information must also be recorded in the patient's chart. All telephone drug orders must be kept as part of the physician's records. Ensure that hard-copy or backed-up computer files are stored safely and securely.

Before calling the prescription in to the pharmacy (if your province allows this practice), *you must always have approval from the doctor*. He or she should place his or

TABLE 5.1	Canadian Telephone Health Advice Services			
Province or Territory	**Program Name**	**Main Number**	**Alternate Number**	**Hearing Impaired**
Alberta	811 Health Link	811	1-866-408-5465	
British Columbia	HealthLinkBC	811		711
Manitoba	Health-Links-Info-Santé	204-788-8200	1-888-315-9257	
New Brunswick	Tele-Care 811	811		1-866-213-7930
Newfoundland and Labrador	811 HealthLine	811	1-888-709-3555	
Northwest Territories	Yukon Healthline	811	1-604-215-4700 (HealthLinkBC) for satellite phones	
Nova Scotia	811 Nova Scotia	811	1-866-770-7763	711
Nunavut	Yukon Healthline	811	1-604-215-4700 (HealthLinkBC) for satellite phones	
Ontario	Telehealth	1-866-797-0000		1-866-797-0007
Prince Edward Island	Telehealth	811	1-866-770-7724	711
Québec	Info-Santé 811	811		
Saskatchewan	HealthLine	811	1-877-800-0002	1-800-855-1155
Yukon	HealthLine811	811	1-604-215-4700 (HealthLinkBC) for satellite phones	

her initials beside the entry that lists the patient's name, date of order, medication name, dosage and/or number, and name of the pharmacy where the prescription is ordered.

Please note that the preceding information regarding prescriptions represents best practices for when physicians renew prescriptions over the phone; however, many physicians will not. Instead, they will ask you to make an appointment for the patient. One reason for this is that the patient may need some follow-up testing, such as with thyroid or blood coagulation problems. In some provinces, telephone prescription renewal is an uninsured service; this means that the physician will not get paid by the province for the time it takes to provide this service. Some physicians will call in the prescription but charge the patient if he or she does not come into the office for an appointment. The charge may be by individual call or by the patient paying a flat fee per annum that covers uninsured services. In some provinces, pharmacies will take telephone prescriptions from physicians only. The rules and regulations around these procedures can be found at your local College of Physicians and Surgeons and are based on previously discussed statutes, such as the *Controlled Drugs and Substances Act* and the *Food and Drugs Act*.

Cancellations

If a patient calls to cancel an appointment, make a note in the patient's paper or electronic chart and on the appointment record. If the physician feels the health and safety of the patient (or others) are at risk, you may be asked to reach out to the patient to reschedule their appointment.

You may have a cancellation list in your office. If you are given enough notice, you can call in another patient to take the cancelled appointment time. If using a manual scheduling system, inform the doctor so he or she can update his or her daily schedule; changes made in an electronic scheduler will be immediately obvious to all staff members that are using the system.

New Patient Inquiries

With the shortage of family practitioners in the country, many individuals do not have a primary care physician (PCP). If your practice is full and you are not accepting new patients, be firm but give the caller an alternative phone number. Some Canadian provinces have new-patient registry systems that are managed by the province. The goal is to match people without permanent primary health care providers with a physician or nurse practitioner who can take them on as a patient. Other provinces, such as Alberta, Saskatchewan, and British Columbia, assist residents in their search for a doctor by providing lists of primary caregivers who are accepting new patients. These lists are provided through the provincial branches of the Canadian Medical Association (CMA) or College of Physicians and Surgeons. In these cases, neither the provinces nor the aforementioned organizations maintain patient registries or take the lead on placing patients with doctors—they provide resources to assist residents in their own search. You could provide callers seeking new doctors the phone number or link to these resources.

Emergencies

The medical administrative assistant will at times be faced with panic situations or emergencies. Use *common sense* and *keep calm*. First, determine if it is a real emergency. Get all the necessary information: the patient's name and number, the type of emergency, duration, and whether an ambulance is required. Examples of symptoms that require an ambulance are uncontrollable bleeding, chest pain, breathing difficulties, change in mental status, or sudden severe pain anywhere in the body. Where possible, the ambulance should be arranged by the person calling the doctor's office. If that person is unable to make the call, be sure to get all necessary information, such as location and directions. You can then call for the ambulance yourself (if you have more than one line, inform the caller that you will put the call on hold and then call the ambulance) or have an available staff member call while you speak with the patient. After you have the instructions from the ambulance service, go back to the patient and report when the ambulance will arrive. In *most* areas, dialing 9-1-1 will give you immediate access to emergency services.

You should have guidelines that outline what is considered an emergency in your office for appointment scheduling. Sudden diplopia (double vision), severe headache, facial or limb paralysis, high fever, burning urination, or blood in urine or stool are some examples. In the health care field, circumstances and conditions can change momentarily. Such guidelines are only that—guidelines. You will need to use common sense. When in doubt, always consult the physician.

Test Results

The medical administrative assistant should use discretion when relaying test results over the phone. If you receive a call requesting test results, it is absolutely essential that you know the caller; otherwise, ask for the person's name and number and discuss the situation with the doctor. Of course, you should never release any results without first checking with the doctor. If test results indicate medical problems, you should make an appointment for the patient to see the doctor. When a laboratory calls your office with verbal results, be prepared to repeat the results back to the caller, and state your name. It is good practice to repeat *all* verbal test results.

Professional Callers

Most physicians will return calls to other physicians, nurse practitioners, and hospital department supervisors, such as the nursing supervisor or bed control coordinator. These types of callers may have follow-up questions that are beyond your understanding or involvement in a patient's care. Not only is it a professional courtesy for the physicians to deal personally with these calls, but it is also an important step in the continuing care of a patient.

Pharmaceutical company representatives may call to secure a face-to-face meeting or to speak over the telephone with the physician. They will seek an opportunity to present their company's new products, provide the clinic with patient samples, and seek feedback from the doctor. Because these representatives are often planning visits in multiple locations across large regions, they may be quite insistent on certain meeting times or days. Be sure to know your office policy around these calls and visits.

Legal offices and third-party insurance providers, including representatives of workers' compensation boards, will call to request information related to their clients' claims. They may be seeking medical reports and historical data related to the case. To satisfy any requests from insurers or lawyers, a consent form for release of the personal health information (PHI) must be signed by the patient. The consent should include specifics on the information to be shared. No information should be shared over the phone without the permission or knowledge of the physician and patient.

Family Members and Personal Calls

Family members often have access to the physician's private line or cell phone; however, if they do use the main office line, ask the physician how these calls should be handled and follow the instructions provided. For instance, should you interrupt the doctor or take a message when a family member calls? Maybe the doctor will take calls from his spouse but not from his siblings—being clear on the expectations will help avoid awkward situations. In most cases, doctors will not interrupt their office day for personal calls. Taking a message on behalf of the doctor will be commonplace in most offices. If the doctor is expecting an important call that warrants an interruption, you will most likely be notified in advance.

Outgoing Calls

Try to limit the number of outgoing calls you are required to make and, when possible, group outgoing calls together during slower periods. You do not want to have your telephone lines engaged unnecessarily because patients need to be able to access your office. Personal calls during working hours are discouraged unless absolutely necessary. Make any necessary personal calls during breaks and away from the reception area.

In the course of your working day, you will have many occasions to make calls on behalf of your employer. You may call laboratories to set up blood tests, diagnostic imaging departments for x-rays, other physicians' offices for referrals, medical suppliers, third-party insurers, health plan payment offices, or pharmacies. In all situations, ensure that you have all pertinent information organized before placing the call. This will save time for both you and the person you are calling, and it will leave a positive impression of you and your office. The following paragraphs offer some advice for carrying out common outgoing call types.

Patient-Related Calls

If you are scheduling diagnostic tests or referrals, have all the patient's sociological information available as well as the types of tests required, and the days and times the patient is available to have the tests performed (see Box 5.4). It may also be helpful to have information about related tests previously performed and the names of the facilities where these tests were administered.

If you need to make a call to the health plan payment office or a pharmacy on behalf of a patient, have the patient's health card number and expiry date available, along with all of his or her sociological information. Similar information will be required when dealing with workers' compensation boards and third-party insurers; however, these providers will require the unique case number assigned to the patient to identify them correctly.

Calls to Patients

Try to handle the majority of patient requests on the first incoming call. This will not only satisfy the patient, but it will also decrease your outgoing calls and keep your to-do list leaner. Technological advances provide many opportunities to locate information in an instant; take advantage of any opportunities to do so.

Because we sometimes rely on others' schedules and are subject to following their processes (as when requesting a specialist consultation), there are times that outgoing patient calls cannot be avoided. When you call patients with information, make sure that you have all the details in front of you, including instructions related to the appointment, contact information for the consultant's office, and directions to the location when appropriate. Many times, you may need to leave a message for the patient. When doing so, you must always remember patient confidentiality. See Box 5.5 for guidelines when leaving a message on a patient's voice mail.

Ordering Supplies

Medical administrative assistants are responsible for keeping sufficient stock of all office and medical supplies. It is likely that the office will use one supplier for office products (paper, printer and fax toners, pens, staplers, telephone message pads) and another for medical supplies (cotton balls, table paper, cotton-tipped applicators, syringes, tongue depressors, sterilization products). The hospital or laboratory with which your employer is affiliated may also be a source for medical supplies. Laboratory and other diagnostic tests, blood collection tubes, urine sample cups, medical swabs, and microscope slides are

---

• BOX 5.4   Information Needed for Diagnostic Testing/Physician Referrals

- Type of test or appointment
- Patient's name, date of birth, health insurance number, phone number
- Urgency of test
- When the patient is available
- Provisional diagnosis if possible

• BOX 5.5   Leaving Voice Mail Messages

1. Make sure that you have reached the appropriate number.
2. If the patient is not identifiable, do not leave a message. For example, a message that states "You have reached 555-1111" does not mean that the patient is still at that number.
3. Leave as little information as needed, e.g., "Please have Mr. Baxter call this number when he arrives."
4. Do not leave appointment times or test results in a recorded message.

---

examples of items commonly ordered from hospitals and laboratories.

Before calling any of these suppliers, ensure that you have an accurate list of your requirements, and follow up your telephone order with a formal purchase order. Use the company's standard order form or website information, such as item numbers, catalogue pages, and units for ordering, so that your order can be processed accurately. Although many companies now have online ordering, placing orders by phone allows you the opportunity to ask questions you may have about your order and to build a mutually beneficial relationship with suppliers.

Answering Services

There are two types of answering services. One is a separate number (usually listed after the office number in the telephone directory), where messages can be left for after-hours callback. The most common type, however, is a direct connection with the doctor's office telephone so that when a call is made to the office, it is picked up by the answering service when the office is unavailable. These answering services are user-friendly to the caller in a world of automation. The patient can speak to a real person. The answering service will take messages and relay them to the office. If the physician is on call, the service will contact the doctor on his or her pager (beeper) or cell phone and relay the message directly. There are certain areas in hospitals that prohibit the use of cell phones; therefore the service will usually call the pager number.

Answering services can be used after hours, at lunch time, or at peak periods to relieve the medical administrative assistant. If a service is used, you must check first thing every morning for all messages, and last thing before you leave to advise the service where the doctor may be reached (if on call) and when the office will be open again.

DID YOU KNOW?

Modern-day answering services called *virtual receptionists* interact with offices in real time. They can escalate emergency calls, book appointments, send appointment reminders, book referrals, and record conversations for medical records. Most answering services now offer virtual reception services in addition to traditional services.

Voice-Messaging Systems

In areas where telephone answering services are not available, many physicians use voice-messaging systems. Some physicians prefer to use answering systems, such as voice mail, rather than have the additional cost of an answering service. The medical administrative assistant will record a message on the system informing the caller what the office hours are and what to do in the case of an emergency. The message must be current, and any extended absences need to include the dates of departure and return. Let your callers know whom they should call in your absence, or have the calls forwarded directly to another administrative assistant when possible. If you have a system that provides extensions to individual staff members, a call can be automatically redirected, and the caller can then leave a message for that individual only. Voice mail requires a password from the staff member to access his or her message.

When programming a standard message that your callers will receive in your absence or when you are busy, plan it carefully. You will change your message often (every morning when you arrive, and every evening when you leave), so, if necessary, write down your standard messages to ensure that they are concise and accurate. When you record them, remember to speak clearly, at a moderate speed, and with a smile in your voice. See Box 5.6 for an example of a standard message.

Some automated answering systems are for information only, and the caller is unable to leave a message. Most telephone systems will have a flashing light that will prompt you that there is a message waiting. Other systems have only an interrupted dial tone that is heard when the receiver is picked up, indicating that you have a message. With this type of system, you will need to check frequently; in a busy office, this is often inconvenient and may result in missed or delayed messages.

• BOX 5.6   Standard Message

"Thank you for calling Dr. Plunkett's office. It is (date), and I am in the office but either away from my desk or on the other line. Please leave a message, and I will return your call as soon as possible. You can call 8-1-1 for nonemergency medical advice. If this is an emergency, please dial 9-1-1 or go to the nearest emergency department."

The Telephone Directory

The medical administrative assistant's best reference source is a telephone directory. Some provinces and cities still offer a paper directory, but if one is not available, web searches offer an easy solution. The Yellow Pages and White Pages are now available online. Government and company websites often provide employee directories and certainly offer a main phone line number and address. A one-stop directory for physicians in your area is the College of Physicians and Surgeons and/or your provincial CMA branch. If you work in an office that refers many patients to many different physicians, it might be reasonable to print a copy of the physician directory.

You should also set up your own office telephone directory, listing in it numbers you call frequently, such as drugstores, hospitals, laboratories, other doctors, ambulance and emergency services, long-term care services, social services, community agencies, and staff members' home telephone numbers. This directory may be set up electronically in word processing or spreadsheet software. Some electronic medical record systems provide features for creating directories. The software may offer functions such as searching, alphabetizing, copying, pasting, and creating labels. You should maintain a hard copy of your directory for use when your computer networks are not available—or some employees just prefer a printed copy.

A Cardex or Rolodex system is still an efficient way to keep reference information such as referring physicians' names, addresses, identification numbers, and telephone numbers. If you have someone in your office who prefers this manual system, you could use any electronically created directory to create a Rolodex by placing the entries in an appropriate template and printing the numbers and addresses. Providing the addresses and phone numbers in typeset, rather than handwritten, form may prevent some errors.

If you have a speed dial feature on your telephone system, store the most frequently called numbers. Have an index of the stored numbers in a convenient location.

Equipment

Several companies offer sophisticated telephone equipment for business and industry. If you work in a private-practice setting with one or two physicians, you will probably have a telephone system with three or four incoming landlines (ringing to the reception area) and a separate landline (private line for the physician), plus perhaps a number for a fax machine. Many institutions use private-branch exchange (PBX) systems, or hybrid PBX systems that include newer Voice over Internet protocols (VoIP). Some health care telephone systems include Centrex, Mitel, and Avaya. Hospitals, clinics, and medical centers generally employ receptionist/switchboard operators, and the equipment used in these settings are multiline devices.

Modern telephones are programmed to allow you to do such things as dial a second number if the first number you called is busy; when the number you have called is free, your telephone will ring, at which time you can complete your call. Call waiting, redial, speed dial, caller identification, call forwarding, and call transfer are other telephone features that assist in the operation of an efficient office.

Fax Machines

Many medical offices still use traditional fax machines. In most cases, faxing has replaced the use of the mail service. For example, many offices fax specialist referrals, prescription information to pharmacies, and third-party billing forms. As is the case when using any communication tool, sending and receiving faxes requires attention to detail. Confidentiality and privacy concerns can be reduced by following the simple guidelines discussed below.

It is good practice to program frequently used numbers into the speed dial function if using a fax machine. This will avoid confidential information being sent to the wrong location if you happen to misdial the number. Always use a cover sheet when sending anything over a fax machine. Most word processing software contains professional fax cover sheet template options that can easily be modified with your office information. This cover sheet should have your doctor's name, address, phone number, and fax number clearly visible on it. It should also contain a confidentiality disclaimer that includes instructions on what to do if a fax is received in error (see Fig. 5.6). Because you will be dealing with sensitive medical information, it is good practice to make notes on your original fax copy of when it was sent and by whom. You should also attach a copy of the printout from your machine that confirms the fax was sent successfully. In some cases, such as when you are faxing to a number for the first time, you may want to make a follow-up phone call to ensure that your fax was received. The Office of the Privacy Commissioner of Canada suggests that passcodes should be used on all fax machines transmitting and receiving personal information, that fax machines should be kept in a closed area where passersby cannot access them, and that purchasing machines that encrypt transmissions should be considered because fax machines can be tapped and monitored like telephones (Office of the Privacy Commissioner of Canada, 2004). In addition to advice that reduces errors when sending faxes, CMPA offers the following advice to those that receive faxes in error:

"1. Contact the sender and advise them of the breach and to help ensure continuity of patient care.

2. Discuss with the sender how best to dispose of the fax. Do not keep a copy of the fax and do not attempt to forward it to the intended recipient (i.e. leave that to the sender).

3. Consider notifying your institution's privacy officer, if applicable." (CMPA, July 2014, para. 7)

Cell Phones

The use of cell phones and other mobile devices in the medical environment has increased substantially; however, there are special considerations for patients, employees, and physicians around their use.

Many offices have cell phone policies in place for the use of personal cell phones during office hours. It is important to keep in mind that these policies are in place mainly for the protection of the patients, physicians, and employees. Distractions in a medical office can lead to decreased patient-care standards; lack of attention leads to mistakes. Personal cell phone use by employees should be restricted to breaks and take place in designated areas as outlined in your office policy. This will reduce errors from inattention and help you maintain your reputation as a professional. If your office policy allows the use of cell phones for business use, be sure that your patients are aware of this policy by posting the policy and obtaining the proper consents when communicating with patients via mobile devices.

Medical administrative assistants need to be somewhat aware of how patients in their office are using cell phones. Patients should be made aware that taking pictures and videos of the activities and information in the office may represent a breach of privacy legislation. There are situations where audio recordings may be of benefit to the patient, but the physician and patient should have a mutual understanding of the benefits and risks, and of the fact that the recording will become a permanent part of the patient record.

For physicians, cell phones and mobile devices represent an important link between them, their colleagues, and online health resources. There may be situations where it seems the office policy does not apply to the physician, and perhaps it does not; the reason for the physician's cell phone use likely is directly related to the patient care he or she is providing. Medical administrative assistants need to be understanding of the differences between personal and professional use of mobile devices. They must be careful not to adopt the perspective that if one person, or one group of people (like physicians), in the office uses cell phones, all cell phone use is acceptable.

278 O'Connor Street
Ottawa, ON K2P 1V4
Phone: 613-212-1212
Fax: 613-212-2121
www.drplunkettsoffice.com

Dr. Plunkett's Office

Fax

To:	Workplace Safety and Insurance Board	**From:**	Jane Smith
Fax:	416-344-4684	**Pages:**	5 including cover
Phone:	416-344-1000	**Date:**	July 11, 2018
Re:	Claim Number 45678-D	**cc:**	N/A

☐ Urgent ■ For Review ☐ Please Comment ☐ Please Reply ☐ Please Recycle

Dear Case Worker:

Please see attached form CMS8 and supporting documentation as requested.

Regards,

Jane Smith

Jane Smith for Dr. J.E. Plunkett

CONFIDENTIALITY CAUTION

This facsimile transmission is intended only for the use of the individual or entity to which it is addressed and contains information that is privileged and confidential. If the reader of this transmission is not the intended recipient, or the employee or agent responsible for delivering the transmission to the intended recipient, you are hereby notified that any dissemination, distributions or copying of the communication is strictly prohibited.

If you have received this facsimile transmission in error, notify us immediately by calling 613-212-1212 for instructions on how to securely and permanently destroy the information therein. If you do not receive all pages of the transmission, please call 613-212-1212 to inform the sender.

• **Fig. 5.6** Sample fax cover sheet.

eCommunications

eCommunications (electronic communications), or **telemedicine**, includes communication that takes place through e-mail, videoconferencing, social media platforms, and texting. The increased availability of eCommunication tools has made health care services more efficient and portable; this improved accessibility is important to those in remote communities or regions where health care services are restricted in some other way. Despite the advantages they offer, these technologies bring increased privacy concerns as well. In response, the CMPA has included eCommunications in its *CMPA Good Practices Guide* and has also published tips on how to avoid medico-legal risks when using any of these platforms. The Royal College of Physicians and Surgeons echoes the recommendations of CMPA, and provincial Colleges of Physicians and Surgeons often expand on these recommendations by implementing specific policies and guidelines for their use. The concerns regarding the privacy of these modern tools and platforms are also evident in health information acts across the country. You should always check with your local branch of the College of Physicians and Surgeons, or its equivalent, for specific policies before you use any eCommunication tools in your office. A clear office policy should be posted and understood by all staff, the employer, and patients.

Besides privacy issues related to eCommunications, related associations address the idea that eCommunications should not interfere with any of the physician's responsibilities as outlined in the CMA's Code of Ethics. The CMA has established a policy called the *Physician Guidelines for Online Communication with Patients* for its members. The policy outlines starting points and best practices related to online patient–physician relationships, retention of online communications, privacy, security, and associated topics (CMA, 2005).

How physicians and other practitioners get reimbursed for the time they spend in online environments is a concern and barrier to use. Many health services payment acts do not yet recognize the time physicians spend on certain patient-related eCommunications.

E-mail

To prevent any medico-legal complications or misunderstandings about e-mail communications, CMPA recommends using a consent form for any type of e-mail communication with patients. The association has created a form that physicians can modify and should review with each patient he or she will use this communication medium with (see Fig. 5.7). In addition, offices should be familiar with regulations set forth in provincial legislation about the necessary encryption, firewalls, passwords, and other technological protections. Physical or locational restrictions, such as what type of device it is or where a device is stored, may be written into such legislation. It is important that the medical administrative assistant understand that PHI sent or received by e-mail is considered a part of the physical medical record and is therefore subject to the same privacy, security, access, and retention rules as other health information collected or encountered.

Videoconferencing

As with any form of eCommunication, physicians and staff wishing to use videoconferencing services in their offices should contact their local College of Physicians and Surgeons to discuss options, guidelines, limitations, consent, and time when it is reasonable to provide health care services in this manner. Many offices will offer this service only under very special circumstances. Medical administrative assistants should become familiar with the videoconferencing platform used in the office so that consultations can run as smoothly as possible. You will also have to consider whether these services are insured by the province and investigate the rules for billing these services. If they are not aware of them, patients requesting videoconferencing services should be informed of any service charges before the consultation takes place. For private offices using videoconferencing only periodically, low-investment software such as Skype, Skype for Business, Zoom, WebEx, GoToMeetings, or other popular platforms that are easily available to the patient may be appropriate choices. The hospital or health authority the physician is affiliated with may also supply videoconferencing resources upon request.

More than any other type of eCommunication discussed, videoconferencing (often referred to as telehealth) is used to bring important health services to those who cannot access traditional health care services in Canada. Within Canada, many formal telehealth networks have been established; they utilize videoconferencing to deliver clinical, administrative, and educational services. It is important to note that these networks are not the equivalent of the telephone health advice services discussed previously. See Box 5.7 for a list of Canadian telehealth networks.

Canada Health Infoway works with the federal government, provinces, and territories to bring digital health solutions to Canadians. It reports that telehealth videoconferencing is now available to 98% of hospitals in Canada because of its efforts (Canada Health Infoway, 2018). Despite this, many remote communities, such as Nunavut, struggle with accessing videoconferencing because they do not have reliable Internet services.

CONSENT TO USE ELECTRONIC COMMUNICATIONS

This template is intended as a basis for an informed discussion. If used, physicians should adapt it to meet the particular circumstances in which electronic communications are expected to be used with a patient. Consideration of jurisdictional legislation and regulation is strongly encouraged.

PHYSICIAN INFORMATION:

Name: click here

Address:

Email (if applicable):

Phone (as required for Service(s)):

Website (if applicable):

The Physician has offered to communicate using the following means of electronic communication ("the Services"):

(Yes/No) Email	(Yes/No) Videoconferencing (including Skype®, FaceTime®)
(Yes/No) Text messaging (including instant messaging)	(Yes/No) Website/Portal

(Yes/No) Social media (specify):

(Yes/No) Other (specify):

PATIENT ACKNOWLEDGMENT AND AGREEMENT:

I acknowledge that I have read and fully understand the risks, limitations, conditions of use, and instructions for use of the selected electronic communication Services more fully described in the Appendix to this consent form. I understand and accept the risks outlined in the Appendix to this consent form, associated with the use of the Services in communications with the Physician and the Physician's staff. I consent to the conditions and will follow the instructions outlined in the Appendix, as well as any other conditions that the Physician may impose on communications with patients using the Services.

I acknowledge and understand that despite recommendations that encryption software be used as a security mechanism for electronic communications, it is possible that communications with the Physician or the Physician's staff using the Services may not be encrypted. Despite this, I agree to communicate with the Physician or the Physician's staff using these Services with a full understanding of the risk.

I acknowledge that either I or the Physician may, at any time, withdraw the option of communicating electronically through the Services upon providing written notice. Any questions I had have been answered.

Patient name:

Patient address:

Patient home phone:

Patient mobile phone:

Patient email (if applicable):

Other account information required to communicate via the Services (if applicable):

Patient signature:	Date:
Witness signature:	Date:

APPENDIX
Risks of using electronic communication

The Physician will use reasonable means to protect the security and confidentiality of information sent and received using the Services ("Services" is defined in the attached Consent to use electronic communications). However, because of the risks outlined below, the Physician cannot guarantee the security and confidentiality of electronic communications:

- Use of electronic communications to discuss sensitive information can increase the risk of such information being disclosed to third parties.

- Despite reasonable efforts to protect the privacy and security of electronic communication, it is not possible to completely secure the information.

- Employers and online services may have a legal right to inspect and keep electronic communications that pass through their system.

- Electronic communications can introduce malware into a computer system, and potentially damage or disrupt the computer, networks, and security settings.

- Electronic communications can be forwarded, intercepted, circulated, stored, or even changed without the knowledge or permission of the Physician or the patient.

- Even after the sender and recipient have deleted copies of electronic communications, back-up copies may exist on a computer system.

- Electronic communications may be disclosed in accordance with a duty to report or a court order.

- Videoconferencing using services such as Skype or FaceTime may be more open to interception than other forms of videoconferencing.

If the email or text is used as an e-communication tool, the following are additional risks:

- Email, text messages, and instant messages can more easily be misdirected, resulting in increased risk of being received by unintended and unknown recipients.

- Email, text messages, and instant messages can be easier to falsify than handwritten or signed hard copies. It is not feasible to verify the true identity of the sender, or to ensure that only the recipient can read the message once it has been sent.

Conditions of using the Services

- While the Physician will attempt to review and respond in a timely fashion to your electronic communication, the Physician cannot guarantee that all electronic communications will be reviewed and responded to within any specific period of time. The Services will not be used for medical emergencies or other time-sensitive matters.

- If your electronic communication requires or invites a response from the Physician and you have not received a response within a reasonable time period, it is your responsibility to follow up to determine whether the intended recipient received the electronic communication and when the recipient will respond.

- Electronic communication is not an appropriate substitute for in-person or over-the-telephone communication or clinical examinations, where appropriate, or for attending the Emergency Department when needed. You are responsible for following up on the Physician's electronic communication and for scheduling appointments where warranted.

- Electronic communications concerning diagnosis or treatment may be printed or transcribed in full and made part of your medical record. Other individuals authorized to access the medical record, such as staff and billing personnel, may have access to those communications.

- The Physician may forward electronic communications to staff and those involved in the delivery and administration of your care. The Physician might use one or more of the Services to communicate with those involved in your care. The Physician will not forward electronic communications to third parties, including family members, without your prior written consent, except as authorized or required by law.

- You and the Physician will not use the Services to communicate sensitive medical information about matters specified below:

  (Yes/No) Sexually transmitted disease
  (Yes/No) AIDS/HIV
  (Yes/No) Mental health
  (Yes/No) Developmental disability
  (Yes/No) Substance abuse
  (Yes/No) Other (specify):

- You agree to inform the Physician of any types of information you do not want sent via the Services, in addition to those set out above. You can add to or modify the above list at any time by notifying the Physician in writing.

- Some Services might not be used for therapeutic purposes or to communicate clinical information. Where applicable, the use of these Services will be limited to education, information, and administrative purposes.

- The Physician is not responsible for information loss due to technical failures associated with your software or internet service provider.

Patient initials_____

- **Fig. 5.7, cont'd**

APPENDIX CONTINUED

Instructions for communication using the Services

To communicate using the Services, you must:

- Reasonably limit or avoid using an employer's or other third party's computer.

- Inform the Physician of any changes in the patient's email address, mobile phone number, or other account information necessary to communicate via the Services.

If the Services include email, instant messaging and/or text messaging, the following applies:

- Include in the message's subject line an appropriate description of the nature of the communication (e.g. "prescription renewal"), and your full name in the body of the message.

- Review all electronic communications to ensure they are clear and that all relevant information is provided before sending to the physician.

- Ensure the Physician is aware when you receive an electronic communication from the Physician, such as by a reply message or allowing "read receipts" to be sent.

- Take precautions to preserve the confidentiality of electronic communications, such as using screen savers and safeguarding computer passwords.

- Withdraw consent only by email or written communication to the Physician.

- If you require immediate assistance, or if your condition appears serious or rapidly worsens, you should not rely on the Services. Rather, you should call the Physician's office or take other measures as appropriate, such as going to the nearest Emergency Department or urgent care clinic.

- Other conditions of use in addition to those set out above: *(patient to initial)*

I have reviewed and understand all of the risks, conditions, and instructions described in this Appendix.

Patient signature _____

Date _____

Patient initials_____

Alberta Telehealth
British Columbia Provincial Health Services Authority
Keewaytinook Okimakanak eHealth Telemedicine
MBTelehealth
Newfoundland and Labrador Telehealth
Nova Scotia Telehealth Network
NWT Healthnet
Ontario Telemedicine Network
Réseaux Universitaires Intégrés de Santé (RUIS) of Québec
Telehealth Saskatchewan
Yukon Telehealth Network

A common theme among many of the noted networks is outreach to and care for remote Indigenous communities. For example, Canada Health Infoway has committed to an initiative called *Closing the Circle of Care Project* with the goal of improving access to and efficiency of health care services for First Nations communities (Canada Health Infoway: Indigenous Peoples, 2018). The Ontario Telemedicine Network partners with Keewaytinook Okimakanak eHealth Telemedicine (KOeTS) to supply videoconferencing services to Indigenous communities. The network reports that 30 new telemedicine systems were provided in 2017 and that 120 systems are now active in Indigenous communities in the province of Ontario (Ontario Telemedicine Network, 2018). Health Canada's eHealth Solutions Unit (eHSU) "works to develop eHealth tools to support the use of health technologies in Canada's First Nations and Inuit communities" (Health Canada, 2005, para. 2). eHSU works to provide the infrastructure, supports, standards, and online access to health information through media such as videoconferencing (Health Canada, 2005). For example, it partners with First Nations of Alberta to offer the First Nations Telehealth Portal.

Social Media

Social media have become important tools for personal and professional communications. Their use in health care brings many advantages, along with complex challenges. These advantages and challenges are well noted by the CMA, CMPA, Office of the Privacy Commissioner of Canada, and Colleges of Physicians and Surgeons, who all provide guidelines and advice for Canadian physicians.

For administrative assistants and others working in medical offices that use social media for professional reasons, there are important responsibilities around maintaining privacy, confidentiality, and professionalism. Posting pictures or information about patients or events without the proper permissions can lead to dire consequences, such as dismissal or legal actions. Even "sharing" or "liking" an inappropriate patient-related post can lead to negative consequences for employees. Because medical administrative assistants are agents of their employers, an awareness of the guidelines provided by the local College of Physicians and Surgeons should be sought. Provincial health authorities may also have specific policies.

When using social media for personal reasons, it is important to maintain your professional image. Posting inappropriate pictures, videos, or comments may affect how potential employers, or references for employment, view you and your application. They may wonder how your image or online behaviors will reflect on them or their practice. This does not mean that you should avoid having an online image. In fact, some human resource specialists now believe your "online campaign" may be as important as your resume and application. This idea adds strength to the argument that you must always consider whether what you are posting online accurately displays how you want to be viewed by people in your related industry.

Texting

Texting is a very insecure means of communication; the use of unencrypted text messages to patients should be avoided. The dangers of texting are that personal information may be sent to an incorrect number, the personal information may be intercepted, the information may be read by someone other than the intended receiver, or the information may be misinterpreted. If your office offers encrypted text messaging and has a clear policy on what type of information can be sent to a patient by text, a written consent signed by the patient should still be sought. It is important to understand that many health care providers and their patients maintain that texting is dangerous and unprofessional; you must be very clear on the expectations of not only your employer but also of those to whom you intend to send a text message.

Texting between employees has become an efficient way to communicate on topics such as hours of work. However, there are still important considerations for both the sender and the receiver. If you are sending text messages and expecting an immediate response, you may be disappointed. Many offices have cell phone policies that do not permit their personal use during working hours. The person you are texting may not have immediate access to a phone. Just because you send someone an "instant" message does not mean he or she can or should instantly respond. If you have important information relating to work, you should strive to speak directly with the person you are seeking out if there is any chance of miscommunication or disruption to the office in any way. For instance, sending a co-worker a text stating that you are sick or late and hoping he or she will pass it on to the employer is an unacceptable practice in most cases.

Summary

Communication has never been easier; we have multiple ways to connect with patients, co-workers, and others in the industry. However, privacy concerns are considerable when we begin to move away from traditional telephone use and toward the convenience and efficiency offered by e-mail, text messaging, and other eCommunication tools. The medical administrative assistant must be diligent in seeking out the rules, regulations, and best practices set forth by the legal and licensing authorities in health care. The administrative assistant must be keenly aware of office policies related to the use of cell phones, smartphones, and other forms of communication and understand the difference between the personal and professional use of each.

Assignments

Assignment 5.1

The following situations are designed for role-play. Choose a partner, decide how you would handle the situation, and write the script. If possible, you should have a prop telephone for authenticity. You and your partner will then act out the scene, with one student playing the role of the administrative assistant and the other the role of the patient. The remainder of the class will observe, and a session to evaluate your performance should follow.

1. Mrs. Scott calls to inform you that Peter John has just rammed his head into a brick wall while pushing his brother on his bicycle. His head is bleeding profusely, and she thinks the child needs stitches. It is 4:30 p.m., and the doctor has just left to do rounds at the hospital.

2. Mary Shultz, who is obviously under the influence of alcohol, calls and insists on speaking to the doctor. The office is full of patients, and the doctor is running behind schedule.

3. Dr. Plunkett has requested that you call Sandy Shaw into the office for a follow-up appointment. Sandy had a minimally abnormal Pap test, and the doctor wishes to repeat the test.

4. Thomas Bell calls and tells you his wife has just collapsed on the floor. He thinks she has had a stroke because her mouth seems to be twisted.

5. The doctor has asked you to hold all calls due to a difficult consultation. Amelia Jackson calls and insists on speaking to the doctor.

6. Julie Harris calls and is at the point of hysteria. Her son, William, has a very high temperature and is convulsing. She lives 5 km outside the city, her husband has taken the car to work, and she does not know any of the people who live in her neighbourhood. The doctor is not in the office.

7. The doctor's husband is on the phone wishing to speak with his wife. You know that he often calls without good reason, but he insists on speaking with the doctor.

8. Mr. and Mrs. Chang have recently arrived from South Korea, and their sponsor has asked Dr. Plunkett to take them into his practice. Mrs. Chang calls you to book an appointment; however, she is not fluent in English, and you are having trouble understanding her.

9. A new patient (Rosa Geary) called two weeks ago, and you booked her for an appointment. She did not come to the office for her appointment. She called the next day with an excuse, and you booked her again. Again, she did not arrive for her scheduled appointment. She is now calling with an excuse and a request for another appointment.

10. Lori Brier (a single parent) was injured at work. Dr. Plunkett examined and treated her and sent the required forms to the appropriate workers' compensation board. Ms. Brier calls. She is very anxious. She has no money for rent and groceries. She says she called the workers' compensation office and was informed that the required documents from her doctor had not been received. You tell Ms. Brier that you sent the forms, but she doesn't believe you—she NEEDS MONEY NOW!

11. Dr. Plunkett has agreed to cover emergencies for Dr. Moore, who is going on vacation. Dr. Plunkett is doing rounds at the hospital when you receive a call from Tiffany Black, one of Dr. Moore's patients. (You don't know anything of her history.) She tells you that she has attempted suicide twice in the past and is considering it again.

12. Gary Brown is schizophrenic and has been receiving treatment in the community mental health unit of the local hospital. You received a call from the hospital last week informing you that Gary had left the hospital and had not returned. Today you receive a call from Gary, and he seems very confused.

13. Fred Jones is calling the office to talk to Dr. Plunkett about his INR results. He wishes to obtain his prescription of anticoagulant for the week. The results are not back from the laboratory yet.

14. Dr. McCarthy is phoning to speak with Dr. Plunkett about a patient he referred. Dr. Plunkett is with a patient. What do you tell Dr. McCarthy?

15. Miranda Cusack, a friend from high school, sent you message on Facebook to request an appointment with Dr. Plunkett. When you did not answer her request, she sent you a text message. She was obviously upset. What do you do?

Assignment 5.2

Search the website of CMPA, CMA, the local hospital, or the local health authority for policies related to eCommunication tools. (Use search words such as *social media, cell phones, mobile devices, electronic communication, telehealth, e-mail,* etc.). Choose one policy or set of guidelines and create a professional-appearing informational poster for your office that summarizes the information. Be sure to give credit to your source(s) by providing a reference citation.

Topics for Discussion

1. An institution calls and states that it has admitted your patient and needs information. You have no documented or prior knowledge of this admission. How would you handle the call?

2. You need to get in touch with a patient on an urgent basis, but all you get is a voicemail greeting that gives only the patient's phone number. What would you do?

3. A concerned mother calls and is sure that her daughter, who is 18, has an appointment with you today. She wants to leave a message for her. You know that the daughter does not want her mother to know about the office visit. How would you handle the call?

4. You have highly confidential information that a referral facility needs immediately. The only way to get it there is by fax machine. How would you ensure that the receiving facility gets the appropriate information?

5. Many phones have call display. You have called Mr. Baxter's home, but the call went to the answering machine, which identified only the telephone number. You did not leave a message, but his wife saw your number on the call display and is calling to see what the call was about. How would you respond? How can you prevent this in the future?

6. A friend and colleague has taken an inappropriate and unsolicited picture of a patient in a long-term care facility. She posted the picture to a social media site because she thought it was "interesting." You do not "like" or "share" the image. When you see your friend, she asks you about it. What advice can you give your friend?

7. You receive a text message from a patient you know personally; he is asking for medical advice. What advice can you give the patient? How would you go about doing this?

References

Canada Health Infoway. (2018). Foundational programs. Retrieved from https://www.infoway-inforoute.ca/en/what-we-do/progress-in-canada/foundational-programs.

Canadian Medical Association. (2005). *Physician guidelines for online communication with patients.* Retrieved from https://www.cma.ca/En/Pages/SearchPage.aspx?k=physician%20guidelines%20for%20online%20communication.

Canadian Medical Protective Association. (July 2014). *Ten ways physicians can prevent privacy breaches with using fax with other healthcare professionals.* Retrieved from https://www.cmpa-acpm.ca/en/advice-publications/browse-articles/2014/10-ways-physicians-can-prevent-privacy-breaches-when-using-fax-with-other-health care-professionals.

Canadian Medical Protective Association. (January 2016). Using electronic communications, protecting privacy. Retrieved from https://www.cmpa-acpm.ca/en/advice-publications/browse-articles/2013/using-electronic-communications-protecting-privacy.

Government of Canada. Health Canada. (2005). *eHealth.* Retrieved from https://www.canada.ca/en/indigenous-services-canada/services/first-nations-inuit-health/health-care-services/ehealth.html.

Guerriere, M. (2017). *Beyond the fax machine.* Retrieved from https://www.telushealth.co/item/beyond-fax-machine/.

Office of the Privacy Commissioner of Canada. (April 2004). *Faxing personal information.* Retrieved from https://www.priv.gc.ca/en/privacy-topics/technology-and-privacy/02_05_d_04/.

Ontario Telemedicine Network. (2018). Indigenous Telemedicine. Retrieved from https://otn.ca/our-partners/indigenous-telemedicine//.

6

Office Correspondence: Mail, Memos, Letters, and Envelopes

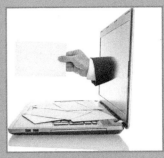

Source: © CanStock Photo Inc./Gajus

This chapter encompasses two topics. The first area of focus is the nature of the mail that will be received in and sent from your office. Descriptions of postal and courier services are provided, and electronic methods for sending and receiving mail are introduced. The second area of focus outlines the types of correspondence you will produce as a medical administrative assistant. Details of memo, letter, and envelope production are provided, along with complementary illustrations that will assist you in reproducing each letter and memo type with ease.

CHAPTER OUTLINE

Introduction

Mail

Postal Services

Courier Services

Electronic Equipment and Software Systems

Memos, Letters, and Envelopes

LEARNING OBJECTIVES

After reading this chapter, you will be able to:

1. Outline how to handle incoming mail
2. Recognize how to handle outgoing mail
3. Identify how to protect the confidentiality of electronic transmissions
4. Describe the varieties of delivery services
5. Describe the different styles of memo format
6. Recognize the various letter styles such as block, modified block, and modified block with indented paragraphs
7. Describe the parts of a business letter
8. Identify the punctuation styles, such as mixed and open
9. Describe how to prepare envelopes

KEY TERMS

Mail porter: An employee assigned to the distribution and collection of incoming and outgoing deliveries for a company or office. In the medical environment, a porter may be used in place of a courier service to transport items to laboratories, pharmacies, or suppliers on a predetermined schedule. For instance, a porter might transport blood tests drawn in an office to a laboratory at the hospital.

Postage meter: Postage equipment that seals the envelope and stamps the appropriate selected postage on the envelope (upper right-hand corner).

Proofread: To review a written work for errors in grammar, punctuation, and format.

Salutation: The salutation is an act of greeting. Dear Dr. Plunkett, To Whom It May Concern, and Dear Sir or Madam are the greetings extended from the letter writer to the recipient.

Introduction

One of your responsibilities as a medical administrative assistant will be the handling of both incoming and outgoing mail (see Fig. 6.1). Part of this responsibility is to prioritize the process. The physician will want to see only the mail that is pertinent to him or her; if you can deal with items independently, you should do so. Guidelines around how mail should be prioritized will need to be discussed with your employer.

It is essential that you become familiar with postal services, delivery services such as couriers, and the electronic systems that serve to reduce your reliance on these services. It is also essential that you are able to accurately format the letters and memos that will be distributed from your office. This chapter, although not exhaustive, will address each of these topics and provide you with an excellent base of knowledge to build upon.

Mail

Much of the patient information that previously would have arrived in your office by mail or priority post is now delivered via electronic sources. Memos, letters, and reports from medical organizations can be sent as email attachments, fax transmissions, or electronic medical and health records. Many medical newsletters and journals are now available on the Internet, which eliminates the need to send them by mail. Despite this, medical

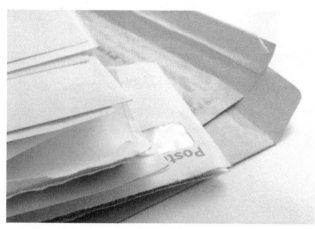

• **Fig. 6.1** Every medical office should have an established policy regarding the processing of incoming mail. (Source: © CanStock Photo Inc./shutterwolf)

• BOX 6.1 **Equipment Useful for Processing Mail**

Letter opener
Date stamp
For Deposit Only stamp
Stapler
Staple remover
Paper clips
Pen/pencil
Highlighter
In larger offices:
    Postage machine with automatic sealer
    Weigh scale
    Postage guidelines

---

offices continue to receive and send moderate amounts of mail through the traditional modalities of mail and courier. How to process this mail will be the focus of the following paragraphs. Box 6.1 lists the equipment you may need to process the mail.

Incoming Mail

Incoming mail may consist of the following:
1. Correspondence (reports from consultants, legal claims, insurance claims)
2. Pamphlets
3. Magazines and medical journals
4. Medical information (from medical associations)
5. Cheques
6. Confidential mail
7. Laboratory, diagnostic imaging, and other diagnostic reports
8. Hospital reports (admission, discharge, operative notes, etc.)
9. Advertisements and drug samples

On receipt of incoming mail, you should open all correspondence, with the exception of envelopes specifically marked "confidential" or "personal." If any letters refer to previous correspondence, retrieve the relevant documents from the file and attach. The administrative assistant should date-stamp each piece of mail, organize it in order of importance, and place it in the doctor's incoming mail tray or on his or her desk.

Prioritizing or sorting should be completed according to the importance or urgency with which the information should be handled. The following is an example of how you might prioritize:
1. Patient information (laboratory, x-ray, and other diagnostic testing reports and consultation reports)
2. Correspondence (special delivery or registered mail first)
3. Cheques
4. Medical information
5. Drug samples
6. Medical journals, magazines, and pamphlets

All cheques must be stamped "For Deposit Only." This prevents the cheque from being cashed by anyone other than the payee (the person to whom the cheque is written). Enclosed cheques should be safely stored and a notation made on the accompanying letter to this effect.

Magazines (with the exception of the doctor's professional journals) can be placed in the waiting room, and inconsequential unsolicited mail can be recycled.

If a return address does not appear on the letter, check the envelope before discarding it. It is good practice to staple the envelope to any letters that arrive in the office. This eliminates the chance of the envelope being discarded, only to find that the return address is not on the correspondence when you are asked to respond to it. Loose enclosures also should be attached to the appropriate correspondence.

After the doctor has read the mail, documents should be initialled to indicate that they have been read, and a notation should be made to indicate what action is required, such as file, discard, or reply. Patient information is usually flagged as "F" for file or "C" for chart to be pulled. By using this system, there is no need to pull the charts for every piece of patient information that arrives in your office.

Outgoing Mail

Outgoing mail consists of the following:

1. Doctor's correspondence (replies to requests, doctor's inquiries, and information reports)
2. Insurance information forms (workers' compensation forms or accident reports)
3. Magazines and medical journals
4. Referral letters
5. Referral requisitions
6. Supply requisitions and purchase orders
7. Patient account statements for uninsured services
8. Files of transferred patients (a photocopy of the complete chart dictated by the doctor should be sent by courier as "confidential")

In many medical offices, it is the medical administrative assistant's responsibility to transcribe the physician's outgoing dictated letters and reports. Some physicians will use a speech recognition system, and the transcriptionist or administrative assistant will proofread, edit, and format the material before mailing it out. The spell-check option on your computer is not enough to ensure accuracy. The spell-check cannot differentiate between *ilium* and *ileum*, *through* and *threw*, or *to*, *too*, and *two*, for example. Proofread the document before giving it to the physician for final approval.

After the document or documents are prepared, they should be appropriately assembled for mailing. A general rule of thumb is to place the original document and any enclosures on top of all other supporting documentation. These are then placed together with an addressed envelope. The completed mail pack should then be secured with a paper clip and placed on the doctor's desk for his or her signature.

When the signed package is returned, fold and insert the document(s) in the appropriate-size envelope and seal it. Make sure that if an enclosure is part of the package, you remember to include it before sealing the envelope.

Remember, it is essential that you retain a *dated copy* of *all* documents. It may be useful to keep general correspondence in a correspondence file or binder. All patient-related documents would be filed in the patient's chart or saved to the patient's electronic medical record (EMR).

Stamps should be available in the office for regular mail. Some larger offices may use a postage meter. If using a postage meter, you need to check daily the amount of postage available. The postage is added to the meter by the post office. This can be done electronically. Larger packages may require a visit to the post office. If you are in doubt about the mailing of any correspondence, consult your local postal authorities.

DID YOU KNOW?

Using postage meters can save offices approximately 15 cents per letter. You can rent meters through Canada Post or one of its Canadian distributors (you cannot buy meters because they are regulated). Meters are available for all business sizes—the largest can process up to 120 letters per minute! (Canada Post, 2018)

Pickup times at the nearest mailbox (or by internal mail in a large organization) should be investigated. It is your responsibility to ensure that urgent mail reaches the box or the mail room in time to be collected that day. Some clinics may have a dedicated mail porter who not only distributes internal mail but also transfers laboratory and other diagnostic samples to hospitals. Their pickup and delivery times also should be noted so that diagnostic samples can be delivered and processed accordingly.

Postal Services

Canada Post offers many types of mail handling services. Important letters and other documents can be sent by registered mail or priority post, which gives overnight delivery, and valuable parcels can be insured. Sealed letters and postcards are sent first class, whereas some newspapers and periodicals are sent second class. Parcels may be sent parcel post; small parcels and printed matter are sent third class. Because Canada Post's services and rates are extensive and subject to frequent change, you should become familiar with its website and confirm services and charges regularly (https://www.canadapost.ca). Canada Post staff can assist you if there is any uncertainty about the method to use in forwarding material by mail.

DID YOU KNOW?

Canada Post issues alerts (red, yellow, and green) to notify customers of postal disruptions, suspensions, and restorations so that you can make appropriate delivery choices. The alerts are listed under "announcements/service alerts" on its website (Canada Post, 2018).

Courier Services

To ensure prompt and safe delivery of special letters and parcels, many businesses use courier services. Although using a courier is more expensive than regular mail services, it guarantees prompt delivery—often overnight. When a courier such as Purolator or FedEx is used, each package is given an identification number. This allows you to trace your package if it does not arrive within the required time frame. It is important that you keep a log of mail that is delivered by one of these services. Courier services are listed in the Yellow Pages of the telephone directory or on the Yellow Pages website (https://www.yellowpages.ca). It is important for the efficient administrative assistant to be aware of the cost of courier services and to use them with discretion.

Most communities have intercity courier and laboratory services that will pick up correspondence, specimens, and drugs to be transported between physicians' offices, laboratories, and hospitals. Medical administrative assistants should know the names and scope of service of such courier services in their locality. If it is necessary to send specimens or drugs by mail, specific rules must be followed. Check with your local postal authorities before placing such materials in the mail. The courier services also will have guidelines for transporting these materials.

Electronic Equipment and Software Systems

Medical offices and hospitals use various types of electronic equipment, including computer network systems, for communication of medical information and general correspondence. It is important to follow guidelines and policies related to eCommunications, as discussed in Chapter 5, when exchanging, creating, or storing information via any electronic equipment and associated software (see Box 6.2 for Email Etiquette for the Professional Office). Because most of these electronic products rely on the Internet, backup procedures should be in place for times of power outage or Internet disruption.

Medical Offices

Medical offices have computer networks and terminals that allow quick and easy communication. Staff may use a variety of stand-alone software products such as email, word processing, and instant messaging. Letters, memos, envelopes, and medical reports can be keyed into computer software programs installed on computer terminals, and prepared electronic documents can be received by other users almost instantly.

Fax machines are still used by most medical offices. Medical administrative assistants may be required to send referrals, letters, memos, or reports by fax to other medical offices or to hospitals. They may also receive similar information and must treat this incoming "mail" in the same manner as mail that arrives by the postal or courier services discussed.

EMRs are used in many medical offices. Medical administrative assistants will interact with these systems when dealing with patient-related information. All office staff members eligible to access the EMR can do so from their respective computer terminals or mobile devices, reducing the reliance on paper medical charts. As for reports and documents received from outside of the office environment, medical administrative assistants may be required to scan the information into the EMR. As with communications received by other methods (post, courier, fax), these reports must be processed appropriately before being scanned into the EMR. Increasingly, EMRs are connecting to laboratories, pharmacies, and patients, further reducing the reliance on mail services.

Hospitals

In addition to the fax machines, scanners, and computer networks and terminals already discussed, electronic health record (EHR) systems are also streamlining the electronic communication of medical information. EHR systems, which are being implemented by all Canadian provinces, greatly reduce or eliminate the need to mail information between hospitals, hospital departments, and other authorized health care providers. Authorized hospital staff members need only to identify the patient in the EHR and choose the notes or reports required. These may include reports from the transcription department because most hospitals are moving toward speech-recognition systems. These electronic systems allow physicians to dictate directly into the EHR or to transfer their completed files to the EHR after they are proofread and edited by the medical administrative assistant. Physicians may use landline communication systems for their dictations, or they may be able to connect via their smartphones or other mobile devices. EHR systems are audited regularly to ensure that patient information is not being accessed by unauthorized personnel.

> **DID YOU KNOW?**
>
> "Laboratory test results for 97 per cent of Canadians are available electronically for access by authorized clinicians" (Canada Health Infoway, 2019, para. 3).

Memos, Letters, and Envelopes

Memos, letters, and envelopes are prepared using computer software such as word processing programs and integrated packages that include spreadsheets, word processing,

TO: (the name of the recipient or recipients)
FROM: (the name of the sender)
DATE: (the date the message is produced)
SUBJECT: (what the message is about)

database, medical billing, appointment scheduling, and others. Some EMRs and EHRs may also have word processing features included. The purpose of the next two sections of this chapter is to provide a reference guide for producing memos, letters, and envelopes.

It is assumed that students have had previous instruction on the appropriate formats and word processing functions used in the production of these documents. However, practice exercises have been included to help reinforce your prior learning. The sample letters and memos shown throughout the chapter are created using the traditional 1.0-line spacing option. Your word processing software may default to a contemporary 1.08 or 1.15-line spacing option—either spacing option is acceptable and will create similar-appearing documents with slightly more space visible between lines when using a contemporary option.

Memos

Memos are the most informal type of written communication. The word *memo* is the short form of the word *memorandum,* which means "something to be brought to mind." Three acceptable memo styles will be reviewed below. Producing the note with the date, name of the sender, name of the receiver(s), and the subject formalizes the message.

Most business organizations send informal messages in a memo form. The most common mode of relaying these messages is through departmental email. Another option is to produce the memo, photocopy or print the required number of copies, and then distribute it either through internal mail or the postal service. Either way, a copy is kept by the sender for future reference and filing. The most common heading style and order of memo headings appear in Box 6.3.

The body of the memo is generally single-spaced but can be double-spaced if the message is short (if double-spaced, indent the beginning of each paragraph by hitting the TAB key on your keyboard one time). Initials of the person who produced the memo appear at the left margin a double-space below the last line of the message. These reference initials are lowercased (check that your word processing program does not automatically capitalize the first letter—if it does, remove this initial capital) and identify the person who typed the document (not the sender or the person who dictated the message).

If four or five people are to receive the memo, key all names on the memo beside "To." If the memo is to be sent in paper format, place a check mark opposite the appropriate name (or highlight the name with a marker) when distributing or mailing the finished memo.

In today's medical office environment, most memos are created and distributed by email. Multiple recipients can be selected from the email address book. The memo can be produced and distributed to all recipients with one keystroke. When sending mail in this manner, speak with your employer about any confidentiality that should be guarded. For instance, should the memo be "blind copied" to individuals (meaning others will not know who received it) or just sent as regular email? Email programs have the ability to notify you that the email has been read. You will have to turn on this email option in your software program to receive delivery and read receipts. Proper language and spelling are to be used when sending memos. The memo should look professional.

Styles of Memo

Headings and body styles of the following memo forms can be interchanged to produce a style that is appealing and acceptable to your employer. Full-block styles are the most popular as they are simple to format and are visually attractive. Other styles require you to set more tabs and use more word processing features; however, once a nicely formatted document is achieved, it can be saved as master copy and used for all future memos.

Style I: Full-Block Style

In a full-block memo style (also called "block" memo style), all headings are placed flush with the left margin. The information that follows the headings (names, date, and subject) should also be blocked or should begin at the same point on your horizontal ruler. This is most easily achieved by hitting the TAB key on your keyboard after the longest line (SUBJECT:). Match the tab location from this line with the other three headings. Type your headings in bold uppercase font. Double-space between heading lines and use a double to triple space before the memo message. Single-space the body (double-space if the message is short) and double-space between paragraphs. The typist's reference initials are typed at the left margin a double space below the last line of the message. They are lowercased.

Note that there is no formal signature line on a memo because the sender's name appears in the memo headings. A memo produced on 8.5-inch paper has 1-inch margins. Style I is shown in Fig. 6.2A. Fig. 6.2B shows the same memo with nonprinting formatting characters/marks (paragraph marks, tab arrows, space indicators, etc.) included. Also known as "show/hide" marks, these symbols are revealed when a word processing function is enabled; this feature helps you with spacing and formatting professional documents. Every ¶ (paragraph mark) you see indicates that the ENTER key on the keyboard has been pressed.

Style II: Right-Tab Style

Headings are placed vertically as in Style I, except that the longest line (subject) is keyed flush with the left margin, whereas the last letters of the heading titles are aligned at the right. To accomplish this, set a right tab on the

Dr. Plunkett's Office
278 O'Connor Street
Ottawa, ON K2P 1V4
Phone: 613-212-1212
Fax 613-212-2121
www.drplunkettsoffice.com

TO: Jane Smith, RN; Dawn Clark, NP; David Yang, ND; Andrea Borne, CHDS

FROM: Dr. Plunkett

DATE: April 20, 20XX

SUBJECT: Vacation Requests

As you all know, summer vacation requests are due by May 1, 20XX. This is a reminder to start your planning process and submit your requests by the deadline provided.

Once I have everyone's requests, I will do my best to grant the preferred vacation time to each of you. Obviously, we cannot all be out of the office at the same time, but we will work as a team to find the best solution for ourselves and our patients.

As outlined in your contracts, no more than seven consecutive vacation days can be granted for the period of June 15 to August 15 of any employment year. Please adhere to this policy unless you have special circumstances that need to be considered. If you do have a special request based on personal circumstances, please book a time to meet with me before May 1.

As always, I appreciate your daily efforts and look forward to everyone enjoying some much-deserved time off with their family and friends.

lp

• **Fig. 6.2** A, Memo Style I: Full-Block Style.

Dr. Plunkett's Office
278 O'Connor Street
Ottawa, ON K2P 1V4
Phone: 613-212-1212
Fax 613-212-2121
www.drplunkettsoffice.com

TO: Jane Smith, RN; Dawn Clark, NP; David Yang, ND; Andrea Borne, CHDS

FROM: Dr. Plunkett

DATE: April 20, 20XX

SUBJECT: Vacation Requests

As you all know, summer vacation requests are due by May 1, 20XX. This is a reminder to start your planning process and submit your requests by the deadline provided.

Once I have everyone's requests, I will do my best to grant the preferred vacation time to each of you. Obviously, we cannot all be out of the office at the same time, but we will work as a team to find the best solution for ourselves and our patients.

As outlined in your contracts, no more than seven consecutive vacation days can be granted for the period of June 15 to August 15 of any employment year. Please adhere to this policy unless you have special circumstances that need to be considered. If you do have a special request based on personal circumstances, please book a time to meet with me before May 1.

As always, I appreciate your daily efforts and look forward to everyone enjoying some much-deserved time off with their family and friends.

lp

• **Fig. 6.2, cont'd** B, Memo Style I: Full-Block Style with Formatting Marks.

horizontal ruler that aligns with the colon after the word *Subject*. The body is single-spaced with the first line of each paragraph indented by hitting the TAB key on the keyboard one time (indicated by the nonprinting character of an arrow) or using the first-line indent function on your horizontal ruler.

Fig. 6.3A and Fig. 6.3B show Right-Tab Style memos with and without nonprinting formatting marks.

Style III: Adjacent-Headings Style

"To" and "Subject" are placed flush with the left margin; "From" and "Date" begin at the centre point (3.25 inches on the horizontal ruler), adjacent to the other headings. This style is a bit more difficult to format because it requires you to set multiple tabs on the same line to achieve symmetry. To accomplish this, you must use the tab dialogue box (see Fig. 6.4) in your word processor to set three different tabs on each of the two lines. Depending on your font choice, left tabs at 1.0, 3.25, and 4.25 should work well. Because this format lessens the room required for headings, you may need to add extra spaces after the headings to balance the memo and make it more visually attractive. If there is a long list of recipients, this style does not work well because there is not enough room to add many names. This memo style is single-spaced, but it can be double-spaced if the memo is short and more spacing would enhance the appearance. Paragraphs would then be indented by hitting the TAB key on your keyboard one time or by using the first- line indent function on your horizontal ruler. Fig. 6.5A and Fig. 6.5B show Adjacent-Headings style memos.

Letters and Envelopes

We will now review letter styles, spacing, punctuation styles, two-page letters, parts of a business letter, and envelopes. The material presented will allow you to observe how medical correspondence is composed in the medical office environment and how medical terminology is applied to communication documents.

Inappropriate format, misspelled words, and improper use of grammar will reflect on your office. Your professional standards as well as those of your physician's office may be judged by the quality of correspondence that you distribute. Be sure to proofread all correspondence before it is sent out. Do not depend on your computer's spell-check function for accuracy.

Letter Styles

Several styles of letters have been used over the years. At one time, the very formal indented style was used extensively. Since the advent of the computer, letter styles have become more simplified, and the indention of paragraphs is seldom used. It is good practice for offices to choose one style, font type, font size, and spacing option and to have all administrative staff use this style consistently.

Full-Block Style

Also called "block" style, this is the easiest style to remember and format; it is the most commonly used format. All lines begin at the left margin. Fig. 6.6A is an example of the block format; Fig. 6.6B shows a letter with formatting marks—spacing guidelines are discussed below.

Modified Block Style

The modified block style is still popular, but it is more difficult to format properly. You need to be very comfortable with using the horizontal ruler and setting tabs in your word processor if you choose to use this format. The body, inside address, and salutation of the letter are identical to those of the full-block style. However, the date line, complimentary closing, writer's name, and writer's title all begin at the centre of the page (3.25 inches on the horizontal ruler when using 1-inch margins). See Fig. 6.7A and B for Modified Block samples, with and without the nonprinting formatting marks.

Modified Block Style with Indented Paragraphs

This style is the same as modified block, but the first line of each paragraph is indented by hitting the TAB key on the keyboard one time. This style has become less common since modern word processing technologies have made the introduction of new paragraphs more obvious with better line spacing options. Fig. 6.8A and B provide examples of modified block letters with indented paragraphs, both with and without formatting marks.

Spacing

A letter properly arranged on the page should, as much as possible, resemble a picture in a frame. This effect is achieved by using proper line lengths and correct spacing between parts of the letter. Overall, spacing should be consistent throughout all letters, unless you are trying to prevent one or two single lines from moving to a second page. In this case, you would first take one to two lines away between the date and the inside address. If you still need a bit of space, remove one space in the signature block (between the complimentary closing and the signature line), provided the writer still has room to sign his or her name. If you are still looking for space, it is likely you should create a two-page letter to accommodate all the letter requirements.

The letterhead usually occupies the first 10 to 12 lines after the 1-inch top page margin (if you turn on your vertical ruler, you can see that the page margin is the shaded area on the ruler). Depending on the length of the letter, you may prefer to begin the date on the fourteenth or fifteenth line (ENTER two to three times after the letterhead). As mentioned above, you can adjust your spacing between the date and inside address according to the length of the letter.

At the end of the last line of your inside address, hit ENTER two times (double-space); this leaves one empty single line space between the inside address and the salutation. Please note the format of the inside address on the sample letters—this format follows current Canada Post

Dr. Plunkett's Office
278 O'Connor Street
Ottawa, ON K2P 1V4
Phone: 613-212-1212
Fax 613-212-2121
www.drplunkettsoffice.com

TO: Jane Smith, RN; Dawn Clark, NP; David Yang, ND; Andrea Borne, CHDS

FROM: Dr. Plunkett

DATE: April 20, 20XX

SUBJECT: Vacation Requests

As you all know, summer vacation requests are due by May 1, 20XX. This is a reminder to start your planning process and submit your requests by the deadline provided.

Once I have everyone's requests, I will do my best to grant the preferred vacation time to each of you. Obviously, we cannot all be out of the office at the same time, but we will work as a team to find the best solution for ourselves and our patients.

As outlined in your contracts, no more than seven consecutive vacation days can be granted for the period of June 15 to August 15 of any employment year. Please adhere to this policy unless you have special circumstances that need to be considered. If you do have a special request based on personal circumstances, please book a time to meet with me before May 1.

As always, I appreciate your daily efforts and look forward to everyone enjoying some much-deserved time off with their family and friends.

lp

• **Fig. 6.3** A, Memo Style II: Right-Tab Style.

Dr. Plunkett's Office¶
278 O'Connor Street¶
Ottawa, ON K2P 1V4¶
Phone: 613-212-1212¶
Fax 613-212-2121¶
www.drplunkettsoffice.com¶

¶

¶
¶
¶

→ **TO:** → Jane Smith, RN; Dawn Clark, NP; David Yang, ND; Andrea Borne, CHDS¶
¶
→ **FROM:** → Dr. Plunkett¶
¶
→ **DATE:** → April 20, 20XX¶
¶
SUBJECT: → Vacation Requests¶
¶
¶

→ As you all know, summer vacation requests are due by May 1, 20XX. This is a reminder to start your planning process and submit your requests by the deadline provided. ¶
¶

→ Once I have everyone's requests, I will do my best to grant the preferred vacation time to each of you. Obviously, we cannot all be out of the office at the same time, but we will work as a team to find the best solution for ourselves and our patients. ¶
¶

→ As outlined in your contracts, no more than seven consecutive vacation days can be granted for the period of June 15 to August 15 of any employment year. Please adhere to this policy unless you have special circumstances that need to be considered. If you do have a special request based on personal circumstances, please book a time to meet with me before May 1. ¶
¶

→ As always, I appreciate your daily efforts and look forward to everyone enjoying some much-deserved time off with their family and friends. ¶
¶
lp¶

• **Fig. 6.3, cont'd** B, Memo Style II: Right-Tab Style with Formatting Marks.

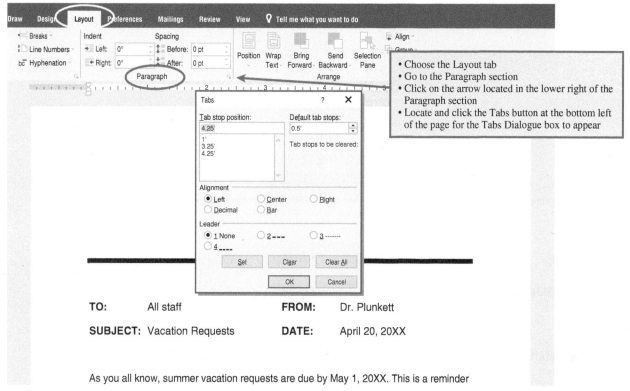

• **Fig. 6.4** Tab Dialogue Box.

guidelines. In particular, two-letter provincial codes are to be used rather than the full name of the province; the six-character alphanumeric postal code stays on the same line as the city and province (place two to three spaces between the two-letter provincial code and the postal code; place one space between the first three characters and last three characters of the postal code). Write out the words *road, street, avenue,* etc.; do not use their abbreviated forms. See Box 6.4 for Canada's two-letter provincial codes.

DID YOU KNOW?

The first three characters of a postal code are known as the *forward sortation area (FSA),* and the last three characters are called the *local delivery unit (LDU)* (Canada Post, 2018a).

Spacing between the inside address, the salutation, the body of the letter (and between paragraphs within the body of the letter), and the complimentary closing is the same—there is one single line space between all of these elements.

The space between the complimentary closing and the writer's name and title is three blank lines—this means you hit ENTER four times, beginning at the end of the complimentary closing, before you begin typing the signature line. This gives the writer enough room to sign the document.

The spacing between the signature block (writer's name and title) and all of the remaining letter elements is one single line space. Review the letter style figures that include formatting marks for a visual representation of the spacing explanations.

Punctuation Styles

Punctuation styles relate only to the salutation and complimentary closing areas of letters. All other punctuation within letters should follow standard grammar and punctuation rules. The two accepted styles of punctuation are open punctuation and mixed punctuation. It is acceptable to use either style of punctuation with any style of letter.

Open Punctuation

Open punctuation means that there are no punctuation marks following the salutation (Dear Dr. Plunkett) or the complimentary closing (Sincerely) of the letter. The full-block letters in Fig. 6.6A and B show the open punctuation style.

Mixed Punctuation

Mixed punctuation style means that punctuation is used following the salutation and the complimentary closing. A colon is placed after the salutation, and a comma is placed after the complimentary closing. The modified block letters in Fig. 6.8A and B show the mixed punctuation style.

Two-Page Letters

When producing letters with more than one page, place the name of the recipient, the page number, and the date at the top of the second and succeeding pages. Left-align and single-space the information. If referring to a patient, add the patient's name and a unique identifier, such as the

Dr. Plunkett's Office
278 O'Connor Street
Ottawa, ON K2P 1V4
Phone: 613-212-1212
Fax 613-212-2121
www.drplunkettsoffice.com

TO:	All staff	**FROM:**	Dr. Plunkett
SUBJECT:	Vacation Requests	**DATE:**	April 20, 20XX

As you all know, summer vacation requests are due by May 1, 20XX. This is a reminder to start your planning process and submit your requests by the deadline provided.

Once I have everyone's requests, I will do my best to grant the preferred vacation time to each of you. Obviously, we cannot all be out of the office at the same time, but we will work as a team to find the best solution for ourselves and our patients.

As outlined in your contracts, no more than seven consecutive vacation days can be granted for the period of June 15 to August 15 of any employment year. Please adhere to this policy unless you have special circumstances that need to be considered. If you do have a special request based on personal circumstances, please book a time to meet with me before May 1.

As always, I appreciate your daily efforts and look forward to everyone enjoying some much-deserved time off with their family and friends.

lp

• **Fig. 6.5** A, Memo Style III: Adjacent-Tabs Style.

Dr. Plunkett's Office¶
278 O'Connor Street¶
Ottawa, ON K2P 1V4¶
Phone: 613-212-1212¶
Fax 613-212-2121¶
www.drplunkettsoffice.com¶
¶

¶
¶
¶
TO: → All staff   → FROM: → Dr. Plunkett¶
¶
SUBJECT: → Vacation Requests → DATE: → April 20, 20XX¶
¶
¶
As you all know, summer vacation requests are due by May 1, 20XX. This is a reminder to start your planning process and submit your requests by the deadline provided. ¶
¶
Once I have everyone's requests, I will do my best to grant the preferred vacation time to each of you. Obviously, we cannot all be out of the office at the same time, but we will work as a team to find the best solution for ourselves and our patients. ¶
¶
As outlined in your contracts, no more than seven consecutive vacation days can be granted for the period of June 15 to August 15 of any employment year. Please adhere to this policy unless you have special circumstances that need to be considered. If you do have a special request based on personal circumstances, please book a time to meet with me before May 1. ¶
¶
As always, I appreciate your daily efforts and look forward to everyone enjoying some much-deserved time off with their family and friends. ¶
¶
lp¶

• **Fig. 6.5, cont'd** B, Memo Style III: Adjacent-Tabs Style with Formatting Marks.

Office of the Chief Medical Officer
2339 Ogilvie Road
Gloucester, ON K1J 8M8
Phone: 613-745-9993
Fax 613-745-9994
www.chiefmedofficer.com

July 31, 20XX

Dr. J.E. Plunkett
278 O'Connor Street
Ottawa, ON K2P 1V4

Dear Dr. Plunkett

It has been brought to my attention by the World Health Organization (WHO) that many cases of latent syphilis are becoming evident in persons who have been treated for gonorrhea.

As you know, treatment for gonorrhea can temporarily mask syphilis but not control it.

We are being asked to ensure that blood be taken for possible syphilis being present concurrently with gonorrhea. By doing syphilis serology when patients are suspected of having gonorrhea, adequate dosages of antibiotics can be administered to control both diseases. This will prevent the later complications of syphilis, including neurosyphilis. It will also prevent the spread of syphilis which is increasing each year.

Your cooperation will be of great assistance. Should you have any questions, please contact my office. I have also enclosed the WHO's latest statistics on this topic for your review and consideration.

Regards

Dr. Peter Lafitte

P.K. Lafitte, MD, FRCP(S)C

jd

Enclosure

• **Fig. 6.6** A, Full-Block Letter with Open Punctuation.

Office of the Chief Medical Officer¶
2339 Ogilvie Road¶
Gloucester, ON K1J 8M8¶
Phone: 613-745-9993¶
Fax 613-745-9994¶
www.chiefmedofficer.com¶
¶

¶
¶
July 31, 20XX¶
¶
¶
¶
Dr. J.E. Plunkett¶
278 O'Connor Street¶
Ottawa, ON K2P 1V4¶
¶
Dear Dr. Plunkett¶
¶
It has been brought to my attention by the World Health Organization (WHO) that many cases of latent syphilis are becoming evident in persons who have been treated for gonorrhea. ¶
¶
As you know, treatment for gonorrhea can temporarily mask syphilis but not control it. ¶
¶
We are being asked to ensure that blood be taken for possible syphilis being present concurrently with gonorrhea. By doing syphilis serology when patients are suspected of having gonorrhea, adequate dosages of antibiotics can be administered to control both diseases. This will prevent the later complications of syphilis, including neurosyphilis. It will also prevent the spread of syphilis which is increasing each year. ¶
¶
Your cooperation will be of great assistance. Should you have any questions, please contact my office. I have also enclosed the WHO's latest statistics on this topic for your review and consideration.¶
¶
Regards¶
¶
Dr. Peter Lafitte¶
¶
P.K. Lafitte, MD, FRCP(S)C¶
¶
jd¶
¶
Enclosure ¶

• **Fig. 6.6, cont'd** B, Full-Block Letter with Open Punctuation and Formatting Marks.

Office of the Chief Medical Officer
2339 Ogilvie Road
Gloucester, ON K1J 8M8
Phone: 613-745-9993
Fax 613-745-9994
www.chiefmedofficer.com

July 31, 20XX

Dr. J.E. Plunkett
278 O'Connor Street
Ottawa, ON K2P 1V4

Dear Dr. Plunkett:

It has been brought to my attention by the World Health Organization (WHO) that many cases of latent syphilis are becoming evident in persons who have been treated for gonorrhea. As you know, treatment for gonorrhea can temporarily mask syphilis but not control it.

We are being asked to ensure that blood be taken for possible syphilis being present concurrently with gonorrhea. By doing syphilis serology when patients are suspected of having gonorrhea, adequate dosages of antibiotics can be administered to control both diseases. This will prevent the later complications of syphilis, including neurosyphilis. It will also prevent the spread of syphilis which is increasing each year.

Your cooperation will be of great assistance. Should you have any questions, please contact my office. I have also enclosed the WHO's latest statistics on this topic for your review and consideration.

Regards,

Dr. Peter Lafitte

P.K. Lafitte, MD, FRCP(S)C

jd

Enclosure

• **Fig. 6.7** A, Modified Block Letter with Mixed Punctuation.

Office of the Chief Medical Officer¶
2339 Ogilvie Road¶
Gloucester, ON K1J 8M8¶
Phone: 613-745-9993¶
Fax 613-745-9994¶
www.chiefmedofficer.com¶
¶
¶
¶
July 31, 20XX¶
¶
¶
¶
Dr. J.E. Plunkett¶
278 O'Connor Street¶
Ottawa, ON K2P 1V4¶
¶
Dear Dr. Plunkett:¶
¶
It has been brought to my attention by the World Health Organization (WHO) that many cases of latent syphilis are becoming evident in persons who have been treated for gonorrhea. As you know, treatment for gonorrhea can temporarily mask syphilis but not control it. ¶
¶
We are being asked to ensure that blood be taken for possible syphilis being present concurrently with gonorrhea. By doing syphilis serology when patients are suspected of having gonorrhea, adequate dosages of antibiotics can be administered to control both diseases. This will prevent the later complications of syphilis, including neurosyphilis. It will also prevent the spread of syphilis which is increasing each year. ¶
¶
Your cooperation will be of great assistance. Should you have any questions, please contact my office. I have also enclosed the WHO's latest statistics on this topic for your review and consideration.¶
¶
Regards,¶
¶
Dr. Peter Lafitte¶
¶
P.K. Lafitte, MD, FRCP(S)C¶
¶
jd¶
¶
Enclosure ¶

• **Fig. 6.7, cont'd** B, Modified Block Letter with Mixed Punctuation with Formatting Marks.

Office of the Chief Medical Officer
2339 Ogilvie Road
Gloucester, ON K1J 8M8
Phone: 613-745-9993
Fax 613-745-9994
www.chiefmedofficer.com

July 31, 20XX

Dr. J.E. Plunkett
278 O'Connor Street
Ottawa, ON K2P 1V4

Dear Dr. Plunkett:

   It has been brought to my attention by the World Health Organization (WHO) that many cases of latent syphilis are becoming evident in persons who have been treated for gonorrhea. As you know, treatment for gonorrhea can temporarily mask syphilis but not control it.

   We are being asked to ensure that blood be taken for possible syphilis being present concurrently with gonorrhea. By doing syphilis serology when patients are suspected of having gonorrhea, adequate dosages of antibiotics can be administered to control both diseases. This will prevent the later complications of syphilis, including neurosyphilis. It will also prevent the spread of syphilis which is increasing each year.

   Your cooperation will be of great assistance. Should you have any questions, please contact my office. I have also enclosed the WHO's latest statistics on this topic for your review and consideration.

                                        Regards,

                                        Dr. Peter Lafitte

                                        P.K. Lafitte, MD, FRCP(S)C

jd

Enclosure

• **Fig. 6.8** A, Modified Block with Indented Paragraphs, Mixed Punctuation, and Formatting Marks.

Office of the Chief Medical Officer¶
2339 Ogilvie Road¶
Gloucester, ON K1J 8M8¶
Phone: 613-745-9993¶
Fax 613-745-9994¶
www.chiefmedofficer.com¶
¶

¶
¶
→   July 31, 20XX¶
¶
¶
¶
Dr. J.E. Plunkett¶
278 O'Connor Street¶
Ottawa, ON K2P 1V4¶
¶
Dear Dr. Plunkett:¶
¶

→ It has been brought to my attention by the World Health Organization (WHO) that many cases of latent syphilis are becoming evident in persons who have been treated for gonorrhea. As you know, treatment for gonorrhea can temporarily mask syphilis but not control it. ¶
¶

→ We are being asked to ensure that blood be taken for possible syphilis being present concurrently with gonorrhea. By doing syphilis serology when patients are suspected of having gonorrhea, adequate dosages of antibiotics can be administered to control both diseases. This will prevent the later complications of syphilis, including neurosyphilis. It will also prevent the spread of syphilis which is increasing each year. ¶
¶

→ Your cooperation will be of great assistance. Should you have any questions, please contact my office. I have also enclosed the WHO's latest statistics on this topic for your review and consideration.¶
¶
→   Regards,¶
¶
→   *Dr. Peter Lafitte*#
¶
→   P.K. Lafitte, MD, FRCP(S)C¶
¶
jd¶
¶
Enclosure ¶

• **Fig. 6.8, cont'd** B, Modified Block with Indented Paragraphs and Formatting Marks.

Alberta (AB)
British Columbia (BC)
Manitoba (MB)
New Brunswick (NB)
Northwest Territories (NT)
Nova Scotia (NS)
Nunavut (NU)
Ontario (ON)
Prince Edward Island (PE)
Quebec (QC)
Saskatchewan (SK)
Yukon (YT)

medical record number (MRN). Precede the patient's name or unique identifier with RE: or SUBJECT:. These can be typed in all capitals or with an initial capital only; they should always be followed by a colon and one to two spaces before typing the patient's name or unique identifier. If using both the patient's name and a unique identifier, place a comma between the two pieces of information. When you are producing a medical note (Consultation; History and Physical), include the type of note on the second and any succeeding pages under the patient name. Add two to three empty line spaces after the second-page header and the body of the letter. Fig. 6.9 shows a two-page full-block letter with mixed punctuation for your review.

Parts of a Business Letter

Letterhead
The essential parts of the letterhead are the name and address of the office; it should also include the telephone number, fax number, email address, and any available web addresses. Some offices create their own letterhead and use the electronic template for correspondence; however, many offices use good-quality bond paper on which the letterhead is preprinted. Medical offices usually use ordinary bond paper for their correspondence (this is physician preference), with the letterhead on only the first page. Many companies have preprinted second-page stationery with only the firm's name printed on it.

Date Line
The date generally is placed three or four lines below the letterhead and includes the month, day, and year. You should type the month in long form—do not abbreviate the month. Follow it with the numeric day followed by a comma and the four-digit year, for example, September 27, 20XX. There is no comma between the month and the day. Most computer programs can insert dates automatically when producing a letter; however, you will need to remember to check the font style and size to ensure that they match the rest of your letter.

Inside Address
This is placed two to four line spaces below the date, depending on the length of the letter. The inside address

consists of the recipient's name, title (if any), street address, city, province, and postal code. Be sure to apply the guidelines discussed previously.

Attention Line—Some letters are sent to the attention of a specific person in the organization. The attention line is double-spaced below the last line of the inside address and placed at the left margin. The position of the attention line is shown in Fig. 6.10. The attention line can be in regular or bold font and can be typed in all capitals or in initial-capital format. A colon and one to two spaces follow the notation.

DID YOU KNOW?

There are over 150 street types and 16 directions used in Canadian postal addresses. In addition to the standard "street" and "avenue," street types include the more unique "ramp," "manor," "wharf," and "dell" (Canada Post, 2018b).

Salutation
The salutation is double-spaced after the last line of the inside address or attention line, if used. When a letter is addressed to a company and contains an attention line, or both, the salutation is usually Gentlemen, Ladies and Gentlemen, or Dear Sir or Madam. When the letter is addressed to an individual, the salutation is Dear Dr. Plunkett, Dear Mr. Smith, Dear Ms. Jones, or Dear Jim.

Subject or Reference Line
Some writers identify the letter's subject in a reference line, which appears a double space below the salutation. The reference line is placed at the left margin (see Fig. 6.10). In the medical environment, letters contain the patient's name and date of birth, MRN, or other unique identifier in the reference line. A good rule of thumb when choosing between using a reference notation (RE:) or a subject notion (SUBJECT:) is to use RE: when relating to a number and SUBJECT when relating to a name. If using both a name and a number, feel free to choose between the two.

Body
The body of the letter begins a double space below the reference line (or below the salutation if there is no reference line). The body is generally single-spaced with a double space between paragraphs. The body of the letter should contain at least two paragraphs.

Complimentary Closing
The closing is placed two line spaces below the last line of the body of the letter. "Yours truly" and "Sincerely" are the most commonly used closings for business letters. Only the first word of the closing is capitalized.

Signature Block
The signature block contains the writer's name and title. A space (not less than three or more than five spaces) after the complimentary closing is left for the signature, and the writer's name is typed below this space. When including a longer title

Dr. Plunkett's Office
278 O'Connor Street
Ottawa, ON K2P 1V4
Phone: 613-212-1212
Fax 613-212-2121
www.drplunkettsoffice.com

November 15, 20XX.

Kenmare Insurance Company
327 Crown Drive
Ottawa, ON K1V 439

ATTENTION: Kenneth Mare

Dear Sir:

RE: Lois Elliott, Accident of February 9, 20XX.

Thank you for your letter of May 6, 20XX regarding Ms. Elliott. I first saw her in the Emergency Department at the Ottawa General Hospital (OGH) on February 9, 20XX at the request of Dr. Phelan. She was involved in a motor vehicle accident (MVA) with an injury involving the forehead. She also had multiple pieces of glass and other foreign bodies in the skin and subcutaneous tissues. She was taken to the operating room the same day, and the procedures of debridement, plastic reconstruction, and removal of the foreign bodies were undertaken.

She was kept in the hospital from February 9, 20XX to February 13, 20XX. During this period, she did well, with good recovery, along with good wound healing. She was reviewed in my office after discharge from the hospital—I saw her on February 20, 20XX. The sutures were removed at this time, and the wounds were healing well. Naturally, the scars were visible. She had a palpable, tender, painful foreign body in the form of a piece of glass in the forehead. We made arrangements to remove this piece of glass as an outpatient at the OGH on March 19, 20XX. She had follow-up appointments in my office on March 30 and June 15, 20XX. Her progress has been satisfactory.

Ms. Elliott was reviewed again in my office today, November 15, for the purpose of requesting this letter. She states she is having occasional headaches and dizziness. If these symptoms continue, we should seek a neurological consultation. With regard to her physical examination today, she has a scar that runs from the right side of her

---

Page 2
Kenmar Insurance Company
RE: Lois Elliott, MRN 123456789
November 15, 20XX

forehead toward the right side of her nose. The scar measures 7-8 cm and is markedly rough and irregular. The area is hyperemic and broken due to instability of the epithelium; I think this will epithelialize in time. She does not appear to have any numbness or tingling, indicating that the nerves of the forehead are intact and her injuries were superficial. Her skull and facial bones are intact and normal. The maxilla and mandible are also intact with good occlusion of the teeth.

In summary, this young lady was involved in an MVA, and the injuries were confined to her forehead. There were abrasions and lacerations that were treated and repaired; some foreign bodies were removed. She is left with a visible, irregular, rough scar on her forehead. She should be reassessed in six months' time.

Sincerely,

Dr. J.E. Plunkett

J.E. Plunkett, MD, FRCP(S)C

lp

Enclosures: History and Physical, February 9, 20XX
Operative Note, February 9, 20XX
Progress Notes (3), February 10, 11, and 12, 20XX
Discharge Summary, February 13, 20XX
Procedure Report, March 19, 20XX
Clinic Notes (3), February 20, March 30, June 15, 20XX

C   Lois Elliott, MRN 123456789

• **Fig. 6.9** Two-Page, Full-Block Letter with Mixed Punctuation and Formatting Marks

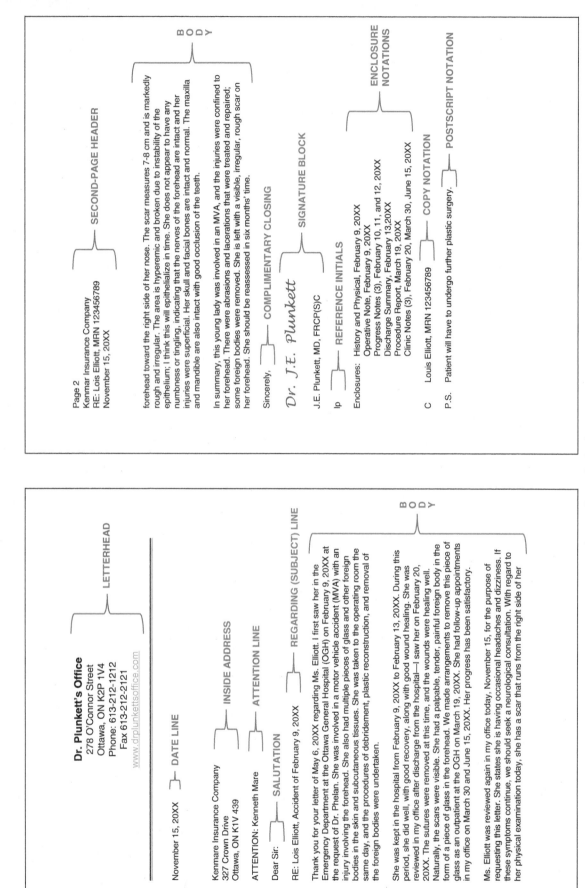

• **Fig. 6.10** Parts of a Business Letter

line, it should be typed on the line directly beneath the writer's name; in this case, no comma is added after the writer's name. For shorter titles, just as with professional designations, place the writer's name and title on the same line with a comma separating them. For instance, a doctor's name is usually followed by his or her degree (but not preceded by "Dr."); for example, "J.E. Plunkett, M.D., FRCP(S)C to match Fig. 6.10." In this example, periods are used with the uppercase abbreviation "M.D." It is noteworthy that, although traditional rules require periods with academic degrees (but not professional designations, such as FRCPC), it is becoming more common to drop the periods so that there is consistency within the signature line.

Reference Initials

Several styles are used to key reference initials. At one time, the writer's initials followed by the typist's initials was the preferred style. However, since the writer's name is already at the end of the letter, only the initials of the person typing or transcribing the letter are required. Initials are placed at the left margin, usually two spaces below the signature block, and do not require any punctuation or other special characters. As mentioned previously, the reference initials are lowercased. The initials help to identify the transcriptionist if any follow-up is needed.

Enclosures

If a document is enclosed with the letter, a reference to the enclosure is made one double space below the reference initials. If more than one document is enclosed, the number may appear after the word *enclosures*. There are many styles of enclosure notations; your office should decide on one to use so that your documents are consistent in appearance. Some styles of enclosure lines follow:

Enclosure
Encl.
Enc.
Enclosures (3)
Enclosure—Policy
Enclosures: Policy
       Operative Note
       Form 234

Copy Notations

If copies of a letter are being sent to people other than the addressee, a copy notation must be included. This ensures that all parties are aware of who will receive the letter. Copy notations are placed a double space below the last line of a letter, that is, below the producer's initials or the enclosure line. Copy notations can be typed with either an uppercase or lowercase "c" and are followed by a tab (0.5 inches on the horizontal ruler) before the recipient's name. See the copy notation in Fig. 6.10 for an example. The copy notation comes before the postscript.

Postscript (P.S.)

The postscript can be used to express an important afterthought. The postscript appears at the very end of the letter, a double space below the last keyed line. Since the advent of computerized word processing, the use of postscripts has become quite rare because the afterthought can easily be incorporated into the letter. However, they are sometimes still used to draw attention to an important fact. Fig. 6.10 shows the placement and format of a postscript.

Envelopes

The two sizes of envelopes most commonly used are No. 8 and No. 10. A No. 8 envelope measures approximately 16.5 cm × 9 cm (6.5 inches × 3⅝ inches), and a No. 10 envelope is approximately 24 cm × 10.5 cm (9.5 inches × 4⅛ inches).

The address on the envelope should duplicate the letter both in name and address and in punctuation style and format.

> ### DID YOU KNOW?
>
> In an address, only house number *one* should be spelled out; all other house numbers should be in Arabic numeral/figure form. For streets, spell out numbers *ten* and below and use figures (with ordinals when appropriate) for numbers above *ten*. For example, One Ninth Avenue, 12 North 27th Street, or 4-132 Green Parkway (place a hyphen between a house number and a civic or street address when both require figures).

Computer programs have a label function. Some programs can produce the labels to a preprogrammed label printer. Others will allow you to create the label-free text.

Most addresses are single-spaced. The address consists of the name of the recipient, the title (if any), street address or post office box number, city or town, and province. The postal code is keyed two to three spaces after the two-letter provincial code on the same line. Regardless of the style of punctuation used, there is no punctuation after the postal code. Nothing should be placed opposite, or in the space below, the postal code. Special mailing instructions, attention lines, and so on are usually placed two or three spaces below the return address (see Fig. 6.11).

When folding a letter for insertion into a No. 8 envelope, place the letter on the desk facing you and fold from bottom to top to within roughly 0.5 cm (1/4 inch); fold from the right one-third to the left, and fold from the left to within roughly 1 cm (0.5 inch) of the right edge. With the envelope opening facing you, insert the left creased edge first with the open side facing toward you.

When folding a letter for insertion in a No. 10 envelope, you may do as follows: with the letter on the desk facing you, fold from bottom to top one-third of the way and from top to bottom to within roughly 1 cm (0.5 inch) of the first creased edge. Insert the last creased edge toward the bottom of the envelope. Or, with the letter on the desk facing you, fold from bottom to top one-third of the way, turn the letter over, and fold the top edge down over the first crease approximately 1 cm (0.5 inch). Insert with the overlap to the top of the envelope. The second method of folding eliminates the risk of the recipient cutting the letter in two with a letter opener.

When folding a letter to fit a window envelope, bring the bottom third of the letter up and make a crease, then

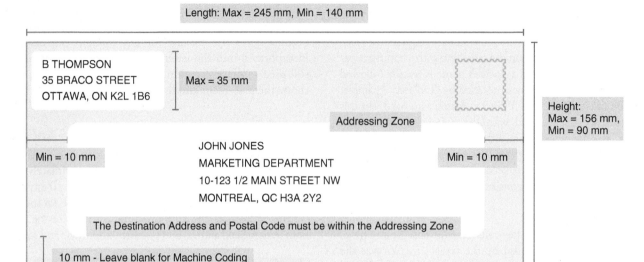

- **Fig. 6.11** Standard Envelope Setup (Source: Canada Post. (n.d.). *How to address mail properly.* Retrieved from https://www.canadapost.ca/web/en/kb/details.page?article=addressing_mail_accu&catt ype=kb&cat=addressing&subcat=accuracy)

fold the top of the letter back to the crease. The inside address should be facing you. Insert the correspondence. The inside address should appear in the window.

Remember to insert any required enclosures before sealing the envelope.

Summary

Although more and more documents are being shared electronically, medical offices continue to send and receive reports, correspondence, cheques, and supplies via mail and courier services. This chapter has offered advice on how to prioritize, organize, and prepare items that may travel via postal or courier service.

You have discovered a variety of memo and letter types, along with the specifics for proper formatting of these documents. All correspondence you create, edit, and format as a medical administrative assistant presents an image of your office, your abilities, and your commitment to administrative standards. You have been presented with tools to help ensure that your image is a professional and knowledgeable one.

Assignments

Assignment 6.1

This assignment is designed as a group project. Choose one of the delivery services—postal or courier—and prepare a report/presentation that outlines an aspect or aspects of the service as assigned by your instructor. You will contact or visit a postal or courier service to discover the details for your assigned topic(s). You may request supplies (waybills, special packages, or other materials) to enhance your presentation and understanding. Prepare a summary of the service(s), including points such as the name of the service, how it is provided, where the service extends (intercity/country to country), the cost(s) of the service(s), preparations necessary before using the service, and so on. Prepare the information in the manner or format outlined by your instructor, and be prepared to share your information with the class.

Assignment 6.2

Complete an Internet search for the topic of EHRs in your province. Write a short summary about the advantages of using EHRs to communicate health information electronically.

Assignment 6.3

Compose a memo using the following information. Once you have determined the specific content, use the information to produce three memos using each of the three different styles mentioned previously. Check for correct spelling, spacing, tabs, indents, and paragraphing. Use the memo samples provided as a guide.

Dr. Plunkett has asked you to send a memo to the Ottawa Hospital Board of Directors informing them that the annual board dinner meeting will be on December 1, 20__, at the Holiday Inn in the Wilfrid Laurier Room. Dinner will be served at 6 p.m.; the meeting is at 8 p.m. Members are asked to be prepared to present their annual reports.

Assignment 6.4

Produce the following letters on appropriate letterhead. For Letter 1 use block style, open punctuation; for Letter 2 use modified block style, mixed punctuation; and for Letter 3 use block style with mixed punctuation.

Letter 1

From Doctor Pelham to Dr. H.A. Schmidt, 33 Block Avenue, Ottawa, Ontario, J5Z 3Y7. Reference Mrs. Lisa Basciano. Mrs. Basciano whom we thought had an acute carpal tunnel syndrome on the right wrist was reviewed in my office today. I presume you have the E.M.G. report with you and those indicate normal tracing with no evidence of any compression of the median nerve at the wrist. Also, clinically today, when I examined her, she seems to have normal sensation but with the occasional pain and tenderness whenever she lifts heavy objects. I think she should be left alone and periodically reviewed.

Letter 2

From Doctor Plunkett to Dr. R.J. Mahon, Bell Clinic, 377 Unger Street, Ottawa, Ontario, J5Z 5X8. Subject Peter J. Scott. Thank you for referring me to see Peter John who certainly has a lesion on his upper lip, as well as a possible intradermal nevus on the temporal areas. I will be making arrangements for the removal of this under local anaesthesia (Loc. or L/A) as an outpatient at the O.G.H. I am enclosing a reference report on this patient.

Letter 3

From Doctor Pelham to Heavenly Haven Home for the Aged, R.R. 3, Kars, Ontario A7W 5S3. Attention: Mr. R.J. Seymour, Administrator. Re: Mr. Mel Thompson. Mr. Thompson was reviewed in my office today, regarding his persistence of having an operative procedure of blepharoplasty done on his lower eyelids. I certainly appreciate the bagginess of his bilateral lower eyelids, and he tells me they are impairing his vision because they are dragging his lower eyelids down. Dr. Blenkan, medical consultant for MoH, did phone me that it has been approved in May 20__ and I could carry out the procedure of bilateral lower blepharoplasty with this approval. I will be making arrangements for him to be admitted to the Ottawa General Hospital and carry out the procedure of bilateral blepharoplasty and reconstruct the orbital septum.

Assignment 6.5

Dr. Plunkett has dictated the following letter (via a speech-recognition program) to Mr. Ronald Gilmour, 3279 Circle Square, Ottawa, J5X 7W4. Mr. Gilmour is about to be discharged from the hospital following a heart attack. Dr. Plunkett has asked you to review the format, proofread the letter (there are errors to correct), and send hard copies to Dr. Pelham and to Dr. E.S. Langan at the heart clinic. Once you have corrected the document (type a new one with your corrections), produce the required copies: one for Dr. Plunkett's office, one for Mr. Gilmour, and one for each of the doctors mentioned.

"Once you are discharge from the hospital, you should continue to ad aktivities according to the schedule I have give you. It would helpful tourself if you established realistic weekly goals of activity or other alternatives of lifestyle that are impotant for your heart's health. For example, make a contract with a family memer that you will loose one kilogram each weak for a month, or you will walk a set distance every day, reduce cigarette consumption by one cigarette perda until you stop. You may help someone else besides yourself. Continue with your activity program even after complete recovery. Whatever formactivity you choose, remember, it must be performed a minim of three times week to be of any benefit. You are well on the way to recovery and if you follow the instructions I have given you, a full recovery and resumption of normactivities is expected."

Topics for Discussion

1. You have mail that arrives in your office stamped "URGENT/CONFIDENTIAL." Your employer is at a conference and will not return to the office for a week. The letter looks important. What would you do?

2. The postal service in your area is running smoothly; however, you notice that the destination area of the package you need to mail is suspended (as indicated on Canada Post website) due to inclement weather. The package is not urgent. What is your best course of action? If you are not sure, who can you consult?

References

Canada Health Infoway. (2019). *Progress in Canada*. Retrieved from https://www.infoway-inforoute.ca/en/what-we-do/progress-in-canada.

Canada Post. (2018a). *Addressing guidelines*. Retrieved from https://www.canadapost.ca/tools/pg/manual/PGaddress-e.asp#1441964.

Canada Post. (2018b). *Addressing guidelines*. Retrieved from https://www.canadapost.ca/tools/pg/manual/PGaddress-e.asp#1441964.

Canada Post. (2018). *Postage stamps and meters*. Retrieved from https://www.canadapost.ca/web/en/products/details.page?article=postage_stamps_meter&ecid=murl07001130.

7

Health Insurance Plans

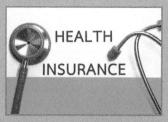

Source: © CanStock Photo Inc./everydayplus

The chapter provides an overview of Canadian health insurance plans. You will discover how patients register and become eligible for services offered by Canada's provincial and territorial plans. The privileges of our system, including the portability of insurance, are explored. You will learn how physicians register and become eligible to work within each government-sponsored plan. How physicians get reimbursed for the services they provide is discussed in detail; this includes how fees are established, where fees and regulations are outlined, and what information and processes are required for claim submission and payment.

Canadian provinces and territories also offer medical insurance coverage to injured workers through workers' compensation plans. You will examine these plans, along with third-party insurance options developed to assist Canadians in managing expenses not covered by Canada's publicly funded plans.

CHAPTER OUTLINE

Introduction

Eligibility

Registration

Insurance Premiums

Extended Health Insurance

Health Card

Reciprocal Medical Billing (RMB)

Travel Grants or Assistance

Visitors From Outside of the Province

Coverage Outside of Canada

Patients From Outside of Canada

Privacy and Confidentiality

Physicians' Fee Schedule

Physician Registration and Payment Options

Introduction to Claims Submission

Service Codes

Procedural Codes

Diagnostic Codes

Time Units

Premiums

Supporting Documentation

Methods of Submitting Claims

Claim Submission

Auditing Claims

Remittance Advice

Remittance Advice Inquiries

Appeals

Workers' Compensation

Making a Claim

Release of Workers' Compensation Information

Third-Party Insurance

How the Ministry of Health Communicates With Medical Administrative Assistants

LEARNING OBJECTIVES

After reading this chapter, you will be able to:

1. Describe provincial and territorial eligibility for a health care plan
2. Recognize the similarities of and differences between provinces and territories
3. Describe the format of the physician's fee schedule and the method for using the information it provides
4. Demonstrate knowledge of submitting health claims
5. Develop the ability to interpret remittance advice and understand the reprocessing of returned claims
6. Describe the implications of error codes
7. Describe physician responsibility, employee responsibility, employer responsibility, and medical administrative assistant's responsibility when processing a Workers' Compensation Board (WCB) claim
8. Describe the process for out-of-province claim submissions
9. Develop an awareness of grants or assistance that may be available for patients

KEY TERMS

Day sheet: A typed or generated list of the patients being seen in the office on a specific day. The medical administrative assistant provides the list to the physician to inform him or her of which patients are attending the office that day. It can also be used by the physician to record the service and the diagnostic and procedural codes related to each patient visit for billing purposes. It can be used as an alternative to encounter forms.

Diagnostic code: The diagnostic code identifies the reason the patient is seen by the provider. The code is usually three to four numeric or alpha-numeric characters. Most services require a diagnostic code when processing a health care claim.

Electronic claim submission: Method of submitting billings for health care services.

Encounter form: A form printed from electronic billing software that includes all the necessary information to bill a claim for medical services. Each individual patient form provides an area for the physician to write the service and the diagnostic and procedural codes for the patient encounter. A medical administrative assistant provides the physician with a form for each patient prior to the encounter (likely placed in the front of the chart) and collects each form for billing after the encounter. These forms can be used in place of a day sheet.

Independent consideration (IC): A service or fee code used by physicians when a service they wish to claim, or perform on behalf of a patient, is not in the physician's fee schedule. The service may be considered uninsured, but under special circumstances and with compelling documentation, the Ministry of Health (MoH) may grant the service. IC claims are normally submitted before a service is performed.

Insurable services: Services provided by physicians, and other health care providers, that are eligible for payment under the government-sponsored health insurance plan of each province and territory.

International Classification of Diseases (ICD): The World Health Organization's globally accepted system for the identification of health trends. "It is the diagnostic classification standard for all clinical and research purposes. ICD defines the universe of diseases, disorders, injuries and other related health conditions, listed in a comprehensive, hierarchical fashion" (World Health Organization, 2018, para. 1). ICD codes are updated regularly, and each version is assigned a sequential edition number. The most recent edition is ICD-11; however, the ICD-9 and ICD-10 versions are still in use.

Master agreement: This document is a collection of several related agreements that outline the obligations, compensations, rules, and regulations of physicians practicing medicine in their province or territory. It is the result of contractual negotiations between provincial and territorial branches of the Canadian Medical Association and ministries of health.

Physician registration number: The physician registration number is a unique number assigned to each physician by the MoH in the province in which they are practising. This number is also known as the *physician billing number.*

Preamble: An agreement that provides the rules and definitions necessary for the appropriate billing of insured services outlined in physicians' fee schedule. A general preamble may provide overarching advice for all physicians, whereas more specific preamble information may be provided for medical specialties when required.

Remittance advice: The remittance advice is an itemized statement of the individual payments made by the MoH for insured services.

Service codes: The service code identifies the service that was provided by the physician or health care provider to the patient. Service codes are found in the provincial fee schedule and must be submitted when processing a health care claim.

Shadow billing: A billing process by which physicians report each patient encounter even when a fee-for-service payment is not being sought.

Tariffs: A system of payment for health care services. It is the monetary value of services, or sets of services, as determined by standardized codes, rules, and regulations and as outlined in physicians' fee schedules.

Introduction

Health care can be expensive, and to minimize these expenses for its citizens, Canada has instituted a universal health care plan. Canada's health care plan includes several foundational elements consisting of accessibility, universality, portability, and comprehensiveness. Accessibility is designed to ensure that all insured persons have a reasonable expectation of health care services available. Universality involves the assurance that all insured individuals receive a comparable level of care from coast to coast. Portability provides for the relocation of a resident from one part of Canada to another with their home province or territory providing coverage until the waiting period for coverage in the new province or territory is effective. Comprehensiveness implies that all necessary medical services are covered under the plan. Additionally, all health care plans in Canada are publicly administered by a non-profit entity that is accountable to the province or territory in which the plan operates. This system of health care is funded primarily through taxation at the federal, provincial, and territorial levels; in some provinces, additional funding streams arise from payroll health care premiums leveraged to support and sustain the system.

This system originated through the enactment of the *Medical Care Act*, introduced by Prime Minister Lester B. Pearson during the 1966/67 session of Parliament. This Act was replaced by the *Canada Health Act* of 1984.

Each province and territory has its own government-sponsored plan, for example, Prince Edward Island's Health PEI, British Columbia's Medical Services Plan (MSP), the Alberta Health Care Insurance Plan (AHCIP), Ontario Health Insurance Plan (OHIP), and Yukon Health Care Insurance Plan (YHCIP).

Most features of each plan—eligibility and enrollment, out-of-province benefits, payment options, and the fact that the plan pays only for *medically necessary* services—closely resemble one another.

Complete information on claims processing, physician and subscriber registration, and eligibility can be obtained through your local Ministry of Health (MoH) office or through each province's or territorial government's website.

This chapter is designed to provide a Canada-wide perspective of health care plans. Topics include registration, health cards, billing plans, claim submission, physician fee schedules, service codes, service fees, and diagnostic codes.

Eligibility

As mentioned previously, eligibility for the health care plan of each province or territory is similar. The following is a listing of the basic provincial and territorial eligibility guidelines and their associated referential websites:

Alberta (AHCIP—Alberta Health Care Insurance Plan)

An applicant must meet the following criteria:
- Legally entitled to reside in Canada with a permanent home in Alberta
- Physically present in Alberta at least 183 days in a 12-month period
- Not claiming or obtaining residency benefits in another province or territory

If one is moving to Alberta from another province, territory, or country, there may be a waiting period before a newcomer is eligible for AHCIP. For more information, refer to https://www.alberta.ca/ahcip-apply.aspx. This card is required, along with photo identification, to access health care services in this province.

British Columbia (MSP—Medical Services Plan)

An applicant must be a resident of British Columbia (BC) and meet the following criteria:
- Be a citizen of Canada or be lawfully admitted to Canada for permanent residence, making BC their home

- Be physically present in BC at least six months in a calendar year or during a shorter prescribed period
- Eligible residents who are outside of BC for a vacation absence are permitted a total length of up to seven months in a year

Coverage may start three months after the arrival date in British Columbia. It is recommended that a newcomer purchase private insurance during the waiting period if coming from another province or territory, or from another country. For more information, refer to https://www2.gov.bc.ca/gov/content/health.

Manitoba (MHSAL—Manitoba Health, Seniors and Active Living)

An applicant is required to meet the following criteria:
- Be a Canadian citizen or have immigration status as outlined by the provincial health act
- Establish residency in Manitoba
- Physically reside in Manitoba for six months out of one calendar year

Coverage for newcomers who meet eligibility requirements will begin on the first day of the third month after arrival in Manitoba. It is recommended that during the wait period for health coverage, you maintain coverage with your previous health plan. For more information, refer to http://www.gov.mb.ca/health/mhsip/index.html.

New Brunswick (Medicare)

An applicant must meet the following criteria:
- Be a Canadian citizen or be legally entitled to reside in Canada and make a permanent home in New Brunswick
- Be an international student who meets the eligibility criteria

Coverage may begin on the first day of the third month when permanent residency is established in New Brunswick. For more information, refer to https://www2.gnb.ca/content/gnb/en/departments/health/MedicarePrescriptionDrugPlan.html.

Newfoundland and Labrador (MCP—Medical Care Plan)

An applicant must meet the following criteria:
- Be a resident of the province
- Be legally entitled to reside in Canada
- An applicant fits into four basic groups: Canadian citizen, permanent resident, international worker, and international post-secondary student

Coverage will normally be effective the first day of the third month following the date of arrival. For information, refer to http://www.health.gov.nl.ca.

Northwest Territories (NWT Health Care Plan)

An applicant must meet the following criteria:
- Be lawfully entitled to be or remain in Canada

- Make NWT their permanent residence. Be physically present in NWT a minimum of 153 days during each calendar year
- Be 19 years of age or older to apply

Coverage will begin on the first day of the third month immediately following the month you became a resident of the NWT. For more information, refer to https://www.hss.gov.nt.ca/en/services/nwt-health-care-plan.

Nova Scotia (MSI Medical Services Insurance)

An applicant must meet the following criteria:
- Be a Canadian citizen or permanent resident, formerly called a *landed immigrant*
- Be a resident who has his or her permanent home in Nova Scotia
- Be physically present in the province 183 days every calendar year

Coverage typically begins on the first day of the third month following the date of established residency. For more information, refer to https://novascotia.ca/DHW/msi.

Nunavut (NHCP Nunavut Health Care Program)

An applicant must meet the following criteria:
- Be a Canadian citizen or permanent resident of Nunavut, which is a person who has Nunavut as his or her primary place of residence
- Persons possessing employment or a student visa valid for one year or more. The visa is required to show a Nunavut address

Coverage begins when eligibility has been confirmed. For more information, refer to https://gov.nu.ca/health/information/nunavut-health-care-plan.

Ontario (OHIP—Ontario Health Insurance Plan)

An applicant must meet the following criteria:
- Be a Canadian citizen or a permanent resident
- Have applied for permanent residency
- Be in Ontario on a work permit and work at least six months for an employer
- Have a permanent home in Ontario and be physically in Ontario for 153 days in any 12-month period

Coverage can take up to three months to begin after approval. An applicant must be physically present in Ontario for at least 153 days of the first 183 days immediately after commencing living in Ontario. For more information, refer to https://www.ontario.ca/page/apply-ohip-and-get-health-card (see Fig. 7.1).

Prince Edward Island (Health PEI)

An applicant must meet the following criteria:
- Be in Canada legally

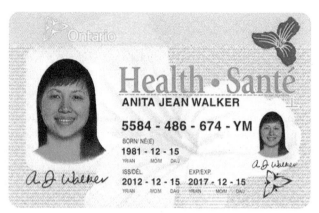

- **Fig. 7.1** Ontario Health Card. (Source: MHLTC, Claims Services Branch, Direct Services Division.)

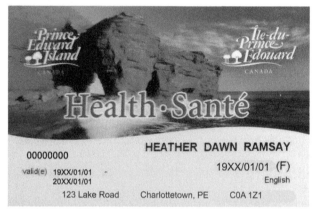

- **Fig. 7.2** Prince Edward Island Health Card. (Source: © 2019 Government of Prince Edward Island.)

- Have his or her permanent home in Prince Edward Island and be present for at least six months plus a day each year, or have received a waiver of this requirement from Health PEI

Coverage begins on the first day of the third month following arrival in PEI if eligibility requirements are met. For more information, refer to https://www.princeedwardisland.ca/en/information/health-pei. See Fig. 7.2.

Québec (Québec Health Insurance Plan, also known as *RAMQ Régie de l'assurance maladie du Québec*)

An applicant must meet the following criteria:
- Be a citizen of Canada
- Maintain permanent residency in Québec
- You must be present in Québec 183 days or more per calendar year.
- Other criteria may meet eligibility, and these could include refugee claimant, temporary seasonal worker, or international student

Coverage for the Québec Health Insurance Plan commences on the first day of the third month following the date you take up residence in Québec. For more information, refer to http://www.ramq.gouv.qc.ca/en/citizens/health-insurance/Pages/health-insurance.aspx.

Saskatchewan (Saskatchewan Health Services—e-Health Saskatchewan)

An applicant must meet the following criteria:
- Permanent residency in Saskatchewan
- Live in the province six months out of the year
- Register for benefits with e-health Saskatchewan

Coverage will commence on the first day of the third calendar month following the date you established residency in Saskatchewan. For more information, refer to https://www.ehealthsask.ca.

Yukon (YHCIP Yukon Health Care Insurance Plan)

An applicant must meet the following criteria:
- Be a Canadian citizen or have immigration status (permanent residency)
- Have a permanent home in Yukon
- Be physically present in Yukon and not absent for more than six months without a signed waiver.

Coverage typically is effective three months after the date residency is established in Yukon. For more information, refer to http://www.hss.gov.yk.ca/yhcip.php. There are two coloured cards, a green one and a blue one. The green card indicates senior benefits for those 65 years or older, or for a married person 60 years of age or older living with a resident who is 65 years of age or older.

The previously listed provincial and territorial websites link to their respective MoH, where the following additional information is outlined:
- Services that are not covered
- Coverage if travelling to another province
- Travelling outside of Canada
- Moving within Canada
- Instructions for registering for coverage
- Instructions for applying for a new card (i.e., name change, lost or stolen card, address change)

NOTE: It is the patient's, not the physician's, responsibility to report an address change to the MoH.

The following persons may be excluded from provincial or territorial health care coverage; their coverage is provided by a federal governing body:
- First Nations living on reserves
- Regular members of the Royal Canadian Mounted Police (RCMP) and the Canadian Armed Forces (however, their family members are eligible for provincial or territorial coverage)
- Federal public service employees
- Federal judges

Employees under designated agencies and corporations:
- Inmates of federal penitentiaries

Individuals *not* eligible for provincial or territorial coverage:

- Tourists and visitors to the province
- Transients (people who are not intending to remain permanently in the province or territory)
- Students from other provinces or on student visas (in some provinces, coverage is available)

DID YOU KNOW?

Estimated as of 2017, overall spending on health care in Canada totals approximately $6000 per citizen.

Registration

To receive health care coverage, an application must be completed and submitted to the provincial or territorial MoH. Some provinces and territories require an in-person initial application because original documents supporting identity are mandatory. Other provinces and territories provide an online application process whereby documents can be digitally uploaded. Application forms and instructions are available on each MoH website listed earlier in the chapter.

Newcomers to Canada

Newcomers to Canada may have to wait up to three months to receive health coverage through their provincial or territorial plan. It is recommended that a newcomer contact the local health ministry upon arrival, and they should investigate private insurance arrangements during the waiting period before government-sponsored insurance commences. In some instances, an individual may be a new Canadian resident who is classified as a protected person. This status is determined by the Immigration and Refugee Board of Canada (IRB). An example of a protected person could be a refugee or refugee claimant. A protected person may be able to apply for permanent residence with this status. Because most provincial and territorial plans require evidence of permanent residence status, health care coverage can be available temporarily through the Interim Federal Health Plan (IFHP) until the provincial or territorial health coverage is accepted. The IFHP provides basic coverage including inpatient and outpatient hospital services; physician services; and laboratory, diagnostic, and ambulance services. Additional supplemental coverages may also include vision and urgent dental care, home care and long-term care, assisted devices, and prescriptions.

Newborn Registration

Each MoH has requirements and a process for registering a newborn. British Columbia offers electronic birth registration through a secure communication network; in Nova Scotia, regional hospitals are equipped with electronic kiosks to register a baby's birth, and a health card is mailed within 10 days to the parent of the newborn. A newborn may be eligible for coverage, even if his or her parent(s) is deemed ineligible, if the infant was born in Canada and is a

TABLE 7.1 Primary Features of Provincial and Territorial Health Cards

Province/Territory	Health Number Format	Term/Expiry	Security
Alberta	9 characters (numeric)	Yes, if temporary resident	Must show photo ID with card
British Columbia	10 characters (numeric)	5 years	Magnetic stripe, bar code, and chip technology
Manitoba	9 characters (numeric)	No, list start date of coverage	No magnetic stripe
New Brunswick	9 characters (numeric)	5 years	Magnetic stripe
Newfoundland and Labrador	12 characters (numeric)	5 years	Bar code
Northwest Territories	1 alpha character followed by 7 numeric characters	3 years on birth date	No magnetic stripe
Nova Scotia	10 characters (numeric)	4 years	Numbers and letters are embossed and tipped with silver foil
Nunavut	9 characters (numeric)	5 years	Health superimposed in four languages
Ontario	10 characters (numeric) followed by 1 or 2 alpha characters representing a version code	5 years	Security background Magnetic stripe and microprint, bar code, photo and signature
Prince Edward Island	8 characters (numeric)	5 years	Magnetic stripe
Québec	4 alpha characters followed by 8 numeric characters (12 in all)	4 to 8 years	Bar code, photo, and signature
Saskatchewan	9 characters (numeric)	3 years (expiry sticker applied to card)	No magnetic stripe
Yukon	9 characters (numeric)	Renewal every year on birth date	No magnetic stripe

Canadian citizen. The parent would need to provide proof that he or she makes a permanent residence in Canada.

Adoption Registration

Newly adopted children will also need to be registered to secure a health card and access health services. As soon as a child physically joins a family, an application for coverage is a best practice. Adoptions that occur inside Canada will require a birth certificate and a notice of placement of the child with the family. Many adoptions involve a child arriving from outside of the country. In these cases, the adoptive authority will provide proof of the adoption through Immigration and Citizenship. An application for citizenship can commence as well as the application for health coverage. In some cases, the three-month waiting period for health care coverage required by the province or territory may be waived.

Insurance Premiums

British Columbia, Ontario, and Québec are the three provinces in Canada where residents pay health insurance premiums. These insurance premiums may be collected directly from individuals, employers, or through payroll deductions.

Health care in the remainder of Canada is funded through taxation revenue streams.

Extended Health Insurance

Government-sponsored health care plans cover basic medical needs. Extended health coverage can cover needs beyond the basic or a percentage of coverage. Some employers offer extended health coverage as an option or benefit of employment. Often both the employee and the employer contribute to these premiums. These benefits can include prescription medications, dental care, physiotherapy, and other allied health services.

DID YOU KNOW?

No one will be refused access to necessary health care due to non-payment of premiums.

Health Card

Each province provides eligible residents with a health card that displays their registration number. Some cards have an expiry date, security features, and photo requirements; in Ontario, a health card may display a version code along with the registration number (see Table 7.1, which displays the primary features for each provincial and territorial health card).

Reciprocal Medical Billing (RMB)

In accordance with interprovincial agreements, all provinces and territories (except Québec) have entered into an agreement to compensate for hospital and physician services needed by residents who require medical attention outside of their home province. This compensation is compatible with the provincial and territorial fees.

Under this agreement, inpatient hospital services are compensated at a rate established by the host province or territory. Outpatient hospital service claims are payable in accordance with rates established by the Interprovincial Health Insurance Agreements Coordinating Committee (IHIACC). The IHIACC was established in 1991 to manage matters arising from interprovincial billing for hospital and physician services.

Using the office's standard billing program, a physician submits a reciprocal medical billing directly to his or her local MoH using the patient's health card number. The physician is compensated in accordance with the rates provided by the physician's, not the patient's, home province or territory. When seeing a patient from Québec, the physician has a few options. He or she can invoice the patient directly according to the physician's MoH rates, provide the patient with a receipt to take back to Québec, and submit to the MoH an application for reimbursement; this is the option most physicians choose. Another option is to invoice the patient directly using the provincial or territorial medical association fee schedule, which typically differs from the MoH. A physician also can bill these patients directly using Québec fee codes and fees, providing a receipt and reimbursement form (see Fig. 7.3 Application for Reimbursement-Québec). Finally, a physician can opt to register with the MoH of Québec and receive a Québec billing number. Physicians who utilize this option usually are positioned close to the province of Québec.

A physician who practices inside of Québec and sees patients from outside of Québec can bill the MoH in the province where the patient is a resident; some provinces will pay according to the fee schedule of Québec, or the physician can bill the patient directly.

To be eligible to receive health care in a visiting province or territory, a patient must provide a valid health card from his or her home province or territory. As the medical administrative assistant accepting the card for service, be sure to examine the card for an expiry date to ensure that the health card presented is valid. Patients who have moved from another province or territory and who require medical treatment before their new province's coverage comes into effect are usually covered by their previous health plan.

When it comes to billing, all areas of the reciprocal claim are identical to those of the health claim, except for the additional information required (see Box 7.1).

Travel Grants or Assistance

Many Canadians must travel long distances to access appropriate health care. A patient will incur additional costs when travelling for health care. Each province or territory outlines a policy surrounding coverage available for residents who must travel to receive health care services not available within the community in which they reside. The specifics of travel grants vary by jurisdiction and are reflective of health services acquired both inside and outside the province or territory. The policy identifies allowances for travel, accommodations, and food. Proof of the need to travel for services is required, and advance approval is the typical protocol. Depending on the policy, partial reimbursement is provided for the cost; in some cases, however, no reimbursement is available. Additionally, maximum allowances are stipulated for associated costs.

The policy and application process detailing eligibility, criteria, and compensation are available through the provincial and territorial MoH web links (see Table 7.2 for the links).

Visitors From Outside of the Province

While working as a medical administrative assistant, you may encounter patients who are visitors from outside your province. As discussed earlier in this chapter, for Canadian residents (excluding Québec) you will complete a reciprocal medical billing claim (unless otherwise directed by the policy set out by your employer) and submit it to the MoH. If the patient does not have a health card with him or her, the patient pays at the time of service and is given an invoice to submit to his or her provincial MoH.

Coverage Outside of Canada

Health care costs outside of Canada may be considerably higher than what the MoH provides. The MoH also covers a limited amount of services outside of Canada. If receiving medically necessary services outside of Canada, reimbursement will be based on Canadian rates and currency. A patient will need to claim the costs for services through his or her local MoH. Written permission may be required to access health services for coverage purposes. It is advisable to arrange private insurance if travelling, working, or studying outside of Canada because many health services outside of Canada charge significantly more than the provincial ministry pays.

Patients From Outside of Canada

A visitor from another country may require medical attention. If he or she is staying with one of your patients, your physician may be asked to see the visitor. Out-of-country visitors are required to pay for the medical service at the time of the

Régie de
l'assurance maladie
Québec ✤✤

APPLICATION FOR REIMBURSEMENT

Before completing this form, read the reverse
side and refer to the information on our website
at **www.ramq.gouv.qc.ca**. Click on **Temporary
stays outside Québec** under Citizens.

FOR OFFICE USE

CHECK THE
APPROPRIATE BOX ▶

Healthcare services received:
☐ in Canada   ☐ outside Canada

APPLICANT'S IDENTITY

HEALTH INSURANCE NUMBER		LAST NAME	LAST NAME AT BIRTH (IF DIFFERENT FROM THE NAME ON THE HEALTH INSURANCE CARD)
LETTERS	NUMBERS	FIRST NAME	DATE OF BIRTH YEAR MONTH DAY SEX M ☐ F ☐

HOME ADDRESS (see over)
NO.   STREET   APT.   MUNICIPALITY

PROVINCE   POSTAL CODE   PHONE NUMBER AT HOME AREA CODE   PHONE NUMBER AT WORK AREA CODE

PERIODS OF TIME SPENT OUTSIDE QUÉBEC

Period during which you received healthcare services

Date of departure from Québec
Year   Month   Day

Date of return to Québec
☐ ACTUEL DATE   ☐ PLANNED DATE   Year   Month   Day

If you spent other periods of **more than 21 consecutive days** outside Québec during the calendar year (January 1 to December 31), please specify:

REASON FOR SPENDING TIME OUTSIDE QUÉBEC (CHECK ONE BOX ONLY)

☐ Vacation or seasonal absence

☐ Work ▶ Employer's name

☐ Studies ▶ Attach a written attestation from the educational institution showing the beginning and end dates of your courses, unless you have already done so.

☐ Receipt of healthcare not available in Québec ▶ Régie's authorization number

☐ Permanent move outside Québec   Date of move Year Month Day

☐ Other ▶ Specify

	1st PERIOD	
Date of departure		Date of return
Year Month Day		Year Month Day

	2nd PERIOD	
Date of departure		Date of return
Year Month Day		Year Month Day

	3rd PERIOD	
Date of departure		Date of return
Year Month Day		Year Month Day

HEALTHCARE SERVICES RECEIVED

Give the reason for which you received these healthcare services

IN THE CASE OF AN ACCIDENT, SPECIFY THE TYPE OF ACCIDENT
☐ Automobile   ☐ Work   ☐ Other (specify)

Date of accident
Year   Month   Day

Describe the services received (examinations, x-rays, surgery, etc.). If you need more space, use a separate sheet.

WHERE DID YOU RECEIVE THESE SERVICES?
MUNICIPALITY   CANADIAN PROVINCE OR U.S. STATE   COUNTRY

If applicable, indicate the number of days you were hospitalized:

REIMBURSEMENT

Amount claimed   ☐ Canadian dollars   ☐ Other currency   SPECIFY: ▶

Have you paid the bills?
☐ No   ☐ Yes   ☐ In full   ☐ In part

AMOUNT PAID (enclose originals of receipts) ▶

TRAVEL INSURANCE

Were you covered by travel insurance when you received the services?
☐ No   ☐ Yes ▶ NAME OF INSURANCE COMPANY   POLICY NUMBER

SIGNATURE AND AUTHORIZATION

☐ I hereby authorize the Régie de l'assurance maladie du Québec to provide to and receive from my travel insurance company all the information and documents required for the assessment and payment of my claims for insured medical and hospital services that I received and, if applicable, that my spouse or children received (family insurance).

☐ I hereby declare, knowing that this declaration has the same value as though it were made under oath in accordance with the *Canada Evidence Act*, that the above information is accurate. I authorize the Régie to request from the health professional or facility any additional information that it may require. If this information is not provided free of charge, I agree to it being obtained at my expense.

If my application results from an automobile accident or a work accident, I authorize the RAMQ to provide the SAAQ or the CNESST with a copy of any documents I may sent to or receive from the Régie.

NAME OF PERSON SIGNING THIS FORM, IF OTHER THAN THE APPLICANT   RELATIONSHIP TO APPLICANT (FATHER, MOTHER, SPOUSE, GUARDIAN ETC.)   SIGNATURE
X   YEAR   MONTH   DAY

1896 266 16/09

• **Fig. 7.3** Application for Reimbursement (RMB)–Québec. (Source: © Gouvernement du Québec, 2003. Retrieved from http://www.ramq.gouv.qc.ca/en/citizens/health-insurance/pages/health-insurance.aspx.)

APPLICATION FOR REIMBURSEMENT

You have **one year** from the date the services were provided to apply for a reimbursement for the cost of medical, dental or optometric services and **three years** for hospital services.

To apply, complete one form per person and indicate the person's Health Insurance Number.

In the case of a child under 12 months of age who has not yet received a Health Insurance Card, indicate the child's last name, first name, date of birth and sex, and enter the father's or mother's Health Insurance Number.

SUPPORTING DOCUMENTS

Please submit the **originals of your bills.**

The following must appear clearly:
- the name, address and signature of the health professional who rendered the services;
- the name and address of the facility where the services were provided, and signature of the authorized person;
- a detailed description of the services received;
- the date of and the fees for each service.

Send the **summary of your medical record** if you were hospitalized, and the **operative report** if you had major surgery.

You must provide **proofs of payment**, e.g. credit card receipts and photocopies of both sides of cashed **cheques**, indicating the name of the hospital or healthcare professional.

In addition, you must attach a French translation of the required documents if they are in a language other than French and English. If it considers it necessary, the Régie may request a certified translation at your expense.

Neither the originals nor photocopies of documents are returned by the Régie.

HOME ADDRESS

This form cannot be used to make a change of address. Please make any necessary changes using the Service québécois de changement d'adresse, available at **https://www.adresse.gouv.qc.ca**.

FOR FURTHER INFORMATION

Go to our website at:

www.ramq.gouv.qc.ca

You may also obtain information by calling:

in Québec
418 646-4636

in Montréal
514 864-3411

Elsewhere in Québec
1 800 561-9749

By mail
Régie de l'assurance maladie du Québec
Case postale 6600
Québec (Québec) G1K 7T3

Opening hours
Monday, Tuesday, Thursday and Friday: 8:30 a.m. to 4:30 p.m.
Wednesday: 10:00 a.m. to 4:30 p.m.

MAILING ADDRESS

Send the *Application for Reimbursement* and all required supporting documents (not stapled), to the following address:

Régie de l'assurance maladie du Québec
SAPHQAT
Case postale 6600
Québec (Québec) G1K 7T3

For more detailed information, visit our website.

Fig. 7.3, cont'd

• BOX 7.1 **Additional Information Required for Reciprocal Claims**

PROVINCE: AB (Alberta), MB (Manitoba), BC (British Columbia), NS (Nova Scotia), etc.
REGISTRATION NUMBER: Ranges from 6 to 12 digits in length
PAYMENT PROGRAM: For *all* reciprocal billing claims entered RMB in place of HCP
PAYEE: *Must* be the provider "P"
SEX: Enter "F" for female or "M" for male

TABLE 7.2 **Provincial and Territorial MoH Travel Policy Links**

Province/ Territory	Travel Policy Link
Alberta	http://www.humanservices.alberta.ca/ AWonline/AISH/7252.html#health
British Columbia	https://www2.gov.bc.ca/gov/content /health/accessing-health-care/tap-bc/travel-assistance-program-tap-bc
Manitoba	https://www.gov.mb.ca/health/mhsip/ travel.html
New Brunswick	https://www2.gnb.ca/content/gnb/e n/departments/health/MedicarePr escriptionDrugPlan/content/medic are/OutOfProvinceHostelFacilities-MealAllowance.html
Newfoundland and Labrador	https://www.health.gov.nl.ca/health/mc p/travelassistance.html
Northwest Territories	https://www.hss.gov.nt.ca/en/services/ medical-travel
Nova Scotia	https://novascotia.ca/dhw/Travel-and-Accommodation-Assistance/
Nunavut	https://gov.nu.ca/health/information/me dical-travel-nunavut-health-care-plan
Ontario	http://www.health.gov.on.ca/en/public/ publications/ohip/northern.aspx
Prince Edward Island	https://www.princeedwardisland.ca/ en/service/apply-online-for-out-of-province-travel-support
Québec	http://www.ramq.gouv.qc.ca/e n/citizens/temporary-stays-outside-quebec/health-insurance/Pages/services-covered.aspx
Saskatchewan	http://publications.gov.sk.ca /documents/13/104474-OOP%20Assessment-Treatment%2 0Program%20for%20Community%2 0Based%20Services.pdf
Yukon	http://www.hss.gov.yk.ca/yhcip-coverage.php

appointment. You will then provide an itemized statement that the patient can submit to his or her own health insurance for reimbursement upon return to the home country. Some out-of-country visitors will not have any health insurance at all.

When billing out-of-country patients, follow the same procedure as when billing for uninsured services, which is discussed in detail in this chapter.

Privacy and Confidentiality

Personal health information is among the most sensitive of personal information. Individuals are understandably protective about sharing medical conditions, yet information flow from one health practitioner to another is necessary to provide quality care. Each province and territory has its own privacy legislation and has a commissioner or ombudsperson responsible for overseeing provincial and territorial privacy legislation. The Office of the Privacy Commissioner of Canada provides detailed information and links to all provincial and territorial privacy laws, including personal health information acts, on its website. The privacy health laws protect how personal health information is collected, kept confidential, and disclosed. Patients are required to consent to the collection of this information.

A valid health card shows that the individual has the right to health care services in the province or territory where it was issued. No person, business, or organization may require someone to show his or her health card to get goods or non-health services. The health card number cannot be collected for credit checks, databanks, or identification. Individuals may choose to use their cards to prove their identity.

The MoH in each province and territory collects information for the following reasons:
- To be sure of eligibility for health coverage and drug benefits, or both
- To process payments for insured services
- To process payments for prescription drugs

The Canadian Medical Association (CMA) views protection of patient health information as a foundational principle of practice for physicians. The CMA addresses this in detail in CMA's Code of Ethics.

As a medical administrative assistant employed in a health care setting, you are a custodian of health information. You will be asking patients to present their health card for validation; it is your responsibility to safeguard the information provided to you. Employers may ask you to sign a confidentiality agreement certifying that you agree to protect this information. Facilities should keep an up-to-date log of authorized insiders—including employees, providers, and others—who have access to personal health information and information systems maintained in the facility.

DID YOU KNOW?

An EKOS Research Associates survey found that 90% of Canadians believe that health care should be the primary focus of national funding decision-making, ahead of the economy and environmental matters.
Source: The Conference Board of Canada

Physicians' Fee Schedule

Each province and territory in Canada is responsible for outlining its own system of payment for physician services. As a medical administrative assistant, you will require extensive knowledge of this standardized system of payment or tariff. The system includes the fees that are paid to physicians for specific sets of **insurable services**, the rules related to billing these services (preamble), codes related to each set of services, payment information in the form of coded statements (remittance advice), and the process to appeal decisions made about a payment. All these components are published together in an agreement, generally called the *physicians' fee schedule* or *provincial schedule*. The schedule may be presented as its own document or be included in a master agreement. Generally, it is divided into separate sections for the preamble, the definitions and guidelines related to services, the codes related to treatment locations or service sites, and the treatment or service codes (also called *fee codes*), along with their associated dollar amounts. Each medical specialty will also have its own section. Diagnostic codes are not included in the fee schedules.

Information in the schedule is the result of a negotiation process between the provincial or territorial MoH and the associated local branch of the CMA (see Box 2.3 of Chapter 2 for CMA branches). The local branch of the CMA represents and advocates for its physician members during this process, which also includes negotiations about benefits, hours of work, billing options, ancillary agreements, incentive programs, rate increases (calculated in the schedule), and other contractual obligations. Fee schedules are available to physicians and their staffs through their medical associations and the responsible MoH. Master Agreements are negotiated approximately every four years; however, updates to fees or fee codes may happen as often as quarterly in some cases. Any updates are provided to physicians and their billing software vendors as they become available. Downloadable versions of the schedules are available online for all provinces and territories, with the exception of Nunavut. See Box 7.2 listing the given names of the physicians' fee schedules for each province. See also Box 7.3, which provides the most current links to each schedule; however, these are subject to change.

Physician Registration and Payment Options

To bill for services provided to patients, all eligible physicians and physician groups must be registered with their provincial MoH. The Ministry assigns a unique physician registration number to the physician to be used when practising in that province. Generally, membership and licensure with the College of Physicians and Surgeons are required before a registration number will be provided. This number is also known as the *physician billing number*. A physician who moves to another province to practise medicine must apply

---

• BOX 7.2   Provincial and Territorial Physicians' Fee Schedules

Alberta	Schedule of Medical Benefits
British Columbia	Payment Schedule
Manitoba	Physician's Manual
New Brunswick	Physician's Manual
Newfoundland and Labrador	Medical Payment Schedule
Northwest Territories	Insured Services Tariff for Physician Services
Nova Scotia	Physician's Manual
Nunavut	(No manual; physicians are salaried)
Ontario	Schedule of Benefits
Prince Edward Island	Schedule of Payments
Québec	Manuel des Médecins— Rémunération à l'acte
Saskatchewan	Physician Payment Schedule
Yukon	Payment Schedule

• BOX 7.3   Links to Physicians' Fee Schedules

Alberta
   https://www.albertadoctors.org/services/physicians/compensation-billing/billing-help/somb#SOMB
British Columbia
   https://www2.gov.bc.ca/gov/content/health/practitioner-professional-resources/msp/physicians/payment-schedules/msc-payment-schedule
Manitoba
   https://www.gov.mb.ca/health/manual/
New Brunswick
   http://www2.gnb.ca/content/gnb/en/departments/health/healthprofessionals.html
Newfoundland and Labrador
   https://www.health.gov.nl.ca/health/mcp/providers/mcpmedpymt.html
Northwest Territories
   https://www.hss.gov.nt.ca/en/resources?search_api_views_fulltext=tariff&sort_by=field_resource_publication_date&sort_order=DESC&=Apply
Nova Scotia
   https://doctorsns.com/contract-and-support/physicians-manual
Ontario
   http://www.health.gov.on.ca/en/pro/programs/ohip/sob/
Prince Edward Island
   https://www.princeedwardisland.ca/en/publication/master-agreement
Québec
   http://www.ramq.gouv.qc.ca/fr/professionnels/Pages/professionnels.aspx
Saskatchewan
   http://www.sma.sk.ca/99/physician-payment-schedule.html
Yukon
   http://www.hss.gov.yk.ca/paymentschedule.php

• BOX 7.4 **Alternative Payment Options and Primary Characteristics**

Enhanced Fee-For-Service: Fee-for-service plus bonuses for complex cases or participation in collaborative care groups or family health care teams.

Salary: The physician is paid a set dollar amount for working a set number of hours. This is time-based, not related to fee-for-service.

Alternative Payment Plans: A variety of complex individual and group contracts that include a combination of fee-based services, time-based services, and bonuses for participating in incentive programs (such as enrolling new patients to their practices).

for registration in that province. Any changes to registered information (such as specialty changes) must be submitted to the MoH in writing.

Registered physicians are required to choose a payment option. Although many new and complex ways of remuneration have recently been introduced, the fee-for-service model is the foundation for all the alternative models and is the basis of the physicians' fee schedules (CMA, 2012). Fee-for-service means that the physician is paid for each individual service provided. For example, if 30 patients attend office hours on a particular day, 30 claims are sent to the MoH. See Box 7.4 for other models that have emerged.

Despite the payment plan option, each physician or group still needs to report on each patient so that the MoH can maintain accurate records and gather statistics. This is done through a process called *shadow billing*, in which a claim is sent to the MoH for each patient (based on the fee-for-service codes in the physicians' fee schedules). The MoH then adjusts the physicians' payments to match their unique contracts. So, regardless of the payment option chosen by a physician, the role of the medical administrative assistant in the billing process is the same.

Although not a common practice, physicians do have the right to opt out of the public health care plan for their province. This means that they cannot apply to the MoH for payment for any services and that their patients have to pay them directly for service provided. The patient can then apply to the MoH to have his or her funds reimbursed. Physicians who opt out are not allowed to charge patients higher fees than those outlined in their provincial or territorial fee schedule.

Introduction to Claims Submission

Once registered, the physician can be set up with an approved billing software (determined by the MoH); the new physician's billing number, the appropriate fee schedule, and the diagnostic codes used by the province or territory will be loaded to the billing software by the software vendor.

The medical administrative assistant needs to understand the billing process and the importance of accuracy in both billing and records maintenance because he or she will be responsible for sending claims (billings) to the MoH. Claims submission is more than a data-entry task. Although billing software programs will pick up and flag most inconsistencies with the fee schedule rules, familiarity with and adherence to the information in the preamble, along with the appropriate use of codes, are necessary for the accurate submission of claims. The paragraphs below outline the information required for all basic claims and provide further explanations about key codes and special considerations.

Required Information

Claims submissions for general medical office billing (billing for hospital services, surgeries, on-call services, and so on are beyond the scope of this chapter) will require the following information, most of which is preloaded to or assigned by your chosen billing software.

- **Provider Registration Number:** Identifies the provider of the service. This is the unique physician billing number that the provider is given by the MoH in their province or territory. The provider registration number or numbers are loaded to the medical billing software. If there is more than one physician in your office, you will need to confirm that you have chosen the correct physician, usually from a drop-down list, before entering claims. See Fig. 7.4 showing a drop-down provider list selection. If you do not choose correctly, the wrong physician will be paid for the services.

- **Health (Registration) Number:** Number that is assigned to eligible residents of a province to cover the individual for medically necessary health services. As already mentioned, provinces and territories now issue health cards with patients' unique health numbers. The cards may have expiry dates or version codes. Once a patient is registered with your clinic, entering his or her health number will generate the remainder of the information so you can ensure that the patient is correctly identified.

- **Date of Birth:** Usually as day/month/year format, but each billing software has its own format. Once a health number is entered to a billing software, the patient's date of birth, sex, address, and other demographic information automatically loads if he or she has previously been registered to your clinic.

- **Accounting Number:** A unique number assigned by a provider to the patient for accounting purposes.

- **Claim Number:** A number generated by the billing software to identify each individual claim saved. Claim numbers are useful when communicating with the MoH about remittance issues or for auditing purposes.

- **Payment Program:** Identifies whether the payment is to be made by the MoH or a workers' compensation board, or whether the billing is to another province. Some provinces have other third-party payment options (e.g., RCMP), or their software may not be set up for any third-party payments.

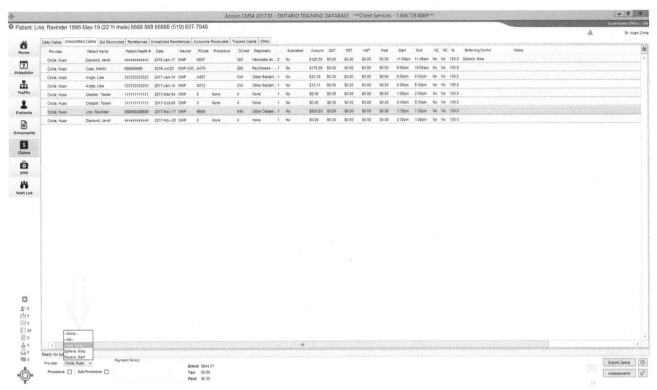

• Fig. 7.4 Provider List Selection EMR. (Source: EMR Accuro.)

- **Referral Provider:** Identifies the health care provider/physician (registration number) who has referred the patient for the service. This section must be completed for *all* types of consultations in any location. Your billing software will have most referral provider registration numbers available; you can type the name of the referring physician into the appropriate field to load his or her billing number.
- **Facility Number or Treatment Location Code:** Identifies the facility name (not individual physicians' offices) where the service is performed. In some cases, there may also be a code for the facility type (hospital, office, detox, etc.). This information may be found in the preamble.
- **Service Code or Fee Code:** Alpha-numeric or numeric codes assigned to all insured medical services. These codes are listed in the provincial fee schedule. When codes are entered to the billing software, their associated fees will automatically load.
- **Fee Submitted:** Amount the provider claims for the service rendered. This amount is found in the provincial fee schedule and will load to the billing software upon entering the appropriate service code.
- **Number of Services (Price per Unit):** Claims are submitted by the number of services provided. Most services (units) are claimed as one service, but for time-based services (psychotherapy), a service or unit is the amount designated by the fee schedule. For example, some services may be for every 15 minutes or part thereof. The

number of services may also be related to the number of times a procedure was performed (wart removal).
- **Service Date:** Identifies the date the service was provided. Be sure to double check that your software has not defaulted to the current date. Date discrepancies during an audit may result in the physician losing income.
- **Diagnostic Code:** Identifies the reason the patient is being seen by the provider. If more than one diagnosis is involved, use the code for the primary diagnosis. Your electronic billing software will have modified ICD codes included.

Further explanations of service codes, diagnostic codes, time units, and other select preamble considerations are provided in the following sections.

Service Codes

Service codes, also called *fee codes,* are numeric or alpha-numeric codes related to specific services or sets of services provided by physicians. Each service code has a specific dollar amount, or fee, assigned to it. To understand what code is applied to each encounter type, the definitions and rules outlined in the preamble of your fee schedule must be consulted. For instance, if three patients attend office hours for the same visit type (not related to their diagnosis), the same service code is billed for their visit. This means that the doctor is paid the same amount for each encounter. However, if another patient attends office hours for a different visit type (defined in

Patient	Visit Type (See Preamble)	Service Code	Fee
Patient A	Limited Office Visit	0113	$36.40
Patient B	Limited Office Visit	0113	$36.40
Patient C	Comprehensive Office Visit	0100	$62.40
Patient D	Consultation	0160	$83.20
Patient E	Limited Office Visit	0113	$36.40

• BOX 7.5 Service Code Sample

the preamble), a different code is applied, and a different fee is charged. In the sample shown in Box 7.5, Patients A, B, and E attend the office for the same visit type (limited office visit). Therefore the service code and associated fees are the same for all three patients. Notice that Patient C presents for a different visit type (comprehensive office visit), which is assigned a different code and fee. Patient D has presented for yet another visit type and is assigned the service code relating to that visit type (definitions for these and other common visit types are noted below).

Factors that account for the differences in service code amounts are as follows: the time it takes to perform the examination, the age of the patient (as with annual health examinations), the complexity of the diagnosis or procedure, the time of day, the urgency, the medical specialty, and others.

Although the service codes, names, definitions, and dollar amounts will vary by province and territory, some of the most common visit types in general practice include the following:

1. **General Assessment or Comprehensive Office Visit**—The patient presents the provider with a complaint, and the provider investigates all systems to make a diagnosis. This visit type usually takes more than 10 minutes of the doctor's time.
2. **Intermediate Assessment or Limited Office Visit**—The patient presents the provider with one complaint or more, and the provider is required to take a history and investigate the related systems. It is less involved than a comprehensive office visit and may take about 10 minutes of the doctor's time.
3. **Minor Assessment or Brief Office Visit**—The diagnosis is fairly simple, and the visit is less time-consuming than an intermediate assessment.
4. **Psychotherapy or Mental Health Assessment**—The patient presents with complaints of a mental, emotional, or psychosomatic nature. The provider investigates through a therapeutic relationship with the patient and then treats accordingly. The service code is usually related to a block of time (15 minutes).
5. **Well Baby Care**—The provider examines a specific system for a diagnosis (less time than a general assessment)

or sees a child up to 2 years of age for periodic health assessment and progress evaluation.
6. **Annual Health Examination**—The patient visits the doctor for a yearly review of physical well-being with no complaint (one visit per year can be charged).
7. **Prenatal Assessment**—The patient presents for a comprehensive assessment after a pregnancy is confirmed. This initial appointment is followed by a number of shorter appointments, unless the expectant mother is referred to an obstetrical specialist for prenatal care.

Only one office visit per patient per day is permitted. If a second billing is attempted, your billing software will send up a cautionary flag. If it is reasonable for a duplicate code to be billed for the same day at a different time, an explanation will need to be provided for manual review of the claim.

Procedural Codes

Procedural codes are a specialized type of fee or service code. They have dollar amounts assigned to them, and they are found in the physicians' fee schedules (usually under their own section for minor diagnostic or therapeutic procedures). Procedure codes can be billed in addition to the fee for an office visit and are normally entered into the same field in your billing software. See Fig. 7.5 for an example. Some common procedures you may be required to bill in a medical office are found in Box 7.6.

Rules related to billing procedural codes are found the preamble. It is essential that you become familiar with the rules because there are many nuances. For example, you can bill the aforementioned Pap smear in addition to a regular office visit, but you cannot bill a Pap smear in addition to an annual health examination; it is already included in the fee.

Diagnostic Codes

Diagnostic codes are an essential component of most medical claims. The list of diagnostic codes is provided to physicians once their independent billing numbers are assigned. As mentioned previously, the codes are loaded into the physician's billing software. They are modified versions of the International Classification of Diseases(ICD) codes governed by the World Health Organization. Most provinces use a three- to five-digit numeric or alpha-numeric

• BOX 7.6 Common Procedures Billed in Medical Offices

Urinalysis
Pap Smear (with or without pelvic exam)
Pelvic Examination (with or without Pap smear)
Injections (allergy, B12, vaccinations)
Dressing Changes
Sutures

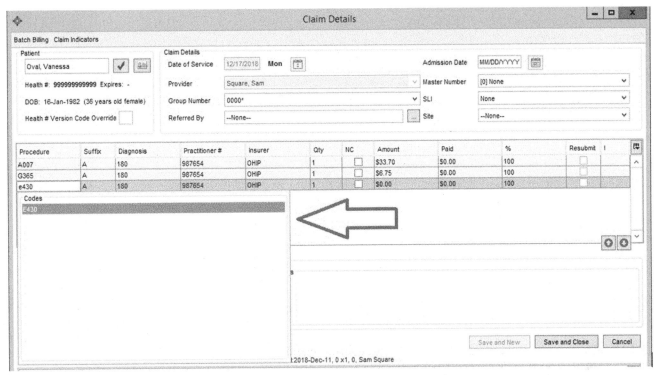

• **Fig. 7.5** Procedural Code. (Source: EMR Accuro.)

code that can be identified simply by keying in the actual diagnosis (i.e., key in *infection*; a pop-up list will appear, and the appropriate diagnosis can be chosen). The computer will then supply the code.

There is no dollar amount attached to a diagnostic code. As mentioned, the purpose of codes is to provide the MoH the reason the patient was seen by the physician. The statistics that result from this data collection are important provincially, nationally, and internationally. The standardized coding system helps governments determine what services are required and where. Diagnostic codes are essential for identifying, reporting, preventing, and mitigating public health risks related to disease.

Time Units

As mentioned previously in this chapter, some services are billed by time units and may require an adjustment to the *number of services* field in your billing software. An example would be a physician seeing a patient for a psychotherapy visit. The physician would bill per 15 minutes, or a major portion thereof (or as outlined in the fee schedule). If the appointment was for one hour, the number of services would be four. If the appointment was for 40 minutes, the number of services would be 3. Therefore if the fee-for-service was $50.00, the physician would receive $200.00 for the 1-hour appointment and $150.00 for the 40-minute appointment.

Another example of a service type that uses time units is detention. Situations that require detention codes (the

doctor is "detained" or held back) are usually unexpected and unpredictable. For instance, a doctor decides to ride in an ambulance with a patient, or the doctor's presence is required on a continuous basis for a period of time (usually in excess of 30 minutes) for examination or treatment (not surgical or procedural). The situations in which detention is an acceptable billing code choice are outlined in physicians' fee schedules.

A physician assisting in surgery may also bill by time units (this information can be found in the preamble of the fee schedule). The time units may increase depending on the length of the service. For example, one time unit may be for every 15 minutes (or part thereof) during the first hour or less. It then increases to two time units for every 15 minutes (or part thereof) after the first hour but on or before the eighth hour, and then three time units for every 15 minutes (or part thereof) after the eighth hour.

In each of these situations, the medical administrative assistant must remember to adjust the *number of services* field in the billing software. This usually involves choosing the correct number of services from a drop-down list in the billing screen. See Fig. 7.6 as an example. You may also be able to type the number into the *number of services* field.

Premiums

There will be times when physicians are required to work outside of their regular office hours, or on holidays, due to

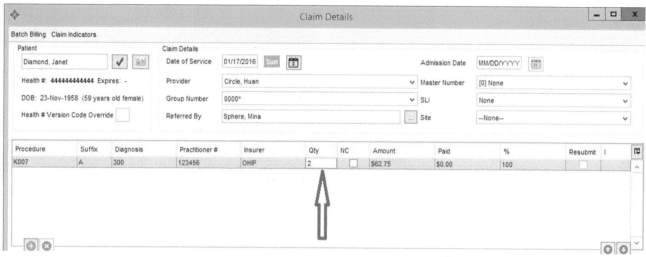

• **Fig. 7.6** Number of Service Claims. (Source: EMR Accuro.)

• BOX 7.7	After-Hour Premiums for Emergency Situations

Time of Day	Premiums Applied
From 1800 to 2400 hours	25% to 50%
From 2400 to 0800 hours	25% to 75%
From 0800 to 1800 hours on Saturday and Sunday	25% to 50%
From 0800 to 1800 hours on holidays	25% to 50%

emergency situations. These may include emergency home visits, resuscitations, visits to long-term care facilities, detentions, assessment of labour, or performance of diagnostic or therapeutic procedures. When these situations occur, after-hours premiums may be added to the claims; these are in addition to the regular fees claimed. The applicable times of day and premium increases, however, will vary by province and territory (specified in the preamble). Box 7.7 outlines some common themes related to the times premiums are applied and lists a range of after-hours premiums from across the country.

There are many factors affecting the application of premiums, and referring to the preamble is essential for proper application. For instance, patients cannot be seen during these hours for the convenience of the physician and patient, special fee codes or documentation may be required, they may not be added with certain fee codes (like those of detention), and so on.

Once you are sure that a premium can be applied, doing so in your medical billing software is quite simple. Usually, a simple tick (see Fig. 7.7) is available that, when applied, will add the premium in a dollar amount and remind you to enter the time and to provide any supporting documentation that is required.

Geriatric premiums may be applied to encounters with elderly patients (usually 75+ years). These encounters may be more complicated or require the physician to spend more time with the patient. Fig. 7.8 shows a claim where

the patient's date of birth automatically adds a premium to the visit code.

Remember the following 5-W's when submitting a claim:

WHAT?—The type of assessment/procedure being billed.

WHEN?—The time the procedure is performed to determine the premium codes and to record correct date.

WHERE?—The location that the procedure/visit was carried out (i.e., office, hospital) (use facility number), other.

WHY? —The reason for visit/procedure to ascertain correct diagnostic code.

WHO? —Which physician is billing the procedure (i.e., attending physician, surgical assistant or anaesthetist).

Supporting Documentation

Certain services, such as independent consideration(IC), must include supporting documentation. IC may be given when a set fee is not listed in the fee schedule. Claims rendered under this heading should contain an explanation of the fee claimed. Some medical billing software will contain a field where the explanation can be added and where the supporting documentation can be attached or uploaded. Other ministries of health may require hard copies of the documentation. When submitting this claim, the field "Flag for Review" or "Manual Review" (field will differ with each software) must be identified (see Fig. 7.9 for one example). This ensures that the MoH will be aware that there is supporting documentation for this claim, and that it may need an independent review by the medical consultant or equivalent.

DID YOU KNOW?

According to the 2016 census from Statistics Canada, 5.9 million people in Canada are over the age of 65. Between 2011 and 2016, the number of people over the age of 85 increased four times as fast as the general population. This increase greatly impacts health care funding and the availability of community services.

Source: Russell, A. (2017, May 5). Is Canada's health-care system ready for our rapidly greying population? *Globe and Mail.* Retrieved from https://globalnews.ca/news/3429041/healthc are-stats-canada-2016-census/

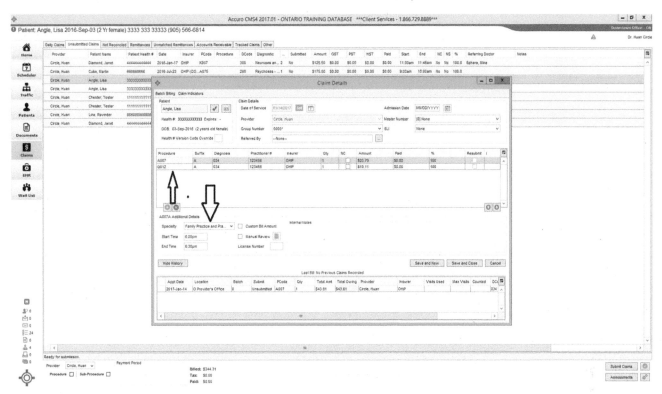

• **Fig. 7.7** After-Hours Premium Claim. (Source: EMR Accuro.)

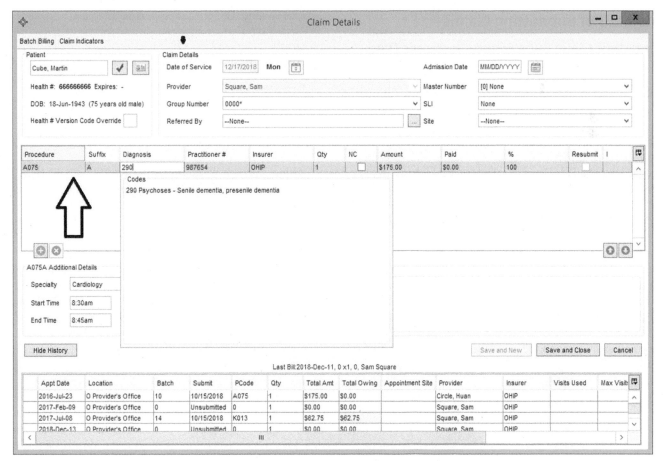

• **Fig. 7.8** Age-Related Premium Claim (Geriatric). (Source: EMR Accuro.)

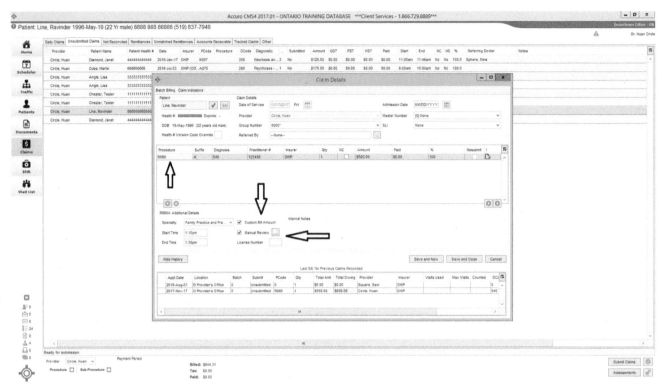

• **Fig. 7.9** Independent Consideration Claim. (Source: EMR Accuro.)

Methods of Submitting Claims

Electronic Claim Submission/Electronic Data Transfer (EDT)

Most billing for health care services is submitted through electronic claim submission using a system approved by the MoH that supports electronic data transfer (EDT). This is a secure web-enabled method of submission using a third-party–compliant billing component of the electronic medical record (EMR). Typically, the MoH has a billing cycle with a claims cutoff date set forth by the provincial or territorial MoH each month for claims to be received and to appear on the upcoming payment period. The EDT is usually available 24 hours a day, 7 days a week. In return, electronic reports reflective of claims processing are generated from the billing communication relayed through the electronic communication channel enabled between the billing party and the MoH after claims are reviewed, such as claims error and remittance advice reporting (see remittance advice section in this chapter). The paid billing will be reconciled in your system. See Box 7.8 showing popular Canadian EMRs.

Claim Submission

As discussed previously, developing familiarity with the format of the provincial or territorial schedule is essential because you may be responsible for managing the billing and associated components in your role.

• **BOX 7.8** **Popular EMRs Used in Canada**

MOIS
Accuro EMR
WOLF EMR
CHS EMR Advantage
Nightingale on Demand
P&P Clinic Information System

Although the billing application within your EMR will vary in appearance and commands, the required fields (as outlined in the Introduction to Claims Submission section) for the MoH to process a billing will be the same because EMRs are designed and approved to match based on MoH claim submission specifications. Some EMRs will allow you to direct-bill from the software by integrating their billing and scheduling modules. These systems will help reduce the need for printing encounter forms (see Fig. 7.10) and day sheets (see Fig. 7.11), reduce billing errors, and greatly increase the efficiency of the billing process. However, some systems still require the medical administrative assistant to bill from the day sheets, encounter forms, or other similar forms. In these cases, claims should be organized in a way that allows you to be the most efficient, yet help you avoid errors. For instance, if you are billing for more than one physician, separate the claims into stacks for each physician and bill one physician at a time. Also separate your day sheets or encounter forms by date, and bill claims for one date at a time. Each of these practices will minimize the number the

Encounter Form

Physician: **Dr. Plunkett**

PATIENT:	**BAXTER, ROBERT**	**CHART NO.: 5786**
DOB:	07-Octobert-1957	Contact Person: Joan Baxter
Health No.:	4892 608 532	Marital Status: Married
Address:	836 Linden Terrace, ON K1S 1Z1	Family Physician: J.E. Plunkett
Home Phone:	613-652-3179	Work Phone: 613-652-1279

ALLERGIES: NKA

DATE OF SERVICE: 06-February-2018   Referring Doctor:

Visit Codes: 1:
               2: *A113A*
               3:

Diagnosis: *concussion*   Diagnosis Code: *850*

Payment Program.

☑ HCP

☐ WCB   Employer:

☐ VAC   Regimental No:

☐ RMB   Province:

☐ OTHER Note:

• **Fig. 7.10** Encounter Form.

times you have to change the date and provider options in your billing software, thus helping you prevent errors.

Once you are organized, you start the billing process by entering the claims into the billing software. It is advisable to enter the billings the same day as the encounter; however, some offices may set aside specific times during the week so that the staff member can concentrate entirely on this important task.

Once claims are entered, they can be sent immediately or stored in the software until you are ready to send them. Claims can be sent to the MoH anytime; however, there are deadlines to adhere to when seeking payments for claims by specific dates. For instance, most MoH pay physicians one to two times per month. As such, you will need to ensure that you understand the specific billing deadlines for your province or territory. A general guideline is that billings submitted by the 25th of the month are paid by the 15th of the next month (CMA, 2012). All claims must be submitted to the MoH within three to six months of the service date, depending on the province. Only under extreme circumstances will the MoH consider making payments for claims submitted after their expiry date. Box 7.9 lists the time limits for submissions for most provinces and territories. The time limits are stated in the units (days, months) outlined in their respective fee schedules, preambles, or other supporting documentation. Box 7.10 shows the basic steps for completing a claim.

Here are two claim examples based on an Ontario billing scenario:

Example 1

Mary Jane Brown came to Dr. Plunkett's office on January 16, 20__, with a rash on her toes. The diagnosis was "tinea pedis."

The procedure for completing the health claim is as follows:

1. The provider name is usually shown on the billing screen. If you are billing for more than one physician, apply the charge when the appropriate physician is identified.

Dr. Plunkett's Office

Clinic Date: Thursday, September 20, 2018   Provider: Dr. J. E. Plunkett

Appointment	Patient	Health Card Number	Reason for Visit	Service Code	Procedural Code	Diagnostic Code
9:00 a.m.	Cheryl Page	9013 157 109	AHE			
9:10 a.m.						
9:20 a.m.						
9:30 a.m.	Walter Page	3100 000 521	constipation			
9:40 a.m.	Rosie Smythe	0178 934 991	elbow pain			
10:00 a.m.	Tim Peters	7031 381 135	ear ache			
10:10 a.m.	Elizabeth Green	3777 220 777	high BP			
10:20 a.m.	Mary Jane Brown	3820 703 795	B12			
10:30 a.m.	Hazel Davis	1781 050 552	Pap			
10:40 a.m.	Sue Jessup	0000 036 408	dizziness			
10:50 a.m.	Evik Shultz	7015 851 901	chest congestion			
11:00 a.m.	Kendra Hall	0110 004 556	back pain			
11:10 a.m.	Sara Downs	0126 759 647	counselling			
11:20 a.m.						
11:30 a.m.						
11:40 a.m.	Lisa Basciano	2719 278 836	rheumatoid arthritis			
11:50 a.m.	Janie Packer	1459 786 324	wart removal			
12:00 p.m.						
12:10 p.m.						
12:20 p.m.						
12:40 p.m.						

• **Fig. 7.11** Day Sheet.

• **BOX 7.9** **Time Limits for Claim Submissions**

Alberta	180 days
British Columbia	90 days
Manitoba	6 months
New Brunswick	3 months
Newfoundland and Labrador	90 days
Nova Scotia	90 days
Northwest Territory	12 months
Nunavut	6 months
Ontario	6 months
Québec	3 months
Prince Edward Island	3 months
Saskatchewan	6 months
Yukon	6 months

• **BOX 7.10** **Basic Steps for Completing a Claim**

1. Identify the provider (if billing for more than one provider)
2. Identify referral provider (if applicable)
3. Identify appropriate patient from database
4. Identify type of billing if it differs from that of health care plan
5. Insert facility number (if appropriate)
6. Insert admission date (if appropriate)
7. Insert service code (software will generate appropriate fee from the service code)
8. Insert number of services
9. Insert diagnostic code
10. Check completed billings with appointment day sheet to avoid any omissions
11. Submit electronically

---

2. Mary Jane's health number and date of birth will be inserted into the billing screen from the registration screen.
3. The payment program is the health care plan (enter HCP), and the provider is to be paid (enter "P"). Most billing software will default to "HCP" and "P."
4. Because the complaint is isolated and fairly simple to diagnose, Dr. Plunkett would charge for a minor assessment. Dr. Plunkett will provide the service code, and the fee will be inserted when the service code field is completed. The service code would be obtained from the Schedule of Benefits under the appropriate section for that provider. Dr. Plunkett would bill under "Family Practice" and "Practice in General" because he is a general health care provider.
5. One service has been performed. This would be entered in the "Number of Services" or "Price per Unit" field.
6. The service date is the day Mary Jane presented her complaint.
7. The diagnostic code would be inserted into that field once the appropriate diagnosis is keyed in or the numeric code is inserted. Dr. Plunkett would provide the diagnosis.

Example 2

While Bob Baxter was cleaning windows, he fell off the ladder, banged his head on a rock, and was knocked unconscious. His wife called an ambulance to take him to

PATIENT BILLING HISTORY
Mary Jane Brown

Patient: **Brown, Mary Jane**

Admitted:

Facility:

Date of Birth: **01- January-1958**

Home Telephone: **(613) 427-3333**

Work Telephone: **(613) 427-2121**

Health Card Number: **3820 703 795** Version No:

Visit Date: **16-January-2018**　　　　　　　　Encounter No:

Service Code	No. of Services	Fee	Diagnosis	Paid	Amount	Account No	Status
A001A	1	21.70	110			476878	HCP Claim

• **Fig. 7.12** Patient Billing Example 1: Mary Jane Brown.

the hospital. Dr. Plunkett admitted Bob and then called in a neurologist, Dr. R.T. Schmidt, for consultation. Dr. Schmidt's diagnosis was concussion. He visited Bob on three consecutive days after the admitting date. The accident happened on Saturday, January 22, 20__.

The procedure for completing the health claim is as follows:

1. The provider number is usually shown in the billing screen.
2. The patient's health number and birth date will be inserted from the registration screen.
3. Because Dr. Plunkett referred Bob to Dr. Schmidt, Dr. Plunkett's personal registration number would be entered in the field "Referred By."
4. Because Bob was admitted to the hospital, the "Facility Number" and "Inpatient Admission" fields must be completed.
5. The service codes are as follows:
   a. A185A—The service is a consultation performed in the hospital by a specialist in neurology. When a provider makes a special trip, the billing code for the assessment component of the visit is taken from the general listing for the applicable specialty. In the fee schedule under neurology (18) you will find A185—Consultation. Service codes used for special trip billings *must* be taken from the general listing's Office Service Codes. A consultation can be charged only when the provider is seeing a patient who has been referred by another provider.

   The suffix for each service code is "A" because the service was rendered by the provider.

   b. C994A—Providers can charge a premium if they respond to calls outside of office hours, or on weekends and holidays, or if they sacrifice office hours. The appropriate codes are listed in the preamble under "Premiums." If the special visit is to the emergency department, the alpha prefix would be "K"; for a visit to a patient's home, the alpha prefix would be "B." However, in this instance, the alpha prefix is "C" because Dr. Schmidt rendered the service to a non-emergency hospital inpatient.
   c. C182A—This is the code used when a neurologist makes subsequent hospital visits to a patient.
6. The appropriate service fees will be applied and totalled from the relevant service codes.
7. Note that under "Number of Services," the number "03" is entered opposite "C182A." This is because Dr. Schmidt visited the patient for three consecutive days. The service date entered is the date of the first visit. (If the visits run consecutively without a break, you can put them together.)
8. The diagnostic code for concussion is 850.

Figs 7.12 and 7.13 are examples of a Patient Billing History for the previous two patients.

Auditing Claims

The MoH will audit claims from time to time to ensure the accuracy of records. The audit process is normally random and may include an MoH representative visiting your office. A list of patients will be presented to you, and their records will be requested. The representative will then match the billings they have received from your office with the notes in the patients' charts, your appointment schedule, or both.

PATIENT BILLING HISTORY
Robert Baxter

Patient: **Baxter, Robert**

Date of Birth: **07-October-1957**

Admitted: **22-January-2018**

Home Telephone: **(613) 652-3179**

Facility: **1768**

Work Telephone: **(613) 652-1279**

Health Card Number: **4892 608 532** Version No: **2**

Visit Date: **16-January-2018**   Encounter No:

Service Code	No. of Services	Fee	Diagnosis	Paid	Amount	Account No	Status
A185A	1	176.35	850			476879	HCP Claim
C182A	3	31.00	850			476879	HCP Claim
C994A	1	60.00	850			476879	HCP Claim

• **Fig. 7.13** Patient Billing Example 2: Robert Baxter.

As part of a random audit, a letter may be sent to a patient asking for verification that he or she was seen by a physician on a certain date, and for a specific reason. Private services such as abortion, organ retrieval, or treatment of sexually transmitted infections (STIs) would not be included.

It is extremely important that the medical administrative assistant ensure that appointment schedules, billing information, and chart documentation are up to date, organized, and accurate to avoid any repercussions from auditing processes. If submitted claim information does not match the information in these other areas of the office, the physician may be required to pay back the funds.

Remittance Advice

The remittance advice is an itemized statement of the individual payments made by the MoH for insured services. If payments are made for programs other than the provincial plan (for example, a workers' compensation board or another province through the reciprocal agreement process), these services and their payment statuses will be identified in the payment identification column. This report can be viewed and/or printed from the EMR. For offices that use day sheets or encounter forms to manage their claims, it is a good practice to store a copy of the remittance advice with the corresponding claim forms submitted. This practice will make for easy and efficient retrieval of the documents if a discrepancy arises and an appeal is necessary.

A Remittance Advice has the following basic divisions (see the blue numbers shown on Fig. 7.14):

1. Header information
2. Claim information
3. Total payment information

Header Information

The header information appears at the top of the form and includes the following (itemized letters in red):
A. Provider's name
B. District office (if applicable)
C. Group/provider's registration number
D. Payment date
E. Page number

Claim Information

The claim information is the main part of the form and relates all data relevant to each claim submission as follows:
F. Provider accounting number—Number assigned by a provider to the patient for accounting purposes.
G. Patient's first and last name.
H. The patient's province of residence.
I. Patient's health card number.
J. The type of payment identification (e.g., provincial health care plan, workers' compensation).
K. The MoH claim number—A unique number assigned by the MoH to identify each claim.
L. Initial service date—The date the service was performed.
M. Number of services.

Ministry of Health

Remittance Advice (1)   Dr. J. Jones   Oshawa   000-12300-01   Page 2   E   D   A   B   C

No.	Accounting Number	Patient's Lastname	Name First	Prov/ Terr	Health Reg. Number	Pay PGM	Claim Number	Service Date	No. Of Services	Sev. Code	Fee Submitted	Amount Paid	EX CD
1	57079111	Schulz	Eric	ON	1234567899	HCP	B928987102	20/03/06	1	A001A	21.70	21.70	
2	78568893	Green	Elizabeth	ON	9877779933	HCP	B639899201	20/03/08	1	A007A	33.70	33.70	
3	76789999	Eggleson	Frank	NB	3457982234	RMB	B389087661	20/03/08	1	G373A	6.75	6.75	
4	57899876	Symons	Dayton	ON	9725356729	HCP	B876523198	20/03/04	1	K007A	62.75	62.75	
5	43523412	Francazano	Paul	ON	8832340421	HCP	B872615435	20/03/09	1	G310A	6.60	6.60	
6	25934567	Fisk	Rena	ON	7779356211	WCB	B345689021	20/03/11	1	Z156A	20.00	20.00	
7	13456789	Nichols	Cynthia	ON	4321145679	HCP	B412356798	20/03/10	1	A003A	77.20	77.20	
8	97654389	Windsor	Haley	ON	9727315693	HCP	B234567821	20/03/11	1	A007A	33.70	33.70	
9	78008007	Arnold	Anita	ON	5558210036	HCP	B432578567	20/03/06	1	A001A	21.70	21.70	
10	54234368	Lake	Gwen	ON	9342322431	HCP	B598753453	20/03/03	1	G372A	6.75	6.75	
11	45678932	Kline	Robert	ON	8933340421	HCP	B25689321	20/04/01	1	K007A	62.75	62.75	

F   G   H   I   J   K   L   M   N   O   P   Q   R

(3) Page Totals   353.60   353.60   S

4,096.50   4,096.50   T

• **Fig. 7.14** Remittance Advice Components.

N. Fee schedule code—Obtained from the MoH Fee Schedule.
O. Fee submitted—The fee submitted by the provider.
P. Amount paid—The amount actually paid to the provider for the service. The fee allowed is usually 100 percent of that specified in the provincial Fee Schedule.
Q. Explanatory codes—The explanatory code will appear in cases in which zero payment, or payment less than 100 percent of the fee allotted, is being issued. Some examples of explanatory codes (sometimes called *error codes*) are listed later in the chapter. More complete or detailed descriptions may be obtained from your MoH claims clerk.

Total Payment Information

R. Page totals—The total amounts billed and paid per page.
S. An aggregate total of previous pages.

Deposits usually are made directly to the provider's account. A cheque number is given if payment is made by cheque.

The last page will state the total claims payable to the provider and any accounting adjustments or interim payments. It is important to check the remittance advice against the office records to make sure all claims are accounted for.

Explanatory Codes

Explanatory codes, also called *error codes,* are used to explain why a claim has not been accepted or paid in full. As mentioned previously, this information is available through the provincial or territorial MoH and, in most cases, is also outlined in the fee schedule. Each province or territory has its own unique explanatory codes; however, the explanations of the codes are similar and coincide directly with the rules outlined in the preamble of each fee schedule. The following are examples of explanatory codes for Ontario, Alberta, British Columbia, and Saskatchewan:

Ontario

AD3 Not allowed with visit.
A36 Claimed by other practitioner.
ADF Code not allowed alone.
EQ2 Specialty mismatch.
M1 Maximum number of services reached.
VH4 Invalid version code.
VK1 Invalid OHIP number.

Source: Ontario Ministry of Health and Long Term Care. (2013*). Resource manual for physicians.* Retrieved from http://www.health.gov.on.ca/english/providers/pub/ohip/physmanual/physmanual_mn.html

Alberta

01 Not Registered—We have no record of this person as being registered with this Personal Health Number.
01B Non Resident—We cannot confirm that this patient is a resident of Alberta. Please contact the patient to obtain the correct billing information.

02 Registration Number/PHN Conflict—The Health Registration Number and the Personal Health Number used are not for the same person.

05A Invalid Personal Health Number—The PHN is invalid or blank.

20B RCMP, Armed Forces, and Federal Penitentiary—Members of the RCMP, the Armed Forces, and inmates at Federal Penitentiaries are not eligible under the Plan.

21 Workers' Compensation Board—Ineligible service. The claim was refused or updated as the claim is the responsibility of Worker's Compensation board or it has been changed as it is an unrelated condition.

41 Documentation incomplete/not received—The report was incomplete or not received.

Source: Alberta Health. (2018). Alberta health care insurance explanatory codes. Retrieved from http://www.health.alberta.ca/professionals/SOMB.html

British Columbia

AB PHN is not on our records.

BF Claim is held for further processing.

CB Number of services and time stated do not correspond.

CW Telephone advice may not be charged when another service was provided on the same day.

ED There is insufficient medical necessity to process this claim.

EG This claim is the responsibility of WordSafeBC.

VN Diagnostic code is missing or invalid.

Source: Government of British Columbia. (2018). *Explanatory codes.* Retrieved from https://www2.gov.bc.ca/gov/content/health/practitioner-professional-resources/msp/claim-submission-payment/explanatory-codes

Saskatchewan

AD Incorrect Health Services Number indicated on claim—Medical Services Branch (MSB) has paid this claim. Please use the number shown on this payment file/list for future claims.

AV This service is not insured.

BE This Payment Schedule service code applies to a specific age or sex.

CY This service is not usually billed by a physician in your specialty.

CT Workers' Compensation Board has advised the MoH that it has paid you or another physician in your clinic for the same service, a similar related service, or a service that includes post-operative care.

DA Only one visit type service is approved during a single patient contact. If there were two separate patient contacts, please resubmit with the reason and time of the second visit.

QC Number of units submitted are incorrect. Either this service does not have units, or the number of units is greater than listed in the Payment Schedule. Resubmit with the correct number of units and fee. Services that do not have units must be submitted on an individual line.

Source: Government of Saskatchewan. (2015). *Payment schedule for insured services provided by a physician.* Retrieved from http://publications.gov.sk.ca/details.cfm?p=23561

Remittance Advice Inquiries

MoH staff attempt to minimize the necessity for inquiries concerning claims payment. However, sometimes discrepancies do occur.

If, after examining the Remittance Advice, you find a discrepancy, the first step is to verify that you have submitted the claim correctly. If you have not, the claim should be corrected and resubmitted. If your claim does not appear to have an error, and you feel that you have been incorrectly paid for the service(s), the next step is to undergo the claims correction process that is appropriate for your region. In most provinces, this means a manual review of the claim in question that begins with completing the proper paperwork for requesting the review. Examples of claims correction forms are a Remittance Advice Inquiry Form and a Request for Review of a Claim (see Fig. 7.15 for a Saskatchewan example). Box 7.11 provides an overview the claims submissions process.

Appeals

If the provider still disagrees with the status of a claim after going through the initial claims correction process, the MoH should be consulted. Appeals of complicated claims may be directed to the MoH's medical consultant, or provincial equivalent, in a district office.

Workers' Compensation

Workers' compensation is the name of legislation designed to provide benefits, medical care, and rehabilitation services to individuals who suffer workplace injuries or contract occupational diseases. The workers' compensation program is administered by the provincial or territorial government. Every province has its own Workers' Compensation program. Most provinces refer to this plan and its administration as the Workers' Compensation Board, or WCB. In some provinces or territories, it has a modified name. For example, in New Brunswick it is referred to as *WorkSafeNB;* in Ontario, it is Workplace Safety and Insurance Board (WSIB); in Nunavut, a shared plan with Northwest Territories is known as *Workers' Safety and Compensation Commission (WSCC);* and in British Columbia, it is referred to

Request for Review of Claim Assessment

Claim Information: All fields must be complete									

Patient's Name				Health Services Number (HSN)		Date of Service			
						Day	Month	Year	

Claim Number	Run Code	Mode	Clinic Number	Doctor Number	Surgical Start Time	Surgical Stop Time	Hospital Care Admit & Discharge Dates:	☐ Team Surgery Dr._____ Dr._____
							A: D:	*Must include all operative reports for adjudication*

Doctor's Name:_____   Phone No: _____

Request: ☐ Change date of service:_____

☐ Billed in error; please retract:_____

☐ Other:

Date:_____   Signature:_____

Please include all service codes billed below:

Service Code	Explan Code	(Shaded area MSB use only)

Medical Services Branch Reply: ☐ No change or original assessment
☐ Adjusted as follows   Date Sent:_____

If you have any questions or concerns regarding this adjudication, please contact our Claims Analysis Unit at: (306) 787-3454. Thank you.

Last updated February 8, 2019

• **Fig. 7.15** Request for Review of a Claim. (Source: eHealth Saskatchewan. (2016). *Healthcare Resources for Physicians.* Retrieved from https://www.ehealthsask.ca/services/resources/establish-operate-practice /Pages/Physicians.aspx.)

• BOX 7.11   **Claim Submission Flow Chart**

Claim submitted
↓
Claim received by Ministry of Health
↓
Claim reviewed by Ministry of Health → Claim rejected
↓↓
Payment to Provider Remittance to Provider
↓
Claim updated & resubmitted
↓
Reviewed by Ministry of Health
↓
Payment to Provider

---

as *WorkSafeBC*. See Table 7.3 for provincial and territorial workers' compensation plans.

For ease of understanding in this chapter, the abbreviation WCB will encompass all references to workers' compensation. WCBs are funded by employers, not the government. Employers are charged a dollar amount based on payroll. It is important to mention that there is not a single rule in all jurisdictions that governs which employers must register, or for which employees the premiums must be paid. Instead, every WCB has its own rules that govern the collection of premiums and the benefits provided. The funding is used to provide compensation to workers who are injured on the job or who contract an occupational disease or illness. The illness can include acute psychological trauma resulting from work. In some provinces, it is optional for small businesses, including small physicians' offices, to pay WCB premiums.

Employers who pay WCB premiums are protected from lawsuits in exchange for financing the provincial or territorial program. In retrospect, employees also give up their right to sue for work-related injuries, irrespective of fault, for guaranteed compensation for accepted claims.

Compensation includes payment for loss of wages that may result from the injury, disease, or condition; future economic loss and non-economic loss awards, or both, for permanent/partial disability; payment of health care expenses; a wide range of vocational and medical rehabilitation services; retraining programs; and survivor benefits in the case of a fatality.

Employers are now much more proactive in finding an employee modified work in his or her area, or in moving the employee temporarily to a more suitable job within the company due to the education and promotion provided by the WCB.

If a worker is not satisfied with the decision rendered by any of the operating divisions at the WCB, the injured worker may need to appeal the decision.

Making a Claim

Employee's Responsibilities

1. Report the injury and get first aid immediately, or if you need further treatment or transportation for treatment,

your employer should arrange for this. Time limits exist in reporting an accident.
2. Report the details of the accident to the employer, even if no further medical treatment is required. If only first aid treatment was needed, no time was taken off work, and pay was not affected, reporting to the WCB is not required.
3. Some employers require an Incident Form to be completed (this form should be available at your workplace).
4. Choose the physician or other qualified health care provider you want to administer treatment.
5. Complete and return quickly any documents required by the WCB. The forms will vary significantly from province to province (as an example, see Fig. 7.16 showing a worker form documenting illness/disease). Be sure all forms are legible (in some provinces, you must use black ink only) and that all information is exact and complete. When an accident is reported to the WCB, the injured worker is assigned a claim number. This number *must* be available for all communication formats with the WCB.

Employer's Responsibilities

1. Make sure first aid is administered immediately, and if care is required beyond first aid, the injury must be reported to the WCB. Some WCBs in Canada specify a window of within 72 hours for reporting an injury.
2. Complete Employer's Report (for example, Fig. 7.17 shows an employer's first report from WSIB-Ontario).
3. Record the details of the accident (date, time, place, type of injury, medical aid given).
4. If necessary, provide transportation to the doctor's office, hospital, or home (within reasonable distance of workplace).
5. Supply any other information required by the WCB.
   All forms are available on the provincial or territorial WCB websites.

Physician's Responsibilities

In all cases in which an injured worker has been treated for a work-related injury, complete and send to the WCB a Health Professional's First Report (as an example, see Fig. 7.18) as soon as the injured patient has been examined. Reports should be submitted within a limited time period of 48 to 72 hours depending on province/territory. All reports can be submitted electronically by employers, physicians, chiropractors, and physiotherapists.

Administrative Assistant's Responsibilities

1. Secure the reason for the visit upon arrival of the injured worker at the doctor's office.
2. Ensure that the Health Professional's Report has been completed and send it to the WCB within 48 hours. This is done after the doctor has seen the patient and has provided the necessary information. Complete the billing portion in the bottom right corner of the form to reimburse the physician for completing the report.

TABLE 7.3   Provincial and Territorial Workers' Compensation

Province/Territory	Workers' Compensation Plan	Link
Alberta	WCB-Alberta	https://www.wcb.ab.ca/
British Columbia	WorkSafeBC	https://www.worksafebc.com/en
Manitoba	WCB-Manitoba	https://www.wcb.mb.ca/
New Brunswick	WorkSafeNB	https://www.worksafenb.ca/
Newfoundland and Labrador	WorkPlace NL	http://www.workplacenl.ca
Northwest Territories	Workers' Safety and Compensation Commission	http://www.wscc.nt.ca/
Nova Scotia	WCB-Nova Scotia	https://www.wcb.ns.ca/
Nunavut	Workers' Safety and Compensation Commission	http://www.wscc.nt.ca/
Ontario	Workplace Safety and Insurance Board	http://www.wsib.on.ca
Prince Edward Island	WCB-PEI	http://www.wcb.pe.ca/
Québec	CSST-Workplace health and safety board	http://www.csst.qc.ca
Saskatchewan	WCB-Saskatchewan	http://www.wcbsask.com/
Yukon	Workers' Compensation and Health and Safety Board	https://wcb.yk.ca/

3. Save the completed form of the Health Professional's Report in the patient's EMR record.
4. Complete and submit an MoH claim using the same procedure as for regular health service claims. Enter "WCB" in the "Payment Program" block.
5. Forward any progress reports completed by the physician related to the WCB claim.

The medical administrative assistant is not required to have considerable knowledge concerning workers' compensation, because reporting work-related injuries is the responsibility of the employer and employee. The doctor is responsible for diagnosing the injuries, and the WCB makes the decision on compensation to the injured worker. The medical administrative assistant should, however, have a general knowledge of the system and be capable of completing all forms related to the doctor's involvement with the WCB.

The medical administrative assistant is responsible for submitting WCB claims under the fee-for-service payment format. The additional information required is listed as follows:
- Identify as a WCB claim
- Patient's Social Insurance Number (SIN)
- Date of original injury
- Claim number (if one has been assigned)

If you have questions or need clarification of information, contact the Workers' Compensation Board directly.

CRITICAL THINKING

A patient attended the office for examination of an injury but did not tell you, or the physician, that the injury was related to his workplace. You billed the visit to the MoH as a regular office visit. Subsequently, you get a phone call from workers' compensation requesting the Health Professional's Report from the patient's recent visit because an Employer's Report had been received. What can you do to rectify the situation? How can you prevent a similar situation from happening in the future?

Release of Workers' Compensation Information

Before releasing any WCB information to a third party you must obtain a release of information. This form is a consent to release of information (as an example, see Fig. 7.19). The form is signed by the injured patient and witnessed by a second party and retained for records.

Third-Party Insurance

In addition to health care plans and workers' compensation, the public may wish to carry additional health care insurance to cover expenses not reimbursed by their respective plans. Extended health insurance is an example of a third-party insurance developed for a group through an employer. Many employers don't offer extended health benefits as a condition of employment, and individuals may seek out third-party insurance directly.

Many private insurance companies issue group and individual policies to cover these additional expenses. London Life Mutual, Blue Cross, Green Shield, and Manulife are examples of third-party private insurance companies.

Benefits Available Through Third-Party Insurance

1. Semi-private or private hospital accommodation (available on an individual pay-direct or a group basis).
2. Extended health care plans (available on an individual pay-direct or a group basis) provide protection against the costs of health services not covered by basic government health plans. The plan can be tailored to the needs of any group.

(Text continues on p. 167)

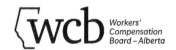

P.O. BOX 2415
EDMONTON AB T5J 2S5

Phone **780-498-3999** (in Edmonton)
1-866-922-9221 (toll free in Alberta)
1-800-661-9608 (outside Alberta)

Fax **780-427-5863** or **1-800-661-1993**

November 2018

WORKER REPORT
of Injury or Occupational Disease   C060

Seven digit claim #:

Worker Details

Past the date of injury: Have you been off work? ☐ Yes ☐ No   ❶ Have your work duties been **modified**? ☐ Yes ☐ No

Last name: First name: Initial:

Mailing address: Apt# _____ ,   Social Insurance #:

City: Province: Postal code: Personal health #:   —

Phone number: Date of birth: *(Year / Month / Day)*   Gender: ☐ M ☐ F

Occupation and job description:

Are you an apprentice? ☐ Yes ☐ No   If yes, date you would have obtained journeyman status: *(Year / Month / Day)*

Date hired: *(Year / Month / Day)*   Are you a partner or director in the business? ☐ Yes ☐ No

Do you have personal coverage? ☐ Yes ☐ No   If yes, coverage number:

Employer Details   ❷ Employer business name:

Mailing address:

City: Province: Postal code:

Contact name: Title: Phone: E-mail:

Accident Details

❸ Date/time of accident: *(Year / Month / Day)*   Time: ___ : ___ ☐ a.m. ☐ p.m. *or* ☐ the injury/condition developed over time

Date/time scheduled shift started (if applicable): *(Year / Month / Day)*   Time: ___ : ___ ☐ a.m. ☐ p.m.

Date/time scheduled shift ended (if applicable): *(Year / Month / Day)*   Time: ___ : ___ ☐ a.m. ☐ p.m.

❹ Date accident/injury reported to employer: *(Year / Month / Day)*

Name of person and their position: Phone number:

If not reported immediately, give the reason:

❺ Describe fully, based on the information you have, what happened to cause this injury or disease. Please describe what you were doing, including details about any tools, equipment, materials, etc. you were using. State any gas, chemicals or extreme temperatures you may have been exposed to:

_____

_____

☐ Cardiac condition/injury?   ☐ Claimed to another WCB? Province: _____

☐ Motor vehicle accident? If you have a police collision report, please send a copy by mail or fax once you have a claim number. Please also complete the WCB Automobile Accident Report.

If you have more information or a list of witnesses, please attach a letter. Please check this box if letter is attached. ☐

Have you had a similar injury before? ☐ Yes ☐ No   **If yes, attach a letter with details.**

Was the work you were doing for the purpose of your employer's business? ☐ Yes ☐ No   Was it part of your usual work? ☐ Yes ☐ No

Did the accident/injury occur on employer's premises? ☐ Yes ☐ No

Location where the accident happened (address, general location or site):

❻ Full name of treating hospital or healthcare professional:

Address:

Phone:

When did you **first** seek medical treatment? *(Year / Month / Day)*   Is any further treatment required? ☐ Yes ☐ No

❼ Did your employer provide health **benefits** to you at the time of the accident? ☐ Yes ☐ No

Will your employer continue paying the **benefit** premium? ☐ Yes ☐ No

C060

REV NOV 2018

Complete all three pages and sign the form before sending.
If your injury is the result of a motor vehicle accident, complete the Automobile Accident Report (L-054).

• **Fig. 7.16** Worker Documenting Injury or Disease. (Source: Workers' Compensation Board ("WCB-Alberta"). (2016). All rights expressly reserved. Retrieved from https://www.wcb.ab.ca/assets/pdfs/wor kers/c060.pdf.)

WORKER REPORT   Page 2 of 3

Worker's last name:	Worker's **first** name:	Initial:

Social Insurance #: | | | | | | | | | Date of birth: *(Year / Month / Day)* | | | | | | |

Injury Details

What part of body was injured? (hand, eye, back, lungs, etc.)   ☐ Left side   ☐ Right side

What type of injury is this? (sprain, strain, bruise, etc.)

Return to Work Details   **Please complete all that apply**

☐ I understand that I have a legal obligation to cooperate with my employer and WCB in arranging my safe return to work. Exceptions: Short-term or some seasonal workers, subcontractors and workers with personal coverage.

8 a. Will/did your employer pay you while off work?   ☐ Yes, pre-accident wages   ☐ Yes, revised rate of pay   ☐ No   ☐ Unknown

Revised rate of pay: $ _____ per _____

b. Date you **first** missed work: *(Year / Month / Day)* | | | | | | | c. If you have returned to work indicate date: *(Year / Month / Day)* | | | | | | |

Current work status: ☐ Regular work duties, *or* ☐ **Modified** work duties   ☐ Regular hours of work, *or* ☐ **Modified** hours of work: _____ hrs per _____

If you are working **modified** duties please describe:

Approximate date you expect to return to work: *(Year / Month / Day)* | | | | |

Is your expected return to work: ☐ Within 2 weeks   ☐ 2-8 weeks   ☐ 2-6 months   ☐ 6+ months   ☐ Unknown

Employment Type Details   **(Complete A or B or C. Select your type of employment.)**

9 **A** Permanent position employed 12 months of the year:

☐ Permanent full-time   ☐ Permanent part-time   ☐ Irregular/casual

or **B** Non-permanent position employed only part of the year (subject to seasonal or lack of work layoffs):

☐ Seasonal worker   ☐ Summer student   ☐ Temporary position

Had this injury not occurred, your last day of employment would have been:

Position start: *(Year / Month / Day)* | | | | | | Position end: *(Year / Month / Day)* | | | | | | ☐ Estimated, *or* ☐ Actual

How many months or days are workers employed in this position? _____

or **C** Special employment circumstance:

☐ Sub contractor   ☐ Vehicle owner/operator   ☐ Welder owner/operator   ☐ Commission   ☐ Piece work   ☐ Volunteer   ☐ Self-employed

Do you incur expenses to perform the work (materials, tools, etc.)?   ☐ Yes   ☐ No   Will you receive a T4?   ☐ Yes   ☐ No

Note: If you have checked any box in 8C please submit a detailed income and expense statement.

Earning Details

a. Your rate of pay at time of accident: $ [   ] per   ☐ Hour   ☐ Day   ☐ Week   ☐ Month   ☐ Year

10 b. Additional taxable **benefits**:

Vacation pay: _____   ☐ Taken as time off with pay   ☐ Paid on a regular basis % [   ]

☐ Shift premium   Please describe:

☐ Overtime

☐ Other

c. Do you have a second job?   ☐ Yes   ☐ No   If yes – Employer's name: Phone:
(Second employer may be contacted)

d. Did you miss time from this second job?   ☐ Yes   ☐ No   If yes, please attach earning information and time missed details.

Complete all three pages and sign the form before sending.

REV NOV 2018

Fig. 7.16, cont'd

Please fill in your name, Social Insurance Number and date of birth at the top of each page of the form in case the pages get separated.

Remember to complete all three pages and sign the form before sending.

WORKER REPORT Page 3 of 3

Worker's last name:	Worker's first name:	Initial:

Social Insurance #:	Date of birth: *(Year / Month / Day)*

Hours of Work Details

11 a. Number of hours (not including overtime): _____ per week

Describe your work schedule (e.g., Monday to Friday, on. Saturday to Sunday, off.):

_____

Declaration and Consent

I declare that the information in the Worker Report of Injury or Occupational Disease form will be true and correct.

I understand that:

- While I am receiving any **benefits** from WCB-Alberta, it is my obligation to inform WCB-Alberta immediately if I return to work of any kind, become capable of working or if there is any other change in my employment status. Work includes but is not limited to any activity in which labour or services are provided, whether or not payment of any kind is received.

- Criminal prosecution may result from any attempt on my part to collect **benefits** by providing false information, failing to provide information regarding my ability to work, or other fraudulent means.

- My employer may request a review or appeal of any decisions made on my claim and may therefore examine my claim **file**. My claim **file** may also be examined by anyone with a direct interest, as determined by WCB-Alberta, or a person or company I have authorized to review my claim **file**. (To provide authorization, use the Worker's Information Release form in the *Worker Handbook*).

- My social insurance number may be used for reporting to Canada Revenue Agency.

- WCB-Alberta may collect information that it considers relevant to determine **benefit** entitlement, including information pre-dating my accident, from any source including physicians, other health care providers, employer(s) and vocational rehabilitation service providers. This information is collected to determine my entitlement to compensation under the *Workers' Compensation Act*.

WCB-Alberta may use and disclose the information collected to determine entitlement, to provide services and **benefits** and, as required or authorized by law. This information may be used and disclosed pursuant to the *Workers' Compensation Act* and the *Freedom of Information and Protection of Privacy Act*.

Date: *(Year / Month / Day)* _____ Name (please print): _____

Signature: _____

Signing the above consent enables the Workers' Compensation Board to process your claim.

NOTE: The information required in the *Worker Report of Injury or Occupational Disease* is collected under sections 33(a) and (c) of the *Freedom of Information and Protection of Privacy Act* for the purpose of determining entitlement to compensation and for determining employers' premium rates. Questions may be directed to the Claims Contact Centre as noted on the front of this form and on the back of the *Worker Handbook*. The information provided to the Workers' Compensation Board is protected by the provisions of the *Freedom of Information and Protection of Privacy Act*.

If your injury was sustained in an automobile accident, fill out and send an Automobile Accident Report along with the Worker Report.

C 0 6 0 REV NOV 2018

Fig. 7.16, cont'd

**wsib
cspaat**
ONTARIO

Mail To: OR Fax To:
200 Front Street West   416-344-4684
Toronto ON M5V 3J1   OR 1-888-313-7373

Please PRINT in black ink

7

Employer's Report
of Injury/Disease (Form 7)

Claim Number

A. Worker Information

Job Title/Occupation (at the time of accident/illness - do not use abbreviations)

Start >

Length of time in this position
while working for you

Social Insurance Number

Please check **if** this worker is a: ☐ executive   ☐ elected official   ☐ owner   ☐ spouse or relative of the employer

Last Name   First Name

Address (number, street, apt., suite, unit)

City/Town   Province   Postal Code

Is the worker covered by a
Union/Collective Agreement?
☐ yes ☐ no

Worker's preferred language
☐ English ☐ French
☐ Other

Sex ☐ M ☐ F

Worker Reference Number

Date of Birth   dd   mm   yy

Telephone

Date of Hire   dd   mm   yy

Fold here for
#10 envelope

B. Employer Information

Trade and Legal Name (if different provide both)

Check one: ☐ Firm Number **OR** ☐ Account Number   Provide Number

Mailing Address

Rate Group Number   Classification Unit Code

City/Town   Province   Postal Code   Telephone

Description of Business Activity

Does your firm have 20 or more workers? ☐ yes ☐ no

FAX Number

Branch Address where worker is based (if different from mailing address - no abbreviations)

City/Town   Province   Postal Code   Alternate Telephone

C. Accident/Illness Dates and Details

1. Date and hour of accident/Awareness of illness   dd   mm   yy   ☐ AM ☐ PM

2. Who was the accident/illness reported to? (Name & Position)

Date and hour reported to employer   dd   mm   yy   ☐ AM ☐ PM

Telephone   Ext.

3. Was the accident/illness:
☐ Sudden Specific Event/Occurrence
☐ Gradually Occurring Over Time
☐ Occupational Disease
☐ Fatality

4. Type of accident/illness: **(Please check all that apply)**
☐ Struck/Caught   ☐ Fall   ☐ Slip/Trip
☐ Overexertion   ☐ Harmful Substances/Environmental ☐ Motor Vehicle Incident
☐ Repetition   ☐ Assault
☐ Fire/Explosion   ☐ Other

5. Area of Injury (Body Part) - **(Please check all that apply)**

☐ Head   ☐ Teeth   ☐ Upper back
☐ Face   ☐ Neck   ☐ Lower back
☐ Eye(s)   ☐ Chest   ☐ Abdomen
☐ Ear(s)   ☐ Pelvis
☐ Other

Left ☐ Shoulder ☐ Right   Left ☐ Wrist ☐ Right   Left ☐ Hip ☐ Right   Left ☐ Ankle ☐ Right
     ☐ Arm   ☐ Hand   ☐ Thigh   ☐ Foot
     ☐ Elbow   ☐ Finger(s)   ☐ Knee   ☐ Toe(s)
     ☐ Forearm   ☐ Lower Leg

6. Describe what happened to cause the accident/illness and what the worker was doing at the time (lifting a 50 lb. box, slipped on wet floor, repetitive movements, etc...). Include what the injury is and any details of equipment, materials, environmental conditions (work area, temperature, noise, chemical, gas, fumes, other person) that may have contributed. **For a condition that occurred gradually over time, please attach a description of the physical activity required to do the work.**

0007A (01/11)   **A guide to complete this form is available at www.wsib.on.ca**   *next page*   Page 1 of 4

• **Fig. 7.17** Employer's Report of Injury/Disease. (Source: © 1998-2018, Workplace Safety and Insurance Board of Ontario. All rights reserved. Retrieved from: http://www.wsib.on.ca/cs/groups/public/documents/staticfile/c2li/mdey/~edisp/wsib012386.pdf.)

**wsib
cspaat**
ONTARIO

7 **Employer's Report**
of Injury/Disease (Form 7)

Claim Number

Please PRINT in black ink

Worker Name

Social Insurance Number

C. Accident/Illness Dates and Details (Continued)

7. Did the accident/illness happen on the employer's premises (owned, leased or maintained)?
Start > ☐ yes ☐ no

Specify where (shop floor, warehouse, client/customer site, parking lot, etc..).

8. Did the accident/illness happen outside the Province of Ontario?
☐ yes ☐ no

If **yes,** where (city, province/state, country).

9. Are you aware of any witnesses or other employees involved in this accident/illness?
☐ yes ☐ no

If **yes,** provide name(s), position(s), and work phone number(s).
1. _____
_____
2. _____

10. Was any individual, who does not work for your firm, partially or totally responsible for this accident/illness?
☐ yes ☐ no

If **yes,** please provide name and work phone number
_____

11. Are you aware of any prior similar or related problem, injury or condition?
☐ yes ☐ no

If **yes,** please explain
_____

12. If you have concerns about this claim, attach a written submission to this form. ☐ submission attached

---

D. Health Care

1. Did the worker receive health care for this injury?
☐ yes ☐ no   If **yes,** when :   dd mm yy

2. When did the employer learn that the worker received health care?   dd mm yy

3. Where was the worker treated for this injury? **(Please check all that apply)**
☐ On-site health care   ☐ Ambulance   ☐ Emergency department   ☐ Admitted to hospital   ☐ Health professional office   ☐ Clinic
☐ Other: _____

Name, address and phone number of health professional or facility who treated this worker (if known)   _____

E. Lost Time - No Lost Time

1. Please choose one of the following indicators.   **After the day of accident/awareness of illness, this worker:**

☐ Returned to his/her **regular job** and **has not** lost any time and/or earnings. **(Complete sections G and J).**
☐ Returned to **modified work** and **has not** lost any time and/or earnings. **(Complete sections F, G, and J).**
☐ **Has** lost time and/or earnings. **(Complete ALL remaining sections).**

▶ Provide date worker first lost time   dd mm yy

▶ Date worker returned to work (if known)   dd mm yy   ☐ regular work ☐ modified work

2. This Lost Time - No Lost Time - Modified Work information was confirmed by:
☐ Myself   ☐ Other   Name _____   Telephone   Ext.

F. Return To Work

1. Have you been provided with work limitations for this worker's injury?
☐ yes ☐ no

2. Has modified work been discussed with this worker?
☐ yes ☐ no

3. Has modified work been offered to this worker?
☐ yes ☐ no

If **yes,** was it ☐ Accepted ☐ Declined
☐ If Declined please attach a copy of the written offer given to the worker.

4. Who is responsible for arranging worker's return to work
☐ Myself   ☐ Other   Name _____   Telephone   Ext.

0007A (01/11)

next page

Fig. 7.17, cont'd

wsib
cspaat
ONTARIO

7 **Employer's Report**
of Injury/Disease (Form 7)

Claim Number

Please PRINT in black ink

Worker Name

Social Insurance Number

G. Base Wage/Employment Information - (Do not include overtime here)

1. Is this worker **(Please check all that apply)**

Start >

☐ Permanent Full Time
☐ Permanent Part Time
☐ Temporary Full Time
☐ Temporary Part Time

☐ Casual/Irregular
☐ Seasonal
☐ Contract

☐ Student
☐ Unpaid/Trainee
☐ Other _____

☐ Registered Apprentice
☐ Optional Insurance

☐ Owner Operator or
(Sub) Contractor

2. Regular rate of pay $ _____   per   ☐ hour   ☐ day   ☐ week   ☐ other _____

H. Additional Wage Information

1. Net Claim Code
or Amount   Federal [_____]   Provincial [_____]

2. Vacation pay
- on each cheque?   ☐ yes ☐ no   Provide percentage _____ %

3. Date and hour last worked
dd   mm   yy
☐ AM ☐ PM

4. Normal working hours on last day worked
From _____   To _____
☐ AM ☐ PM

5. Actual earnings for last day worked
$ _____
☐ AM ☐ PM

6. Normal earnings for last day worked
$ _____

7. Advances on wages:
Is the worker being paid while he/she recovers?   ☐ yes   ☐ no   If yes, indicate: ☐ Full/Regular   ☐ Other _____

8. **Other Earnings (Not Regular Wages):** Provide the **total of additional earnings** for each week for the 4 weeks before the accident/illness.

＊ For Rotational Shift workers - If the shift cycle exceeds 4 weeks, please attach the earnings information for the last complete shift cycle prior to the date of accident/illness.

▼ Use these spaces for any other earnings (indicate Commission, Differentials, Premiums, Bonus, Tips, In Lieu %, etc..).

Period	From Date (dd/mm/yy)	To Date (dd/mm/yy)	Mandatory Overtime Pay	Voluntary Overtime Pay	Commission	Commission	Commission	Commission
Week 1			$	$	$	$	$	$
Week 2			$	$	$	$	$	$
Week 3			$	$	$	$	$	$
Week 4			$	$	$	$	$	$

I. Work Schedule (Complete either A, B or C. Do not include overtime shifts)

☐ **(A.) Regular Schedule** - Indicate normal work days and hours.

Sunday	Monday	Tuesday	Wednesday	Thursday	Friday	Saturday

▶ **Example:** Monday to Friday, 40 hours

S	M	T	W	T	F	S
	8	8	8	8	8	

or,

☐ **(B.) Repeating Rotational Shift Worker** - Provide

NUMBER OF DAYS ON	NUMBER OF DAYS OFF	HOURS PER SHIFT(s)	NUMBER OF WEEKS IN CYCLE

▶ **Example:** 4 days on, 4 days off, 12 hours per shift, 8 weeks in cycle.

or,

☐ **(C.) Varied or Irregular Work Schedule** - Provide the total number of regular hours and shifts for each week for the 4 weeks prior to the accident/illness. (Do not include overtime hours or shifts here).

	Week 1	Week 2	Week 3	Week 4
From/To Dates (dd/mm/yy)	/	/	/	/
Total Hours Worked				
Total Shifts Worked				

J. It is an offence to deliberately make false statements to the Workplace Safety and Insurance Board. I declare that all of the information provided on pages 1, 2, and 3 is true.

Name of person completing this report (please print) _____   Official title _____

Signature _____
Please print form & sign before returning to the WSIB

Telephone _____   Ext. _____   Date   dd   mm   yy

THE WORKPLACE SAFETY AND INSURANCE ACT REQUIRES YOU GIVE A COPY OF THIS FORM TO YOUR WORKER

0007A (01/11)   *next page*   Page 3 of 4

Fig. 7.17, cont'd

wsib cspaat
ONTARIO

7 **Employer's Report of Injury/Disease (Form 7)**

Claim Number

Please PRINT in black ink

Worker Name

Social Insurance Number

K. Additional Information

Start >

Fig. 7.17, cont'd

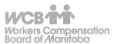

Workers Compensation Board of Manitoba

Phone 204-954-4100
(Toll free 1-855-954-4321)
333 Broadway, Winnipeg R3C 4W3
wcb.mb.ca

Doctor First Report

Claim Number	4

Worker Information

Last Name	First Name	
Address		City
Province	Postal Code	Phone Number	Date of Birth (dd/mm/yyyy)
Gender		Weight	Height
Job Title		PHIN	

Employer Information

Name	Address
City	Province	Postal Code

Injury Details

Date of Incident	Area of Injury
Worker's Description of Incident or Injury	

Examination Findings and Diagnosis

Date of Examination	ICD Code	Diagnosis
Subjective Complaints		
Objective Findings (include ROM, muscle testing & neurological status)		
Describe any pre-existing condition that may affect recovery		
Tests Performed (e.g., X-Ray, CT Scan, MRI, etc.) Attach results	Location	Date

Treatment Plan

Description	Date of next visit

Work Abilities

Will worker be disabled from work beyond the date of incident as a result of the injury? ☐ Yes ☐ No	When can worker return to regular duties? Date ☐ Unknown at time of examination
Is worker capable of alternate or modified work? ☐ Yes ☐ No If yes, outline restrictions:	Duration of restrictions weeks

Physician Information

Physician Name	Address		
Physician Signature	City	Province	Postal Code
	Phone Number	Fax Number	Date

WCB 4036

• **Fig. 7.18** Health Professional's First Report. (Source: Workers Compensation Board of Manitoba. All rights reserved. Retrieved from https://www.wcb.mb.ca/sites/default/files/resources/6334%20WCB%20 Doctor%20First%20Report%20LR.pdf.)

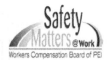

Worker's Authorization For Release Of Information – FORM B

Print, complete and submit this form by mail, fax or in person to:
P.O. Box 757, 14 Weymouth Street, Charlottetown, PE, C1A 7L7
www.wcb.pe.ca

Phone: (902) 368-5680
Fax: (902) 368-5696

Case ID#:	
Worker's Name:	Phone Number:
Address:	City:
Province:	Postal Code:

☐ I hereby authorize the Workers Compensation Board to discuss my claim with the following named authorized representative(s). I understand this authorization will remain in effect until I notify the WCB that it is no longer in effect.

1.	
2.	
3.	
4.	

Worker's Signature:	
Date Signed:	

Personal information on this form is collected in accordance with section 31 of the *Freedom of Information and Protection of Privacy Act* for the purpose of administering claim file releases. For further information about the collection of personal information, please contact the Workers Compensation Board's FOIPP Coordinator at P.O. Box 757, Charlottetown, PE, C1A 7L7 or telephone (902) 368-5680.

Case files for workers will be released in accordance with section 83 of the *Workers Compensation Act* and the Workers Compensation Board Policy, POL-04, Access To Information – Worker Claim Files.

Do not email sensitive information.

CL-05
March 2018

• **Fig. 7.19** Worker's Authorization for Release of Information. (Source: Wssorkers Compensation Board of Prince Edward Island. Retrieved from http://www.wcb.pe.ca/DocumentManagement/Document/frm_workersauthorizationforreleaseofinformationformb.pdf.)

3. Prescription drug plan (available on a group basis), to help protect group subscribers and their families against the costs of prescribed drugs and injectables.
4. Vision care plan (available on a group basis), to provide payment toward the purchase of eyeglasses and contact lenses.
5. Dental plan (available on a group basis).
6. Nursing home plan (available on a group basis).
7. Allied health services such as chiropractic and massage therapy services.
8. Health plan for visitors (on an individual or a family basis), designed to provide visitors to Canada with protection against unexpected costs of hospital care.
9. Health plan for Canadians while travelling outside of Canada (on an individual or a family basis), designed to protect people from unexpected costs of medical bills incurred while on business or vacation anywhere outside of Canada.

A general knowledge of what is available through third-party insurance companies is an asset. Although each private company offers its own plan, most benefits offered are very similar.

How the Ministry of Health Communicates With Medical Administrative Assistants

The MoH communicates with medical administrative assistants in various ways. The following is a list of some of these ways:
1. Provincial Fee Schedule—The current fee schedule typically is available online through the MoH website in a downloadable PDF format. See the provincial and territorial links provided earlier in the chapter.
2. Bulletins—These are available when changes such as updates in rules or fees are made.
3. Brochures/Posters/Forms—Available for a variety of subjects. Additional copies are available from your local ministry office. Also available are all forms mentioned earlier in this chapter.
4. Claim Submission Manuals—Available in an online downloadable format from the local MoH. This manual assists administrative assistants in completing claims.
5. Some provinces use interactive voice response (IVR), which is available to registered providers, to validate health card numbers or time-limited service codes. The IVR system is accessed by a touch-tone phone.

Summary

As this chapter demonstrates, the Canada health care system is not a single entity; it comprises several agencies at the provincial/territorial and federal levels. The federal bodies oversee the administration and governance of health care and the transfer of payments to the provinces and territories. The provinces and territories are responsible for the delivery of health care services. These various levels of government work in harmony to build the cohesive system that forms the health care landscape of Canada.

All of the preceding information will prove helpful once you begin your work as a medical administrative assistant. It is intended as a basic outline only. As in all professions, additional on-the-job training must be gained before you are proficient in your field.

Remember that your local MoH office is available for any assistance it can provide.

Assignments

Assignment 7.1

With the assistance of your instructor, locate the physicians' fee schedule for your province or territory. Find the section that relates to General Practice (this may also be called *Family Medicine, Family Practice,* or something similar). Locate five of the seven common visit types (or similar visit types) mentioned in the Service Codes section. These were 1) general assessment or comprehensive office visit, 2) intermediate assessment or limited office visit, 3) minor assessment or brief office visit, 4) psychotherapy or mental health assessment, 5) well baby care, 6) annual health examination, and 7) prenatal assessment. Remember, you will have to refer to the preamble for definitions of each type. Note the associated fee code, dollar amount, and rules or guidelines related to the visit type.

If you have access to an EMR, your instructor will provide the information you require to practice adding these and other visit types to your EMR.

Assignment 7.2

With the assistance of your instructor, locate your provincial or territorial Health Professional's Report for workers' compensation. Using the following information, complete the Health Professional's Report and the MoH claim.

On February 16, 20__, Tim Peters was involved in an industrial accident. Dr. Plunkett was doing rounds at the hospital (no. 1220), and Tim was transported to the hospital for examination. On examination, it was discovered that he had a severe sprain in his left ankle. The doctor recommended bed rest for one week, after which time he felt Tim would be able to return to work. Dr. Plunkett feels that three weeks of physiotherapy (twice weekly) will be required to restore the muscles in the ankle.

Tim Peter's social insurance number is 416 274 963. He is employed at Smith and Smith Limited, 372 Parkview Drive; insert your province or territorial location. A claim number has not yet been issued. Dr. Plunkett first saw Tim at 1535.

Topics for Discussion

1. A patient arrives in the office for a visit. He has travelled over 300 kilometers for this visit and is complaining to you of the cost to him. How would you handle this situation?
2. Your office health care claims are sent by EDT. It is almost the end of your billing cycle, and the computer system has crashed. You still have to submit your claims. Is there anything you can do?
3. Your physician has given you a billing to submit. He saw the patient on a Sunday at 1730 in the hospital. He has given you the service code and diagnosis. What further details do you need to complete this billing?
4. Mr. Thomas has been sent to your office with an injury that occurred at work. What do you need to complete this billing?
5. Your physician has brought you some hospital billings that were found in his home office. You notice the dates are two days past the cutoff timeline for your province. What will you do?

Assignment 7.3

Your instructor will provide you the material required to complete this assignment.

Assignment 7.4

If your class is interested in more detailed information about third-party insurance, appoint a group to arrange for representatives of private insurance companies to visit your class to expand on the benefits offered by their particular organizations.

References

World Health Organization. (2018). *Classifications.* Retrieved from https://www.who.int/classifications/icd/en/.

8

Financial Records

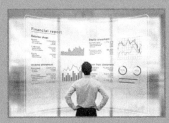

In a medical environment, patient records are commonly our primary focus. Alternatively, financial records are of substantial importance from both the business and regulatory perspectives. The topics covered in this chapter will identify typical tasks associated with the development and management of standard financial records.

CHAPTER OUTLINE

Introduction

Managing Finances in the Medical Office

Banking

Payroll

LEARNING OBJECTIVES

After reading this chapter, you will be able to:

1. Describe how to perform basic bookkeeping procedures
2. Describe how to manage accounts payable and receivable
3. Describe how to manage petty cash
4. Describe how to administer banking procedures
5. Describe how to direct payroll activities using standard deduction tables
6. Describe how to comply with Canada Revenue Agency remittance activities

KEY TERMS

Accounts receivable: The money due to the office.

Accounts payable: The money owed or paid out by the office.

Disbursement: The money that is being paid out.

EMV chip technology: A method of payment using tools such as a card with an embedded microchip.

Invoice: An itemized list of prices and charges owed.

Remittance: The money that is being paid to the facility.

Remote deposit capture (RDC): This permits deposit of cheques anytime, from the office with a computer or with a mobile app and a compatible scanner.

Statement: A financial accounting sheet.

Transaction: An exchange or transfer of goods, services, or funds.

Introduction

It is essential for any business to keep accurate and complete financial records. Large organizations such as hospitals, clinics, and health service organizations employ accountants and have a separate finance department because their accounting systems are very complex. Generally, a small service organization maintains an adequate set of accounting records to enable an accountant to complete the financial statements and process the proprietor's income tax returns.

The system of recording and summarizing business and financial transactions and analyzing, verifying, and reporting the results is known as *accounting*. The financial records maintained by the staff in a medical office will be transferred to an accountant for processing.

Your role as a medical administrative assistant in most instances will require organized and accurate record keeping for financial transactions for accountant processing. This chapter will explore the standard records and processes to follow for accurate financial reporting.

Managing Finances in the Medical Office

Businesses in Canada are required to maintain and retain organized financial records. According to current taxation laws, these financial records are retained for a period of six years from the end of the year they relate to.

As explored in Chapter 7, most doctors in Canada receive compensation by submitting invoices generated through the billing component of their electronic medical records (EMR) system, reflective of services provided to patients. Under this fee-for-service model, each provincial or territorial health insurance plan reimburses the physician. From a business perspective, each patient visit is considered a financial transaction. Comparatively, each office supply order is also a financial transaction because a payment for this service is required. Record keeping for all of these transactions is essential for effective operational management.

The medical administrative assistant at a physician's office or medical facility may be responsible for maintaining a bookkeeping system, including accounts receivable and accounts payable. Accounts receivable is the money due to the office. Accounts payable is the money owed or paid out by the office. A medical administrative assistant in a solo, partnership, or group proprietorship practice should be knowledgeable about single-entry bookkeeping, writing cheques, bank deposits, petty cash records, completing patients' accounts and statements, and bank reconciliations. As a recommendation, manage these basic accounting functions at a quieter time or in a private location within the office away from patient view.

Financial management refers to the day-to-day operations as well as the long-term direction of the medical office. For accurate financial management, reporting is used for external and internal purposes. When used for internal purposes, financial reports help with forecasting by management for planning and projecting outcomes. See Fig. 8.1 showing financial business components.

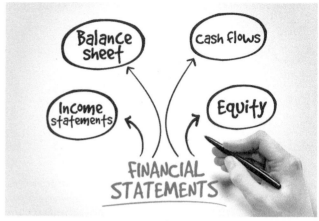

• **Fig. 8.1** Financial Records and Statements. (Source: © CanStock Photo Inc./dizanna.)

In medical offices today, accounting procedures are automated and include medical plan and third-party billing, reconciliation, cash receipts disbursements, cheque preparation, and so on.

Computerized Accounting Systems

Primarily, financial billing matters are managed through the EMR system in the office. Additional financial tracking and record keeping, such as payroll and expenses, are performed using an electronic bookkeeping system. A needs-based analysis is considered when selecting an electronic system for bookkeeping tasks. Small-business accounting systems like QuickBooks can perform several tasks, such as monitoring cash flow and tracking inventory and expenses; they can prepare cheques and perform bank reconciliation and payroll functions.

Many accounting systems have customizable options specific to the medical field. Here are three items to keep in mind when selecting a system:
1. **Costs.** Consider the expense of the basic accounting software or web application compared with the benefits it provides.
2. **Usability.** How many users need to access the software? Do you prefer a cloud-based system you can access anywhere or desktop software? Is a mobile app required?
3. **Features.** What do you need the accounting software program to do? Do you need both accounts receivable and accounts payable tools?

Disbursements Journal

In a single-entry bookkeeping system, a multicolumn journal is maintained to record all expenditures. Review Fig. 8.2. This is a cash disbursements journal. Using the journal, you record where the money is spent. The payment entry is extended into a column that groups similar payouts. The accountant who sets up your doctor's accounting records will suggest basic column headings for disbursements. On a typical day in the doctor's office, you might record the following transaction in your disbursements journal.

Disbursement Journal

Date	Number	Description	Category	Amount
2/24/2020	100	Scotia bank	Fees	$155.65
2/26/2020	101	City Power & Light	Electricity	$85.00
2/27/2020	102	Medical Insurance	Insurance	$100.00
2/27/2020	103	Office Supplies	Office Supplies	$1,200.00
2/27/2020	104	Courier	Office Supplies	$23.00
2/27/2020	105	Petty Cash	Office Supplies	$68.00
3/3/2020	108	ISP	Internet	$123.00
3/3/2020	109	Litware, Inc.	Office Supplies	$99.00
3/3/2020	112	Medical Equipment	Office Supplies	$100.00
Totals				$1,953.65

• **Fig. 8.2** Disbursement Journal.

February 27, 20__, Courier Services for $23.00. This transaction has been recorded in Fig. 8.2 using the procedures outlined in the next paragraph:

The date is entered into the first column, on line five of the table; following along horizontally, the item "number" (104) is entered—the "description" (Courier) is entered in the next column, followed by the category (Office supplies) of the expense, and finally the "amount" ($23.00) is entered.

DID YOU KNOW?

Bookkeeping is the only English word to contain three sets of double letters back-to-back-to-back without the use of hyphens.

Accounts Payable

A safe and convenient way to handle the payment of accounts is payment by cheque. Alternatively, electronic funds transfer (e-transfer) using an online banking feature

available to the business is also a supported method of payment. These methods are appropriate because an office will not have large amounts of cash on hand and you can eliminate the possibility of theft and loss. Pay attention to the terms of payment listed on invoices received in the office. Some suppliers offer discounts if the bill is paid within a period set by the supplier, such as a 2% reduction if paid in 15 days. Be aware of all payment terms because a fee may be added to the invoice if the bill is paid late. Set up a routine schedule to review your accounts payable to ensure that you both comply with the terms included on the invoice and avoid overpayments.

Mailing a cheque or utilizing an e-transfer of funds rather than making a personal visit to pay cash is usually a more efficient business practice. Never put cash in the mail. Depending on the office setup, manual handwritten cheques similar to those shown in Fig. 8.3 may be used by the business. A business cheque consists of both the cheque and a perforated stub, which is retained and serves as a place to record the details of the payment. Many practices have migrated to a computer-generated

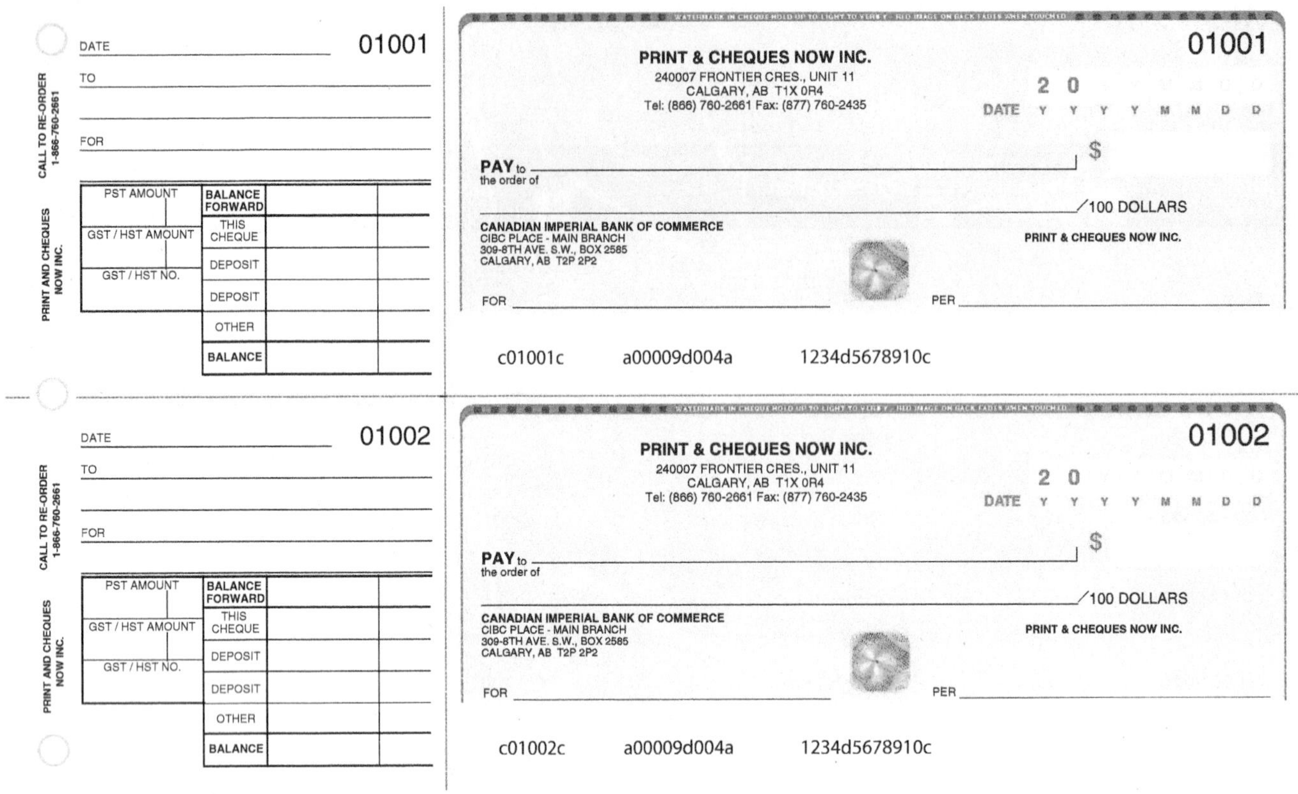

• **Fig. 8.3** Business Cheques. (Source: Print and Cheques Now Inc.)

cheque entry. When using a manual cheque preparation system, a running balance is kept on the cheque stub. This allows you to double-check your accounting accuracy. The cheque number, amount, name of person to whom the cheque is issued, and purpose of the cheque also appear on the stub. On the actual cheque, the amount of the cheque in figures, as well as in words, and the payer's signature must be recorded.

In a computerized system, the cheque is written and automatically posted to the chosen account. The program then balances the account.

CRITICAL THINKING

The accountant for your facility has prepared the year-end financial operating statement reflective of business activity. You are reviewing these documents and notice a calculation error. Would you address it or leave it for someone else to notice? If you decide to address it, how would you approach this?

Accounts Receivable—Patients' Charges

Not all services provided by a medical facility are covered by the provincial or territorial billing schedule, and coverage does vary throughout Canada dependent on the service provided and by whom. When a physician performs an uninsured service, an invoice is generated to bill the service directly to the patient or others using the private billing feature offered through the practice's EMR. Patients need to be aware of uninsured services charges. As a best practice, offices will prepare an annual newsletter or post information about

---

• BOX 8.1 Uninsured Services

Telephone advice
Prescription renewal by telephone (at patient's request)
Tax disability forms
Long-distance phone calls or fax (at patient's request)
Transfer of medical records
Private insurance forms
Return to Work form
Third-party medical examinations (adult)
Drivers' medical examinations
Employment physicals
University/college physicals
Camp physicals
Photocopies
Summary of records requested by a third party
Procedures that are not deemed medically necessary

---

these services and the revolving cost associated. It is the policy of many facilities to require payment up front for uninsured services prior to the services rendered. Ensure that this information is conveyed to patients in written form. The provincial or territorial College of Physicians and Surgeons has policy recommendations on how to manage uninsured billing procedures. Be sure to provide an invoice to all patients paying for uninsured services. The office may choose to waive fees for uninsured services on compassionate grounds due to a patient's inability to pay. The EMR will keep an accurate, reliable record of all charges and payments for all patients. See Box 8.1 for a listing of common uninsured services. The list may vary depending on province and territory.

Dr. JE. Plunkett
Petty Cash Record

Balance $100.00

Date	Receipt No.	Description	Amount Deposited	Amount Withdrawn	Charged To	Received By	Approved By
January 2, 20xx	1011	Deposit to petty cash	$100.00		petty cash		Mary Baker
Total	1		$100.00	$0.00			

• **Fig. 8.4** Petty Cash Record.

As previously explained, the office submits a fee for each patient to the local health ministry and is reimbursed for these charges when his or her monthly medical insurance payment is received. This amount is usually deposited directly into the physician's bank account or facility business account.

At the end of each month, the administrative assistant should review the outstanding billing accounts of uninsured services and send a statement from the private billing report in the EMR system to those who show a balance owing. A statement of account form generated from the EMR may vary in its format, but the information statement is generally the same (see itemized list that follows):

1. Name of statement
2. Originator's name, address, and telephone number
3. The date the statement is issued
4. Name and address of the debtor
5. Date of each service
6. Explanation of the service
7. Amount of the charges
8. Amount of any payment received
9. Balance owed
10. Notification of service charge for overdue accounts

Petty Cash

Medical offices maintain a small petty cash fund to purchase stamps, coffee supplies, and so on. It is essential that an accurate record be maintained for the petty cash. This does not have to be elaborate, but simply a record of the amount received to replenish the fund and a record of what payments were made from the fund (see Fig. 8.4). A petty cash voucher is usually a small form that is used to document a disbursement from the petty cash fund. The voucher is referred to as a *petty cash receipt*. The petty cash voucher should provide space for the date, amount disbursed, name of person receiving the money, reason for the disbursement, account to be charged, and the initials of the person disbursing the money from the petty cash fund. A voucher can be numbered for reference and control. As a best practice,

Petty Cash Voucher	No. 100
Amount_____	Date _____
Paid to _____
For _____
_____
Approved by _____

• **Fig. 8.5** Petty Cash Voucher.

receipts and other documentation detailing the disbursement should be attached to the petty cash voucher. See Fig. 8.5 for a sample petty cash voucher.

Steps for Managing Petty Cash

To ensure sound financial practices, follow the steps outlined below when managing petty cash:

1. Secure a storage box with a lock to store cash funds; select a box large enough to store cash and receipts.

2. Determine which staff member is responsible for managing the petty cash fund and replenishing it. As a best practice, it is usually a medical administrative assistant because most employees will have contact with the assistant on a regular and consistent basis.

3. Place the storage box away from common access.

4. Establish a withdrawal limit. Some organizations set a $30 or $40 withdrawal limit. Higher amounts require accounting procedures.

5. Create a petty cash log. This will detail the initial cash deposit; all withdrawals from the fund are recorded as expenses, which are logged along with the dates of all transactions. Divide the log into columns showing the deposits in one column and the expenses in another.

6. Replenish the funds as needed. For instance, if a fund is normally $100, replenish it when the amount on hand drops below $20.

7. Account for all withdrawals from the petty cash fund. This procedure usually involves a receipt for the expenditure. Add the receipts together to verify that the total fund amount matches the petty cash expenditures. The receipts should add up to the difference between the cash on hand and the expenditures.

DID YOU KNOW?

Sometimes a health practice is faced with unpaid accounts. After several unsuccessful attempts to collect the overdue account, a decision must be made whether to put the account into the hands of a collection agency or to write off the account as a bad debt. The facility accountant generally makes this decision and takes the necessary action.

Let us assume that on January 2, 20__, a cheque for $100 was issued to establish a petty cash fund. The entry would be: year at the top of the "Date" column; date, January 2; explanation—cheque no. 124 to establish petty cash; received, $100; balance, $100.

Banking

When a business ownership structure has been established, a bank account is necessary to track and record the financials. A business chequing account is set up to manage expenditures and permit cheque writing, electronic transfers, payroll funding, and deposits. Most financial institutions in Canada offer a selection of business bank account packages. The medical administrative assistant may be asked to research what is available in terms of products and services and to make recommendations. These services include monthly transaction allowances, overdraft protection, and associated fees. Fig. 8.6 shows a bank account small-business application.

As we know, some services necessitate direct billing and will require a payment by cash, credit, debit, or cheque. Each facility will establish a policy surrounding the receipt of payment and the format accepted. The use of EMV chip technology (Europay, MasterCard, and Visa) is globally popular for accepting payments. This technology features payment tools such as cards, which have embedded microprocessing chips that store and protect cardholder data. See Fig. 8.7 showing a financial institution–issued debit/credit card with the chip technology. To use this technology, the office would acquire a point of sale (POS) payment terminal to process these payments (see Fig. 8.8).

Banking Responsibilities

The three main banking duties required of the medical administrative assistant are as follows:
1. Making deposits
2. Cheque preparation
3. Reconciling the monthly bank statement

We discussed cheque writing earlier in this chapter. We will now examine depositing checks and reconciling the bank statement.

Making Deposits

Deposits will mainly consist of the revenue generated by insured and uninsured direct billing. The health ministry will deposit the fee-for-service payments directly into the business account registered for accepting the deposit. In a complementary care setting such as chiropractic, physiotherapy, or massage therapy, the *main* source of revenue is through direct billing to patients/clients or to individual insurance companies. When you receive a cheque, it is a good safety measure to use a "For Deposit Only" stamp on the back of the cheque (see Fig. 8.9). This is a form of endorsement.

If the cheque is lost or stolen but has this stamp on the back, it cannot be cashed. Each time you receive a cheque, you deposit it in the practitioner's business account.

A deposit slip similar to that in Fig. 8.10 may be used; it is completed before the deposit is presented to the bank teller. Most offices use a deposit book (see Fig. 8.11) rather than deposit slips because the slips can be easily misplaced. The deposit information remains part of the book, therefore eliminating this risk.

It is never wise to accept a post-dated cheque. You cannot deposit a postdated cheque until it is due, and collection on a post-dated cheque returned "not sufficient funds" (NSF) can sometimes cause problems.

Technology allows for remote deposit capture (RDC) through financial institutions. This permits deposit of cheques anytime; they can be sent from the office with a computer and a compatible scanner. Additionally, it allows for the deposit of several cheques at one time. It makes life easy for bank customers because deposits are faster and more convenient. Remote deposit is less labor-intensive for banks; the customer creates the image so the bank does not have to. As a word of caution, because you are not bringing cheques to the bank, you have to follow rules about how to handle the cheques after you scan them. Ask your remote deposit service provider for suggestions on how to stay compliant.

Bank Reconciliation

Each month, a bank account statement is available in paper or paperless electronic format that can be downloaded directly into your accounting software program, which typically has a reconciliation feature, depending on your account setup. Banks are not required to return cancelled cheques to customers; many have stopped this practice or charge a fee for this service. Your office may also use a manual system for reconciliation.

The goal of reconciliation is to compare your records of the business account with those of the financial institution. This is achieved by starting with the beginning balance and adding all deposits and subtracting all cheques and associated debits from the account.

In a manual system, divide a sheet of paper in two and write "Bank Balance" on one side and "Chequebook Balance" on the other, or you could also use a spreadsheet system as shown in Fig. 8.12.

ABCBank

Bank Account Application

Business
Name: _____   Date: _____

Business
Address: _____
Street Address

_____
City   *Province*   *Postal Code*

Phone: _____   Email: _____

Sole Proprietor: ☐   Partnership: ☐   Corporation: ☐

Business Number: _____

Authorized Users

Full Name: _____   Title: _____

Employer's
Entity: _____   Authorization
Level: _____

Full Name: _____   Title: _____

Employer's
Entity: _____   Authorization
Level: _____

Full Name: _____   Title: _____

Employer's
Entity: _____   Authorization
Level: _____

Previous Banking

Institution: _____   Branch: _____
Address: _____   Manager: _____

Disclaimer and Signature

I certify that my answers are true and complete to the best of my knowledge.

Signature: _____   Date: _____

• **Fig. 8.6** Business Bank Account Application.

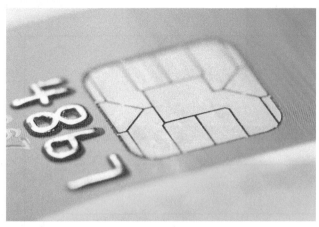

• **Fig. 8.7** EMV Chip Technology Card. (Source: © CanStock Photo Inc./icemanj.)

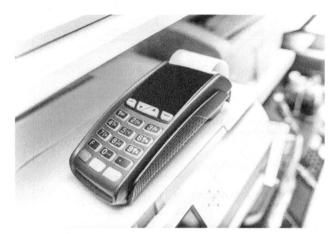

• **Fig. 8.8** Contact Payment Terminal. (Source: © CanStock Photo Inc./believeinme.)

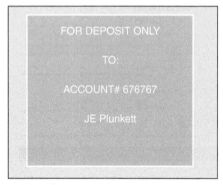

FOR DEPOSIT ONLY

TO:

ACCOUNT# 676767

JE Plunkett

• **Fig. 8.9** "For Deposit Only" Stamp.

On your statement, you see five items that are not checked off. Item (1) is a service charge for $3.50; item (2) is a credit memo for $127.50 for interest you received on your term deposit; item (3) is a debit memo for $200 interest charged on a loan; item (4) is a $5.70 charge for safety deposit box rental; and item (5) is a debit memo for an NSF cheque from Thomas Bell for $165.40.

The procedure to record these items is as follows:

No. 1 The bank has charged you for the service, but you have not recorded the charge on your books. Subtract $3.50 from the chequebook side.

No. 2 A savings deposit at the bank has earned $127.50 interest. The bank has recorded it in your account; now you have to enter the amount in your records. Add to the chequebook side.

No. 3 The bank has made a loan to the business. Two hundred dollars for interest on the loan is deducted from your bank account. You must make an equal deduction from your chequebook record.

No. 4 The bank charges $5.70 yearly for rental of a safety deposit box. The bank has charged your account; you must charge your records with the same amount.

No. 5 A patient, Thomas Bell, gave you a cheque for $165.40. You deposited the cheque in the bank and added the amount to your records. When you received your bank statements, you discovered that Mr. Bell did not have sufficient funds in his account to cover the cheque. It was therefore returned to you. The bank did not add $165.40 to its records. You must therefore subtract the amount from your records.

Items (1), (3), and (4) would be entered in your cash disbursements journal after your statement is reconciled. Although you would not write cheques for these items, you would have to subtract the amounts from your chequebook stubs to keep your running balance accurate. As for item (2), you would record it on your chequebook stub in the deposit space and label it "interest earned." Item (5) would require a follow-up with the patient's record of charges and payments, indicating that the cheque was returned NSF. The amount of the cheque would have to be deducted from the chequebook stub, and an adjustment to Mr. Bell's account would have to be made.

When you examine your chequebook stubs, you discover that three cheques you have written have not been cashed. The cheques are to Smith Office Supplies, $732.60; Jones Medical Service, $1072.91; and the Receiver General of Canada, $427.50.

You have deducted all these cheques from your chequebook. However, because they have not been cashed, the amounts have not been deducted from your bank account. See items (a), (b), and (c) in Fig. 8.12.

Your bank statement was mailed on January 12, and on January 11 you made a deposit of $543.21. You notice that the amount does not appear on your statement. You have added this deposit to your chequebook; you must now add it to your bank statement (d).

Your bank statement and your chequebook balance are now in agreement.

Many offices do not require the completion of a formal printed reconciliation statement. However, you should be aware of the correct format. Based on the information used in Fig. 8.12, a formal keyed bank reconciliation statement would resemble that shown in Fig. 8.13.

At the end of every month, a computerized printout of the general ledger, balance sheet, income statement, and bank reconciliation statement should be available. Often, a comparative income statement and bank statement are completed to show the previous year versus the current year to date.

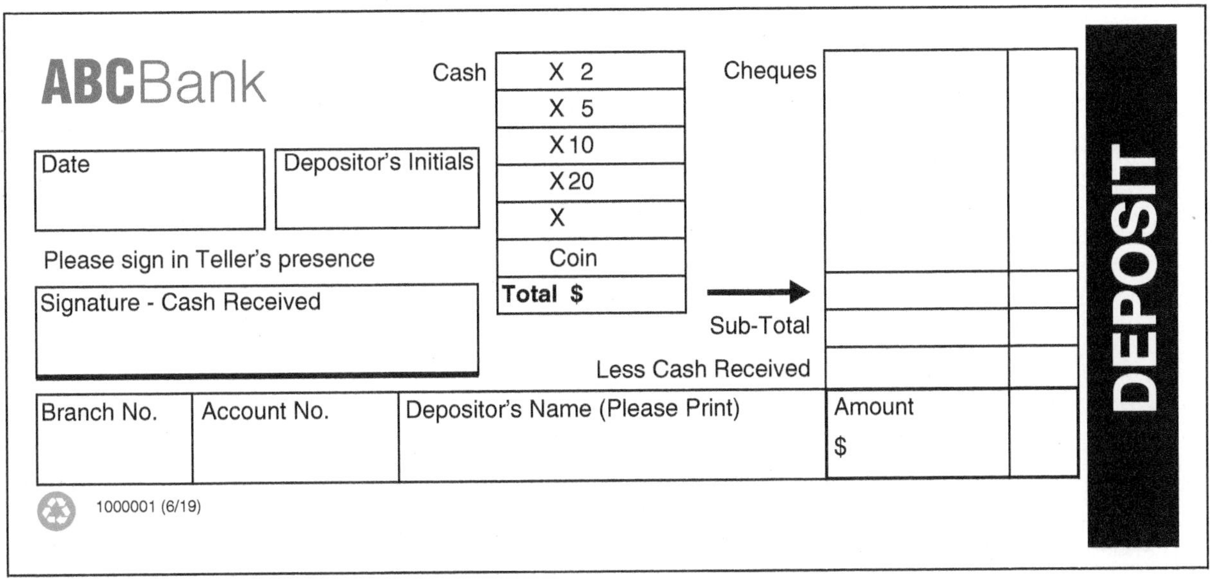

• **Fig. 8.10** Deposit Slip.

DID YOU KNOW?

The words *debits* and *credits* come from the Latin words *debitum* and *creditum*.

Payroll

Payroll refers to employees receiving pay, and to information specific to employee payroll. Processing payroll is an important function of any business and necessitates an understanding of current regulations.

A business with compensated employees is required to open a payroll account with the Canada Revenue Agency (CRA). The business also collects required information from employees, such as their social insurance number (SIN) and their completed electronic federal and provincial TD1 personal tax form found at https://www.canada.ca/en/revenue-agency/services/forms-publications/td1-personal-tax-credits-returns/td1-forms-pay-received-on-january-1-later.html. The electronic forms are revised annually. The TD1 form is used to determine the amount of tax to be deducted from an individual's employment or other income, such as pension. The employee is provided the link for the TD1 form so he or she can complete it and submit it to the employer.

Generally, there are three mandatory deductions: income tax, Employment Insurance (EI), and Canada Pension Plan (CPP). Exemptions involving source deductions exist in Canada. For example, income tax may not be deductible as outlined under section 87 of the Indian Act. An individual who meets the requirements of this act will complete a TD1-IN form. For more information regarding exemptions, refer to https://www.canada.ca/en/revenue-agency/services/aboriginal-peoples/information-indians.html#wb-info.

In the province of Québec, the payroll source deductions include Québec income tax, employer and employee contributions to Québec Pension Plan (QPP), and Québec Parental Insurance Plan (QPIP).

The Government of Canada prepares payroll deduction tables for all three deductions. Guides are no longer published but are available in electronic format at https://www.canada.ca/en/revenue-agency/services/forms-publications/payroll/t4032-payroll-deductions-tables.html. Like the TD1 form, these tables are updated annually. Shown by province or territory, they are based on the new tax year starting on January 1 of each year. The tables are based on monthly, bimonthly, semi-monthly, and weekly payroll periods. Employers are also responsible for a contribution with each employee payroll for EI and CPP. Currently, EI contribution is 1.4 times the employee deduction. CPP and the employer match the employee deduction.

To follow this section of the chapter, download or access a copy of the CPP, EI, and Income Tax Deduction tables using the link provided earlier. These tables are included with most accounting programs.

Before beginning the instructions for payroll, please read the general information section at the beginning of the CPP, EI, and income tax tables. It is essential that anyone working with payroll be familiar with the instructions provided. Because the tables are required to compute any payroll, reprinting the guidelines in this text is unnecessary.

In a large organization, payroll is fairly complicated and requires several employees to process the employee paycheques each pay period. However, in a small organization of, say, 10 or less, the payroll procedure is fairly simple. Many offices use a computerized payroll system. However, for you to understand a payroll process, we are providing information on the manual procedure.

Let us assume that in your office you are the only salaried employee. The doctor does not have a registered nurse. A part-time janitor looks after cleaning and maintenance duties and is paid on an hourly basis.

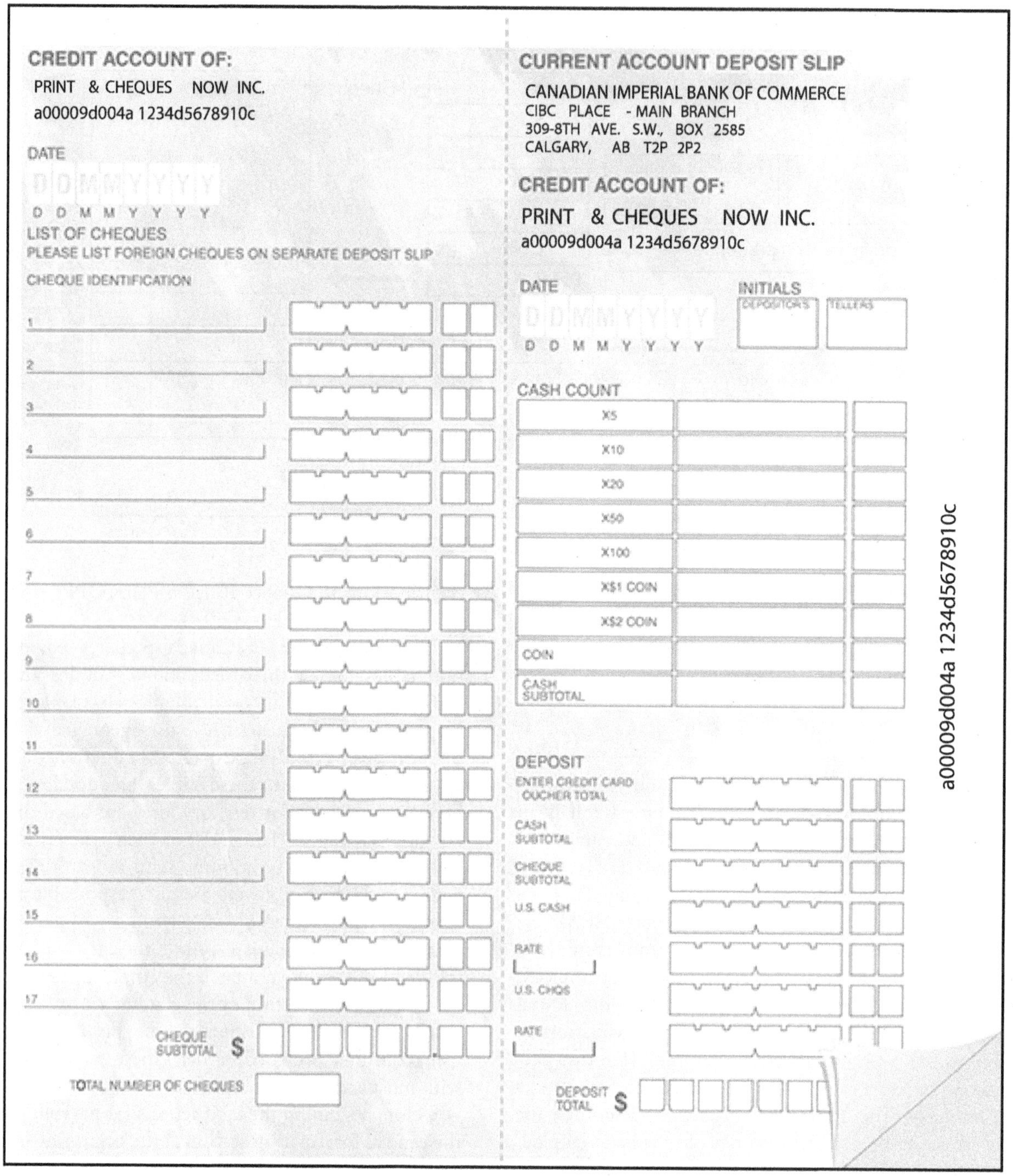

CREDIT ACCOUNT OF:

PRINT & CHEQUES NOW INC.

a00009d004a 1234d5678910c

DATE

D D M M Y Y Y Y

LIST OF CHEQUES

PLEASE LIST FOREIGN CHEQUES ON SEPARATE DEPOSIT SLIP

CHEQUE IDENTIFICATION

CHEQUE SUBTOTAL $

TOTAL NUMBER OF CHEQUES

CURRENT ACCOUNT DEPOSIT SLIP

CANADIAN IMPERIAL BANK OF COMMERCE
CIBC PLACE - MAIN BRANCH
309-8TH AVE. S.W., BOX 2585
CALGARY, AB T2P 2P2

CREDIT ACCOUNT OF:

PRINT & CHEQUES NOW INC.

a00009d004a 1234d5678910c

DATE

D D M M Y Y Y Y

INITIALS
DEPOSITOR'S TELLER'S

CASH COUNT

	X5		
X10		
X20		
X50		
X100		
X$1 COIN		
X$2 COIN		
COIN		
CASH SUBTOTAL		

DEPOSIT

ENTER CREDIT CARD VOUCHER TOTAL

CASH SUBTOTAL

CHEQUE SUBTOTAL

U.S. CASH

RATE

U.S. CHQS

RATE

DEPOSIT TOTAL $

a00009d004a 1234d5678910c

• **Fig. 8.11** Deposit Book. (Source: Deluxe.)

January 13, 20xx

Bank Balance		$2,769.20
Outstanding Cheques		
a. SOS	$732.60	
b. Jones	1,072.91	
c. R. G of		
Canada	427.5	2,233.01
		536.19
d. Jan 11 Deposit		543.21
Bank Balance		**$1,079.40**

Chequebook Balance	$1,326.50
1) Service Charge	−3.50
	1,323.00
2) Interest Earned	127.50
	1,450.50
3) Loan Interest Paid	−200.00
	1,250.50
4) Safety Deposit Box	−5.70
	1,244.80
5) NSF Cheque Thomas Bell	−165.40
Chequebook Balance	**1,079.44**

• **Fig. 8.12** Bank Reconciliation.

J.E. Plunkett
Bank Reconciliation Statement
January 13, 20xx

Balance as per bank statement, January 13		$2,769.20
Add: Deposit of January 11 not recorded by bank		543.21
		$3,312.41
Deduct Outstanding Cheques:		
#236 SOS	$732.60	
#239 Jones Medical Service	1,072.91	
$244 Receiver General of Canada	427.50	
Adjusted Bank Balance		
		2,233.01
		$1.079.40
Balance as per Chequebook, January 13		1326.50
Add interest on term deposit		127.50
		$1,454.00
Deduct: Debit memo for safety deposit box rental	$ 5.70	
Bank interest on loan	200.00	
Monthly service charge	3.50	
NSF Cheque	165.00	374.60
		$1,079.40

• **Fig. 8.13** Bank Reconciliation Statement.

The first step is to complete a TD1 form, which lists your total exemptions and places you in one of the categories in the Income Tax Deduction table represented in columns, which indicates the amount of income tax deductible. The CPP, EI, and tax are calculated according to the pay period, which can be weekly, bi-weekly, semi-monthly, or monthly.

Employee Payroll Statement

An important part of any payroll system is the employee payroll statement. The statement may be attached or electronically available with the employee's payroll date. Fig. 8.14 is an example of an employee payroll statement.

You will note that it gives a complete account of hours worked, earnings, each deduction, and the net amount of

the paycheque. For practice, after you have completed Mr. James's payroll sheet for the two-week period ending January 15, fill in his employee payroll statement on Fig. 8.14.

Payment of EI, CPP, and Income Tax Deductions

Each month, an employer must submit to the Receiver General of Canada in trust the amount of money deducted from employees' payroll, combined with the employer's contribution to CPP and EI. A Statement of Account for Source Deductions, similar to Fig. 8.15, must be completed to accompany the payment. These forms are not available for download online because they arrive pre-printed with specific information unique to the business through the Government of Canada. Use this link, https://www.canada.ca/en/revenue-agency, and search under Forms. The medical administrative assistant should calculate the total amount required for CPP, EI, and income tax and insert the figures in the proper areas of the form. The form can be remitted electronically under the My Payment section, located under the Business Account available through the CRA. Payment can also be made through the pre-authorized

Paystub

EMPLOYER NAME

TELEPHONE

ADDRESS

EMPLOYEE NAME

SIN

ADDRESS

PERIOD ENDING

PAY DATE

EARNINGS	RATE	HOURS	CURRENT AMOUNT	YEAR AMOUNT
Regular				

Gross pay		

DEDUCTIONS		
HST/GST		
EI		
CPP		
Other:		
TOTAL DEDUCTIONS		

NET PAY		

• **Fig. 8.14** Payroll Statement.

debit, online, or telephone-banking options provided by the financial institution; always ensure that you keep a copy for your records. Let us assume that for the month of March, $67.52 has been deducted from your employees for EI, $173.64 for CPP, and $437.98 for income taxes. The calculations for your payment would be as follows:

EI	Employee contribution	$ 67.52
	Employer contribution	
	(47.52 × 1.4) =	$ 94.53
	Total EI submission	$162.05
CPP	Employee contribution	$ 173.64
	Employer contribution	$ 173.64

| | Total CPP submission | $347.28 |
| Income Tax | (amount deducted according to tax schedule) | $437.98 |

Other Payroll Deductions

Apart from the standard deductions, additional deductions may be part of the payroll process within an organization; these are sometimes referred to as *voluntary deductions*. These can include the following:

• **Extended health care.** Medical, dental, and/or vision health premiums are voluntary deductions that are held back

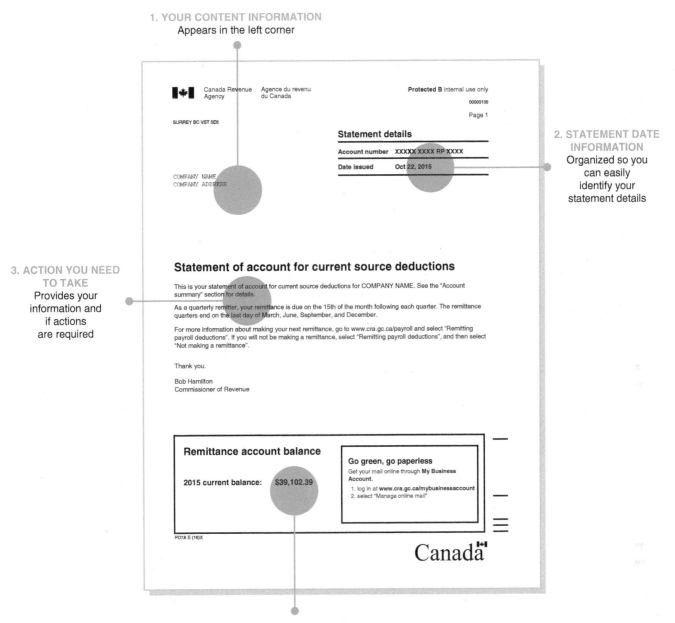

1. YOUR CONTENT INFORMATION
Appears in the left corner

2. STATEMENT DATE INFORMATION
Organized so you can easily identify your statement details

3. ACTION YOU NEED TO TAKE
Provides your information and if actions are required

4. YOUR CURRENT BALANCE
Provides you with your current-year balance

• **Fig. 8.15** Statement of Account for Current Source Deductions. (Source: Reproduced with permission of the Minister of National Revenue, 2019.)

from an employee's paycheck, assuming that the employee is participating in the health insurance program.

• **Long- and short-term disability.** This coverage ensures employees could still receive a percentage of their salary in the event of a health issue that leaves them unable to work and therefore disabled; this deduction type would be used to collect employee premiums toward this insurance.

• **Pension.** This is in addition to the CPP deduction; the organization has set up an additional pension for employees upon retirement who have met specific requirements such as length of service. In many organizations, the employee contributes, as does the employer.

• **Life insurance.** The employer may offer through deductions term life insurance for the employee and their dependents.

• **Union dues.** If working in a unionized environment, like a hospital, the union will collect a set payroll deduction from each employee.

Summary

Accurate bookkeeping can make or break a business. This is also true in a medical facility, and it is precisely why we business side of the medical facility to stay afloat. Sound financial management practices help keep revenue matters on track, avoid regulatory complications, and assist with planning for the future of the facility.

This chapter focused on the important components of managing office finances from a task and function take the time to develop the financial management skills presented in this chapter. Cash flow is necessary for the standard protocol. By taking the time to organize financial records, you will be able to locate what you need when you need it. Practising these skills will enable you to be a contributing member of the team, and this skill set will present diverse opportunities as well as expand employability prospects.

Assignments

Assignment 8.1

Create a disbursement journal. Locate the disbursement journal template found on the Evolve companion site under the file name *Assignment 8.1_Disbursement*. Before starting, review Fig. 8.2 as an example of the format to follow. Record the transactions listed below as entries in your disbursement journal (use consecutive cheque numbers, starting at no. 124):

The column headings found on the disbursement journal indicate the information required; date (as specified below), number (cheque number), description (as shown in brackets below), category (office supplies, payroll, entertainment, rent, electricity, government remittance, internet, donation, or drawing for personal use), and amount of the disbursement cheque. Use your judgement to select an appropriate category of the disbursement.

January

2. Establish petty cash fund for $100

2. The doctor entertained at a dinner party and spent $50 (Romeo's Cafe)

2. Paid Purolator $17.62 for delivery of laboratory reports

3. Purchased letterhead and envelopes $78.29 (ABC Supplies)

3. Paid January rent $1200 (Medical Services Inc.)

4. Paid automobile credit card charges for gas and oil $71.65 (Jay's Gas Bar)

5. Paid your wages $750, and janitor's wages $320 (Don James)

5. The doctor withdrew $350 for personal use

8. Sent cheque to Power Company for $147

8. Made $100 contribution to the United Way

9. Paid Internet service provider $56.50

11. Paid Campbell's Florist $65 for roses sent to the doctor's wife for anniversary

12. Paid your wages $750, and janitor's wages $320 (Don James)

12. The doctor withdrew $350

13. Submitted cheque to the Receiver General of Canada for income tax $290; employment insurance, $15.18; Canada Pension $12.92

13. Reimbursed petty cash $47.41

Examine your entry on January 2 for the dinner party. If a businessperson entertains for the purpose of promoting the business, the expense is tax-deductible. However, a businessperson must not charge personal expenses against the business. You may have entered the $50 dinner expense under "Travel and Entertainment," assuming it was a business engagement. Or you may have assumed it was a personal engagement, in which case the entry would be made under "Drawings."

Assignment 8.2

Write cheques for the first four entries in your cash disbursements journal. The beginning balance on cheque no. 123 is $4062. Assume that on January 2 you deposited $1069. (Extra cheque form can be found on the Evolve companion site under the file name *Assignment 8.2_Cheque*.)

Assignment 8.3

Create a petty cash record and a sample petty cash voucher. From the Evolve companion site locate the file name *Assignment 8.3.1_Petty_Cash_Record* and *Assignment 8.3.2_Petty_Cash_Voucher*. Record the following transactions for January in the petty cash record and complete a sample petty cash voucher for one of the transactions listed as well:

January

2. Bought paper clips, $2.29

4. Pkg 10 red pens, $3.56

8. Purchased sugar, cream, and coffee, $13.35

10. Bought stamps, $30.00

13. Doctor's lunch, $9.50

When the cash in your petty cash box gets low, it is time to replenish the fund. You should have $41.30 in your cash box to agree with the balance column in your petty cash record. To bring your petty cash up to $100, you would write a cheque made out to cash in the amount of $58.70, have the signing authority at the office sign it, and then cash it when you go to the bank.

The petty cash box is generally a small metal box approximately 20 cm × 15 cm × 8 cm (8 inches × 6 inches × 3 inches) and is kept in the administrative assistant's desk or a file cabinet. You should be able to lock the drawer containing the petty cash box. You should always ask for receipts when making payment from the petty cash box to verify the amount of cash paid out. Occasionally, fellow workers may ask to borrow money from the cash box. If you are responsible for petty cash, it is advisable to refrain from making such personal loans.

Assignment 8.4

Locate and enter the following information on a deposit slip see Evolve companion site file name *Assignment 8.4 Deposit Slip*. Date, January 13, 20__; cash $152.60 consisting of 9 one dollar coins, 4 two dollar coins, 3 fives, 6 tens, 3 twenties, and 60 cents in coin; cheques for $13.42 from E.C. Westran, $35 from C.S.A. Insurance Co. (for writing a patient history), $116.28 from W.C. Post, and $52.50 from R.A. James; account no. 6681-35; name of account, Dr. J.E. Plunkett (you made the deposit).

Assignment 8.5

Using the following information, on a blank piece of paper divided into two sections, one section titled bank balance, the other section titled cheque book balance prepare rough draft bank reconciliation statement for Dr. Plunkett. Refer to Fig.8.12 as an example. Make manual calculations based on the information provided below.

a. The bank reported the balance of $2751.16. Your records show a balance of $2823.70. A cheque issued to us from J.P. Sands for $50.75 was returned NSF. Cheque no. 42 is still outstanding. The bank charged $2 for service. Cheque nos. 46 and 53 are outstanding. The account was debited $10 for interest on the demand loan. Cheque no. 55 for $127.50 is outstanding. Cheque stub no. 40 revealed an error: the cheque was recorded as $36 when it should have been $72. The amounts of cheque nos. 42, 46, and 53 are $19.75, $75.80, and $68.30, respectively. Bank deposit made but not recorded on bank statement $295.14. Bond interest paid by bank $37.50. Safety deposit charges $7.50. Date the statement November 30, 20__.

Assignment 8.6

Prepare an automated bank reconciliation statement for Dr. Plunkett using the following information. From the Evolve companion site locate the file under the name *Assignment 8.6_Bank_Reconciliation*. Date the statement April 1, 20__.

Cash account $2140 and March 31 bank statement $2012. Deposit entered in books on March 30 was not taken to the bank until March 31 (amount $530). The bank sent a credit memo for $215 for interest earned on Canada Savings Bonds. The amount is shown on the account. However, the memo has not yet been received. Bank service charges $6. A patient's cheque for $50, included in the March 27 deposit, has been charged back by the bank on the statement as NSF. The patient is J. Wren. Cheque no. 502 was made out to cash for $35 to reimburse the petty cash; this cheque is recorded in the cash payments journal as $53. The following cheques were not returned by the bank with the March statement: no. 521 to R. Smith for $10; no. 523 to J. Jones Ltd. for $50; no. 524 to Metrics Limited for $100 (certified on March 27); no. 525 to P. Brown for $75; and no. 526 to J. Smith and Company for $90.

Assignment 8.7

Prepare payroll. You will complete a payroll statement for yourself and the janitor for the week of January 15, 20__. From the Evolve companion site locate the form under the file name *Assignment 8.7_Payroll_Statement*. Let us assume that you are single with no dependents; your mandatory deductions are income tax deduction, employment insurance (EI), and Canada Pension Plan (CPP).

You are paid a weekly salary of $750 and work 40 hours. The janitor, Mr. Don James, earns $17 an hour. Mr. James lives at 321 Jane Street, Manotick, K2E 7Z3. Mr. James is paid every two weeks. Mr. James's social insurance number is 472 237 942.

You are paid ever week, were not previously employed, were hired on the first day of June this year, and have not received an increase in your salary. Your vacation is negotiable. Use your regular street address and Ottawa as the city in which you live.

Now calculate the earnings and deductions portion of the payroll. Mr. James has worked the following hours over the past two weeks. Week ending January 8: Sunday 4 1/2 hours, Tuesday 5 hours, Thursday 6 hours, Friday 4 hours. Week ending January 15: Sunday 8 hours, Monday 8 hours, Tuesday 5 hours, Wednesday 8 hours, Thursday 5 hours, Friday 5 hours. Mr. James is paid time-and-a-half for hours worked from 41 to 49 inclusive, and double time for hours above 49. Mr. James pays $28.35 each pay period for group insurance. Mr. James also contributes $10 each week to his registered pension plan. CPP deduction $72.50, EI $34.70 and income tax $113.45. Calculate to find the net pay (take home pay after deductions).

Your $750 salary is paid every week. You pay $35 each week to a registered pension, $22 for group insurance. CPP deduction $61.30, EI $27.40 and income tax $88.45. Calculate to find your net pay.

Assignment 8.8

Dr. Plunkett has asked you to write a letter to Thomas Bell informing him that his cheque for $32.50 was returned NSF and asking him to make arrangements to rectify the situation. (Use your imagination.)

Dr. Plunkett has asked you to write a letter to Thomas Bell, informing him that his cheque for $32.50 was returned NSF and asking him to make arrangements to rectify the situation. (Use your imagination.)

Mr. Harris has not yet paid his account in full. It is now four months overdue. Dr. Plunkett sends a statement of account the first month, a reminder notice the second month, an inquiry the third month, and an appeal the fourth month. You have completed the statement of account. Compose correspondence to send to Mr. Harris and the outstanding balance of $37.50. Remember the account is four months overdue.

Topics for Discussion

1. What information would you ask financial institutions when looking to set up a business chequing account?

2. Have you managed computerized bookkeeping systems in previous employment experiences? If yes, what system did you use? If not, research two systems and compare them.

3. Mr. Bell pays by cheque for his completed Medical Form. His cheque comes back NSF, and he has another form that needs to be completed. How would you handle this situation? What policies do you recommend that the office have surrounding NSF cheques and direct bill payments?

4. Services such as circumcision, mole or tattoo removal, etc., that are not medically necessary may not be covered from your provincial or territorial billing schedule. The patient is billed directly for this service. How would you explain this fee to a new patient? What methods could you use to ensure that patients are aware of these fees?

5. What challenges do you envision related to supervising payroll for an office? How can they be managed?

6. What additional voluntary deductions might be held from an employee's paycheque?

7. Research what expenses are prohibited from being used as a petty cash expense.

9

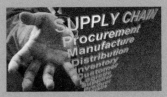

Source: © CanStock Photo Inc. /buchachon

Managing Office Supplies

Having the right supplies on hand is critical for the day-to-day operation of a medical facility. These supplies need to be available for staff to work effectively and efficiently. This chapter examines and guides you through the requirements of supply management, ordering protocol, and inventory control.

CHAPTER OUTLINE

Introduction
Office Supply Management
Supply Chain Management

Purchasing and Inventory Control
Cash Discounts
Sales Taxes

LEARNING OBJECTIVES

After reading this chapter, you will be able to:

1. Identify the common supplies found in a medical office
2. Identify the components of supply chain navigation and best practices
3. Describe the ordering and tracking methodologies for medical supplies, medications, laboratory specimen containers, cleaning products, and general office supplies

4. Understand the safety procedures for handling hazardous materials, medications, and supplies
5. Identify purchasing and inventory control measures
6. Identify cash discounts, sales tax, and terms of purchase

KEY TERMS

Autoclave: A container using high pressures and temperatures for steam sterilization.

Cold chain: Refers to the steps taken to ensure that vaccinations are stored using the optimal cold temperature, in compliance with handling guidelines.

Controlled drugs: These are drugs that have been identified through the Comprehensive Drug Abuse Prevention and Control Act (1971), including all depressant and stimulant drugs, and other drugs of abuse or potential abuse. This act controls all distribution and use of these drugs.

Dispensing: Preparing or delivering medicines.

Narcotics: Substances deemed to possess a high potential for abuse, which may lead to severe psychological or physical dependence.

Supply chain management (SCM): Supervising all aspects of the flow of goods and services, from the acquisition of raw material to the point of consumption.

Workplace Hazardous Materials Information System (WHMIS): This system was created by federal, provincial, and territorial legislation to identify hazardous material, inform employees about the risks, and make sure that workers have the opportunity to use the material safely through education.

Introduction

When evaluating the successful operation of your medical office, it may seem like a stretch to assign importance to having a good stock of supplies. There is no mistaking that having the necessary supplies available promotes productivity. Items such as staplers and examination table paper, or the lack thereof, can bring productivity to a standstill or, at the very least, delay the process. Typically, the workflow schedules do not allow for these delays.

For staff members to accomplish what they need to during their workdays, supplies and equipment are essential. By extension, some supplies, such as masks and gloves, protect the safety of medical staff and patients. Without these, we could compromise safety and send a message that this aspect of medical care is not important.

Highlighted in this chapter is the awareness that you will develop as you focus on the role and responsibility of supply procurement and management.

Office Supply Management

An important function operationally is supply management. The role of supply manager typically is played by the medical administrative assistant. The goal of supply management is to ensure that adequate supplies are readily available for all facets of the practice. See Fig. 9.1 illustrating a common checklist of supplies developed for an office. When the physicians arrive in the office, they will expect that everything needed to provide patients with appropriate medical care is available.

In any medical environment, operational costs are part of the landscape. Operational costs include supplies, staffing, and leasing the physical office space. Medical office supplies fall under the umbrella of operating costs. The administrative professional's responsibility related to supplies is multilayered and includes a systematic approach to sourcing, costing, organizing, and tracking supplies. You should ensure that you consistently have supplies available and that reordering of stock is completed before supplies are exhausted. It is advisable to produce a list of supplies stored in a specific area and to post it in an easily visible place. This serves as a good reminder to check for depleted stock.

Managing supplies, when carefully monitored and tracked, supports a critical administrative function.

Supply Chain Management

Medical practices today often use technology to automate their medical supply management process and to eliminate manual inefficiencies. Utilizing a tool as simple as a spreadsheet to list and track supplies and suppliers can help control costs and keep inventory at optimal levels. Remember, a medical office is a business, and financial costing requires effective management.

Supply Chain Management

Supply Chain Management (SCM) is defined as supervision of all aspects of the flow of goods and services, from the acquisition of raw material to the point of consumption. Of course, medical administrative assistants are not involved with all aspects of SCM; however, there are stages of involvement, as outlined below:

1. **Automate the Process.** Make technology work for you. Maintain a spreadsheet listing the required supplies, and update it based on current stock. Depending on the volume of the practice and the ordering frequency required, the physical monitoring of supplies is scheduled on a regular basis, either weekly, biweekly, or monthly. Assign a responsible person on staff to manage this.
2. **Supplier Procurement.** Select key suppliers and establish alliances with them. Two-way communication, whereby the buyer and seller jointly manage the relationship, is often most effective. Create a mechanism and a platform that enable the relationship to stay consistently positive. This will enhance the value of the medical facility over time. This approach not only ensures the availability of supplies but also promotes cost containment; providing feedback to suppliers often improves their systems to better meet your supply needs. They can, in turn, provide volume discounts and highlight items for promotion through relationship management.
3. **Order Processing.** Purchasing and procurement relationships provide an opportunity to negotiate significant savings. Put any of these agreements in writing to ensure that anyone ordering from your office will know about the agreed-upon terms of purchase. When placing an order, secure a copy of the transaction. Use the preferred ordering method or portal as provided by the supplier, whether it is paper-based or online.
4. **Reconciliation of Orders.** Have a practice in place to check that the correct supplies and amounts are received, and at the right price. As mentioned, this can be an automated procedure through an online platform or a manual means of checking the packing slip against actual items received.

DID YOU KNOW?

Logistics is in part the detailed coordination of supplies. In Canada, over 750,000 people are employed in logistics. It is considered the second or third largest employment sector in Canada.

Stats source: The Logistics Institute Canada

Medical Supplies

Doctors use large quantities of various medical supplies in their practices. Following is a list of the necessities. These will vary, of course, depending on the specialty of physician you are working with.

- Dressings
- Disposable needles
- Surgical gloves
- Sutures
- Tongue depressors
- Thermometers
- Disposable speculums

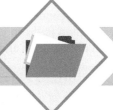

Supply Checklist—Dr. Plunkett's Office

Medical

- ☐ Syringes—all sizes and types
- ☐ Antiseptic wipes (including alcohol, betadine, iodine, and witch hazel)
- ☐ Clinical swabs
- ☐ Cotton balls
- ☐ Tongue depressors
- ☐ Bandages, gauze, dressings, tape
- ☐ Surgical sutures and removal kits
- ☐ Thermometers for body temperature
- ☐ Medical scissors, instruments
- ☐ Speculums (ear and vaginal)
- ☐ Spirometer
- ☐ Death certificates

Equipment

- ☐ Chairs for waiting room
- ☐ Vital sign and blood pressure tools
- ☐ Tables: exam, treatment, and instrument
- ☐ Medical linens, exam paper, gowns
- ☐ Cabinets for medical supplies
- ☐ Autoclave for sterilization
- ☐ Audiometer/Tympanometry
- ☐ Body weight scales
- ☐ Emergency equipment and supplies
- ☐ Laboratory—centrifuge, vacutainers
- ☐ Refrigerator/freezer
- ☐ Sharps container

Office/Cleaning

- ☐ Computers, monitors
- ☐ Printer and paper
- ☐ Desks and chairs
- ☐ Pens, markers
- ☐ Staplers, paper clips
- ☐ Envelopes, letterhead
- ☐ Tape rubber bands
- ☐ Sticky notes, various sizes
- ☐ Tissue, paper towel
- ☐ Cleaning wipes
- ☐ Soap (hand)
- ☐ Trash bags
- ☐
- ☐

Medications/Vaccinations

- ☐ Local anaesthetic for procedures
- ☐ Analgesics
- ☐ Anti-seizure
- ☐ Anaphylaxis treatment
- ☐ Poison treatment
- ☐ Drug Samples—clinical evaluation packets
- ☐ Measles, mumps and rubella MMR
- ☐ Tetanus
- ☐ Mantoux testing
- ☐ Diphtheria, Pertussis, and tetanus DPT
- ☐ Chicken Pox
- ☐ Hepatitis B
- ☐
- ☐

This list is a sample and does not cover all items required in a medical office. Most offices will design their own checklist depending on type of practice and supply requirements.

• **Fig. 9.1** It is the medical administrative assistant's responsibility to ensure a steady stock of supplies.

- Adhesive

This list is not intended to be complete but rather to provide some common items to consider in terms of medical supplies; each office's needs and usage will vary.

Office and Paper Supplies

The medical administrative assistant requires a variety of items to perform daily office duties. The physician generally has pre-printed stationery, such as letterhead, envelopes, statements, and prescription forms. In addition, a supply of pens, pencils, paper clips, staples, notepads, photocopier paper and toner, erasers, plain bond paper, file folders, and requisition and business forms should always be available. It may be helpful to flag supplies at a point where reordering should take place. This can easily be done by fastening a note indicating "Reorder now."

Paper supplies will be ordered in the same way, with a preferred supplier identified by your SCM practices; these paper products can include:

- Examination paper (for the examination tables)
- Disposable gowns
- Drapes
- Paper towels

As a best practice, if there are two or more employees in the office, you may want to designate one person as being responsible for ordering supplies. On a busy day, it can be very disruptive to patient care if the supplies are not available.

Contact your local hospital or other external diagnostic centre to secure their requisition forms if a paper-based copy is required.

Vaccines and Medications

Vaccinations are ordered through your local public health unit. Be sure to learn about the ordering procedures specific to your local unit. As a vaccine provider, you must carefully follow supply-handling procedures as well, such as adherence to the cold chain. The cold chain refers to the steps that must be taken to ensure that vaccinations are stored following the optimal cold temperature stipulations outlined by the manufacturer. Remember, vaccines are biological products, so patient safety is essential. Be sure that all staff members who handle vaccines are aware of these standards. According to the standards outlined by Health Canada, a practice of assigning a vaccination coordinator at a health care facility is a best practice. Because most vaccinations require storage protocol, be aware of these guidelines, and if you do not know them, ask. Vaccines have a limited shelf life with expiration dates listed on each container. Follow these basic steps for vaccine handling:

1. Prior to ordering vaccines, check the optimal storage handling guidelines. Make sure your office storage equipment is sufficient to meet these requirements. The local health unit can provide detailed information.
2. Most vaccines are stored in the refrigerator at an optimal temperature of approximately 5°C, or in the freezer at approximately –23°C. You should check your onsite office refrigerator setting on a daily basis and document the temperature readings. The public health unit may ask for your records. If the temperature readings deviate from the recommended range, you may have to discard vaccines that are no longer effective and cannot be administered. A best practice is always to have a portable cooler on hand for the transportation of vaccines and for backup storage in case the refrigerator is not operating.
3. Check the vaccine stock on a regular basis—weekly, biweekly, or monthly—for expiry dates and ordering needs.
4. Stay on top of the demand for vaccines, and be aware of changing needs during specific times of the year. For instance, school-aged children may be seen just prior to school startup in the fall to update their vaccination records; be aware of the influxes and order ahead. Inventory management is essential to ensure that the required vaccines are on hand for the physician or nurse to administer.
5. To follow the proper protocol for discarding expired or spoiled vaccines, always check with the local health unit; do not simply throw them out.

If you are responsible for ordering medications, remember that drugs deteriorate over time. Keep in mind the shelf life of the medication and the amount your office uses when ordering to avoid unnecessary waste and expense. Develop a consultative approach to determine onsite medication needs. Ask physicians for a list of the medications they want on hand at all times. Do not make quantity purchases without following a consultative process, and determine whether the office has enough storage room. Some medications have storage recommendations; be aware of these by reading the instructions, and adhere to them. For instance, exposure to light compromises specific medications and testing materials. A best practice is to store medications away from public access in one location, not scattered throughout the office. Ensure that inventory control measures such as supply handling are followed, as mentioned earlier in the chapter.

Physicians will receive medication samples from pharmaceutical representatives. The samples are known as *clinical evaluation packets*. According to the College of Physicians and Surgeons of Ontario, "Many physicians receive drug samples from representatives of the pharmaceutical industry. Drug samples are one means of determining whether a drug is effective and useful for a particular patient. As well, drug samples can benefit patients with limited financial resources and who do not have other means to access the drug" (CPSO Prescribing Drugs, 2017, p. 6). Relationships with pharmaceutical representatives are usually an ongoing association and provide benefits to the practice. At times, the physician may ask you to contact the representative when he or she wishes to stock specific clinical sample packets in the office. For ease of contact, keep an electronic contact list for all pharmaceutical representatives.

Most offices do not stock narcotics or controlled drugs. A narcotic is a substance deemed to have a high potential for abuse, which may lead to severe psychological or physical dependence. For example, opioids are considered a narcotic. The use of controlled substances is regulated by the government and is categorized as having a higher than average potential for abuse or addiction. It is not necessary to be a narcotic for a substance to be controlled. For instance, Ritalin® and Valium® are considered controlled substances in Canada. Typically, medications kept in the office include vaccines for influenza and other common diseases, Adrenalin, various ointments and creams, antibiotics, aspirin, Novocain, penicillin, and so on. Controlled drugs need to be stored in a securely locked cabinet with strict dispensing documentation witnessed by the physician and another health professional (usually a nurse). Offices post signs indicating that no narcotics are kept on the premises. Because most doctors' offices or clinics are not open 24 hours a day, this also eliminates the risk of someone breaking in. Documentation guidelines advise the following for physicians and nurses in offices where controlled and/or narcotic substances are administered:

1. Establish the patient's identity; request two or three pieces of identification.
2. Document the medication name, quantity, and strength administered in both the patient and medication record.
3. Monitor the patient for reactions, and document tolerance.
4. Maintain an accurate count of controlled and/or narcotic substances onsite at all times.

As a medical administrative assistant, you are not to administer medications.

In the past, when a drug's shelf life expired, the drug was usually flushed down the toilet. It is no longer acceptable to dispose of drugs in this manner because of the harm it may cause to the environment. Outdated drugs must be incinerated. Many drug companies will collect outdated drugs and have a disposal company incinerate them. Private offices will empty the drugs from the smaller containers into one large disposal container. This container is then taken to a pharmacy for appropriate disposal. Larger medical clinics often have a pharmacy in the building. When disposing of drugs (solid or liquid), you should wear appropriate safety apparel (gloves, goggles, apron).

Used needles are placed in a sharps container. A sharps container is shown in Fig. 9.2. When the container is full, the lid is snapped shut, and it is taken to the pharmacy or to a service provider for disposal. Ensure that disposal is carried out in an environmentally safe manner.

Laboratory and Specimen Collection Containers

Medical offices routinely collect specimens for laboratory analysis. These include culture swabs, urine, sputum, stool collection containers, and blood collection tubes. These kits

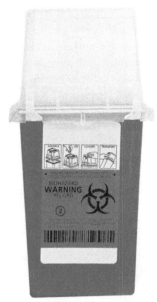

• **Fig. 9.2** A sharps container. (Source: © CanStock Photo Inc./ StephanieFrey.)

and containers are usually sourced from a local laboratory using a formal ordering process. Be sure to contact your local laboratory to determine the protocol, and monitor these containers as you would any other office supplies. Establish a supply chain relationship with your local laboratory.

Be informed about the handling and storage requirements of specimen collections retrieved at your office and follow the guidelines for the transportation of specimens. For instance, a urine specimen not refrigerated shortly after collection begins to grow bacteria and will show as a false positive for bacterial growth on a laboratory analytical report.

Electronic medical records (EMRs) are capable of creating a laboratory testing requisition to accompany a patient or a specimen to the laboratory. The EMR will also track and flag results not received and requiring follow-up. Make sure that you establish a follow-up protocol for specimens sent to the laboratory.

Toiletries, Cleaning and Chemical Products

Items such as soap, paper towels, toilet paper, cleansers, and cleaning cloths are necessary to maintain a clean, sanitary, and safe environment. A local cleaning and maintenance supplier can provide you with these items as well as with safety instructions.

Medical supply companies provide options for ordering disinfectants and specialized chemical mixtures for instrument soaking prior to autoclave sterilization. An autoclave is a container that uses high pressures and temperatures for steam sterilization (see Fig. 9.3). Handle all materials according to industry standards and the manufacturers' instructions.

The Workplace Hazardous Materials Information System (WHMIS) is designed to identify hazardous materials, inform employees about their risks, and educate individuals on how to use certain materials safely in the work environment (see http://www.whmis.ca for more details). This is a national communication standard set by the department of occupational health and safety. Health Canada states, "The key elements of the system are hazard classification, cautionary labelling of containers, the provision of (material) safety data sheets and worker education and training programs" (Health-Canada, 2018, p. 1).

Bleach cleaner, toilet bowl cleaner, correction fluid, liquid handwashing soap, spray for Pap smear slides, and photocopier toner are some examples of materials identified as hazardous under the WHMIS system. The type of hazard is identified by a symbol, as illustrated in Fig. 9.4. Keep all cleaning supplies separate from drug supplies.

A WHMIS program is required in all workplaces that may have controlled products. Employers are obligated to provide workers with information regarding health and safety hazards in their workplaces. Additionally, employees have the right to know of potential dangers that can affect their work and health. Regulations and laws that address workplace safety are a collaboration between the federal, provincial, and territorial governments.

When using hazardous materials, the employee should have gloves, goggles, a mask or apron, or both, available as well as access to and knowledge of appropriate disposal methods. An eyewash station also should be available, if needed. This station can be installed onto a faucet for quick access.

DID YOU KNOW?

Do not store drugs and supplies in the same location. Many drug substances need environmental control such as temperature monitoring to maintain their potency.

Equipment

Arrangements should be made with equipment suppliers to have all equipment (i.e., computers, printers, fax machines, photocopiers, scales, autoclaves) serviced on a regular basis and in compliance with functional requirements. To have an efficient office, equipment must be in good working order. Some office suppliers will generate reminders when toner needs to be reordered. Bear in mind that toner is very

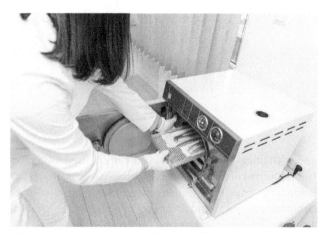

• **Fig. 9.3** An autoclave. (Source: © CanStock Photo Inc. /jalephoto.)

Symbol	Name	Symbol	Name	Symbol	Name
	Exploding bomb (for explosion or reactivity hazards)		**Flame** (for fire hazards)		**Flame over circle** (for oxidizing hazards)
	Gas cylinder (for gases under pressure)		**Corrosion** (for corrosive damage to metals, as well as skin, eyes)		**Skull and Crossbones** (can cause death or toxiciy with short exposure to small amounts)
	Health hazard (may cause or suspected of causing serious health effects)		**Exclamation mark** (may cause less serious health effects or damage the ozone layer*)		**Environment*** (may cause damage to the aquatic environment)
	Biohazardous Infectious Materials (for organisms or toxins that can cause diseases in people or animals)				

* The GHS system also defines an Environmental hazards group. This group (and its classes) was not adopted in WHMIS 2015. However, you may see the environmental classes listed on labels and Safety Data Sheets (SDSs). Including information about environmental hazards is allowed by WHMIS 2015.

• **Fig. 9.4** WHMIS symbols. (Source: WHMIS 2015 - Pictograms, Canadian Centre for Occupational Health and Safety [CCOHS], 2015. Reproduced from https://www.ccohs.ca/oshanswers/chemicals/whmis_ghs/pictograms.html. Reproduced with the permission of CCOHS, 2019.)

expensive; do not order unnecessarily. Prescription pad forms, if used in the office, are often obtained through various print suppliers. The EMR is capable of printing a prescription the physician prepares as well; it can electronically forward the prescription to the local pharmacy.

Purchasing and Inventory Control

The medical administrative assistant should have a systematic approach to record keeping of supplies ordered, the name and address of the supplier, the cost of the item, and the date on which the order was placed. This information can be used for reference when reordering as well as for cost comparisons. It will also give you a general idea of how long a quantity of a certain item lasts and when it will be necessary to reorder. It is good practice also to identify the amount of time between when an order is placed and when it arrives in your office. You should make routine reference to your order book to ensure that your supply room is always adequately stocked. The use of bookkeeping and accounting software such as QuickBooks® allows businesses to create purchase orders and invoices electronically and to store them in an accessible, standard location for quality control.

The Purchase Order

In most office environments, ordering will be completed electronically using the portal provided by the supplier. In some cases, you may also order by phone or by fax. A copy of the

---

PURCHASE ORDER

JOHN E. PLUNKETT
PHM.B., M.D., C.M., F.R.C.P., F.A.C.P.
INTERNAL MEDICINE
278 O'CONNOR ST.   OTTAWA, ONT.

TO: Readymade Office Equipment
225 Rideau Crescent
Ottawa, Ontario
J3X 7X6

DATE: Sept. 25, 20___
ORDER NO.: 3754
REQ'D BY: A.S.A.P.
SHIP VIA: Paxy Transport
TERMS: 2/10/n/30

ITEM NO.	QUANTITY	DESCRIPTION	UNIT	UNIT PRICE		TOTAL	
1	1	Pedestal Desk	1	$525	00	$525	00
2	500	Hanger Files	100	25	00	125	00
		Total				$650	00
		Add G.S.T. 7%				45	50
		Add P.S.T. 8%				52	00
		Total Invoice				$747	50

• **Fig. 9.5** Purchase order. (Source: Plunkett's Procedures for the Medical Administrative Assistant.)

order will serve as a record. In some organizations, it may be necessary to complete a purchase order (see Fig. 9.5). The preparation of the purchase order is needed for approval of the purchasing request.

A copy of the purchase order should be kept in a pending file until the material is received. If quoted prices have been received prior to the order, the amount should appear on the purchase order. It is good practice to obtain the name of the salesperson you spoke with when placing the order as well as a confirmation or service number.

The Packing Slip

A packing slip (see Fig. 9.6) will be enclosed with your shipment of supplies or sent electronically. The items and quantities listed on the packing slip should be compared with the contents of the package. After it has been confirmed that there are no discrepancies in the shipment you received, the packing slip should be compared with the order record to confirm that your supply requirements have been met.

The Invoice

The invoice (see Fig. 9.7) is a statement of the amount owed for goods shipped by the supplier. The quantities on the invoice should match those documented on the packing slip. If you were quoted prices prior to shipment, the prices on the invoice should match those on your order record.

PACKING SLIP

READYMADE OFFICE EQUIPMENT
225 Rideau Crescent
Ottawa, ON J3X 7X6
Telephone: (613) 387-5567
Fax: (613) 387-5568
Toll Free: 1-800-772-8893

INVOICE NO. 337815-33　　　　　DATE: ___/09/29

SOLD TO:　　　　　　　　　SHIP TO:
Dr. John E. Plunkett　　　　Dr. John E. Plunkett
278 O'Connor St.　　　　　278 O'Connor St.
Ottawa, ON J5Z 2X8　　　　Ottawa, ON J5Z 2X8

CUSTOMER ORDER NO. 3754

ITEM NO.	QUANTITY ORDER	QUANTITY SHIP	DESCRIPTION
1	1		1 Pedestal Desk
2	500		400 Hanger Files
			100 Hanger Files on Backorder

Customer Signature

• **Fig. 9.6** Packing slip.

INVOICE

READYMADE OFFICE EQUIPMENT
225 Rideau Crescent
Ottawa, ON J3X 7X6

INVOICE NO. 337815-33

DATE: ___/09/29

SOLD TO:
Dr. John E. Plunkett
278 O'Connor Street
Ottawa, ON J5Z 2X8

SHIP TO:
Dr. John E. Plunkett
278 O'Connor Street
Ottawa, ON J5Z 2X8

CUSTOMER ORDER NO. 3754

ITEM NO.	QUANT. ORDER	QUANT. SHIP	DESCRIPTION	UNIT	UNIT PRICE		TOTAL	
1	1	1	Pedestal Desk	1	$525	00	$525	00
2	500	400	Hanger Files	100	25	00	100	00
			Sub Total				$625	00
			Add G.S.T. 7%				43	75
			Add P.S.T. 8%				50	00
			Total Invoice				$718	75

Customer Signature

• **Fig. 9.7** Invoice.

If there are any discrepancies in price or quantity, or both, the supplier should be contacted.

CRITICAL THINKING

Why would a medical office need both a purchase order and an invoice for the same order? Are you wasting your time preparing a purchase order when the supplier will create an invoice anyway?

Cash Discounts

Suppliers often allow a cash discount on purchases to encourage prompt payment; the cash discount is referred to as the "credit terms." Consult with possible suppliers about their terms. The credit terms on a purchase may be "2 percent 10 days, net 30 days," meaning that if payment is received within 10 days after purchase, 2 percent can be deducted from the total cost; otherwise, payment is due within 30 days of the purchase. The terms are written "2/10/n/30" and expressed as "2, 10, net, 30."

Sales Taxes

The harmonized sales tax (HST) is a consumption tax utilized in Canada. It is used in provinces where the federal goods and services tax (GST) and the regional provincial sales tax (PST) have been combined into a single value-added sales tax. Many variations exist in the types of goods that are taxed. The medical administrative assistant is not expected to know the federal and provincial sales tax laws but should be aware of the types of medical supplies that are *not* taxable. Information can be obtained by contacting your provincial or territorial government sales tax branch. Most suppliers are aware of sales tax implications on the goods they supply and will add tax where applicable. However, if you know which items are taxable, you may wish to add the tax onto your purchase order.

Summary

The health care supply chain involves the flow of many product types. Health care facilities strive to be mindful of safety regulations, supply costs, and the expectation of quality service, as well as health care as a business entity. Supply management and inventory control are a component of this business entity.

Supply utilization management is an emerging practice that will enable health care organizations to consider their supply chain expenses carefully to reap new and better supply savings while meeting the needs of their patient base.

In your role, you will be directly or indirectly involved with supply management, and this chapter provided you with foundational learning related to ordering procedures, inventory controls, and hazardous material protocol for safety standards.

Assignments

Assignment 9.1

Prepare a table-format outline for office supplies. This table is used for supply monitoring and tracking in Dr. Plunkett's office. Be sure to use a heading for each column and row. Consider all the possible ways this table may be used, and by whom. Before submitting it for evaluation, consider whether the table is complete, concise, and easily understood. Submit it to your instructor for feedback.

Assignment 9.2A

Research three medical supply companies in your local area. In a chart, provide pricing from each supplier for the following: 200 disposable needles, 500 disposable thermometer probe covers, 12 dozen pairs of surgical gloves, 20 dozen 5 cm × 10 cm gauze dressings, and 10 adhesive rolls (245 cm × 5 cm). This chart will form a comparison between suppliers for SCM. Provide contact information for each supplier. Submit the chart to your instructor for evaluation.

Assignment 9.2B

Choose one of the three companies you have included on your chart and complete a purchase order for the items listed in Assignment 9.2A. The purchase order forms are found on the website companion. Confirm the taxation percentages in your location, or your instructor will provide them. The following terms are also to be included: 2 percent if paid in 20 days and net due in 60 days; the companies have their own delivery services.

Assignment 9.3

Contact your local health unit and determine the ordering procedures for vaccines. Determine the storage and disposal requirements for vaccines. In a memo to Dr. Plunkett, outline what you have discovered. Submit to your instructor for evaluation.

Assignment 9.4

Search online for business accounting software. List the software's capabilities and describe how they will assist with supply chain management in Dr. Plunkett's office.

Topics for Discussion

1. Should a purchase order have terms and conditions applied to it? Why or why not?
2. Which five supply items would you consider vital for a medical office to function? Which items would you consider essential, and which items would you consider not so essential?
3. In terms of medical equipment standards, how would you determine the safety of equipment prior to recommending the procurement of the equipment?

References

College of Physicians and Surgeons of Ontario. (2017). *Prescribing Drugs*. Retrieved from https://www.cpso.on.ca/Policies-Publications/Policy/Prescribing-Drugs.

Health Canada. (2018). *Workplace Hazardous Materials Information System*. Retrieved from https://www.canada.ca/en/health-canada/services/environmental-workplace-health/occupational-health-safety/workplace-hazardous-materials-information-system.html.

10

The Procedures Manual

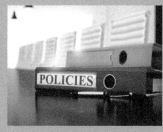

Source: © CanStock Photo Inc./tashatuvango

Procedures are a vital component of any efficient office. Structure and order are the domains in which the medical administrative assistant is relied upon. Aspects of this structure are documented in a dynamic tool known as a procedures manual. This chapter will take you through the process and describe of the important components of compiling a manual reflective of the medical environment.

CHAPTER OUTLINE

Introduction

Description of Procedures Manual

The Importance of the Procedures Manual

Components and Style

Uses

Format

Documenting a Procedure

Creating Checklists and Templates

LEARNING OBJECTIVES

After reading this chapter, you will be able to:

1. Identify and recognize a procedures manual and detail its importance for organizational success
2. Develop the knowledge to create procedures manuals by considering format and best practices for efficient office use

3. Describe the uses of a procedures manual and the creation of procedure documentation

KEY TERMS

Building blocks: Features in word processing software for creating headers, footers, and tables helpful for template creation.

Policy: The rules of an organization.

Procedure: The specific action to take.

Procedures manual: The procedures manual describes the necessary steps involved in completing any and all jobs relating to the business and position, or both.

Standard operating procedures: A set of systematic instructions.

Succession planning: A process for identifying and developing new leaders who can replace old leaders when they leave.

Template: Sample document with specific components already completed.

Introduction

Many administrative professionals are challenged initially when thinking of compiling a formal recording of all procedures. Questions often range from "How do I begin?" to "How do I document what happens in the office?" Consider this: Have you ever started a new job and wished there was a manual to consult to help you figure out a process? As with any major project, the best approach is to view it in pieces or small compartments and build from there.

One of the goals in developing a procedures manual is making it easy for someone to step into your role temporarily while you are on vacation or suddenly absent. The manual serves as a quantifiable measurement of all the tasks you perform on a daily basis.

The processes outlined in this chapter contribute to your office efficiency and will enhance your professional image as viewed through the lens of both your employer and the patients. When patients enter an office, they expect an atmosphere that is calm and well managed. A procedures manual is often paramount in achieving the perception of office calm.

Description of Procedures Manual

Procedures manuals provide an outline of instructions, procedures, and policies essential to the operational activities of a health care organization. Policy refers to a principle of action enacted or proposed by an organization; in simple terms, policy determines the rules of the organization. Procedure refers to the specific action to take. The adoption and creation of a procedures manual is advantageous in ensuring consistency and quality (see Fig. 10.1). Additionally, a procedures manual provides responses for possible challenges and solutions for common problems. The solutions facilitate a consistent approach to a challenge. Some organizations opt for a paper copy, whereas many others support the manual in a digital format.

The Importance of the Procedures Manual

Well-written policies and procedures allow facility staff to understand their roles and promote accountability within defined limits. Policies and procedures guide operations without the need for oversight that is heavily driven by management. The procedures manual provides a format for standard operating procedures (SOPs). SOPs are a set of systematic instructions compiled by an organization to help workers carry out complex routine operations. SOPs drive the results of the facility, controlling costs and increasing productivity. The manual also assists with new-employee onboarding and succession planning. Succession planning is a process for identifying and developing new leaders who can replace former leaders when they leave. The best practices provided support employee development.

Some of the disadvantages surrounding the use of a procedures manual include the difficulty in keeping it up to date, the challenge of interpreting ambiguous language, and the lack of the human element for relationship management in an office.

Components and Style

If you are one of many employees and you are responsible for producing a procedures manual, you will gather information prior to creating the manual. In collaboration with management, interview and observe each employee to describe the procedures involved in completing their particular job. In large facilities, each department has its own procedures manual.

The manual should adhere to the following criteria:

1. It should have a table of contents or easily followed directory in a digital format.
2. It should outline job descriptions or position profiles. This supports a division of work as well as acquainting new employees with their role and the roles of their colleagues. This does not replace a new employee handbook. In smaller organizations, the new employee handbook is integrated with the procedures manual.
3. It should contain checklists and templates, including daily checklists so everyone knows the steps to go through as a guideline. Letter and document template samples are helpful for the creation and management of such documents.
4. It should contain emergency procedures.
5. It should contain contact information—whom to contact and when.

Fig. 10.2 is a reminder of questions to address in a procedures manual.

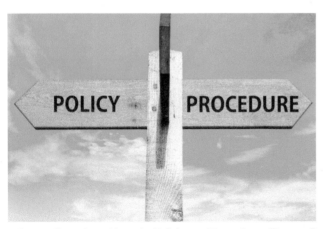

• **Fig. 10.1** Procedures Manual—Policies and Procedures. (Source: © CanStock Photo Inc./stanciuc.)

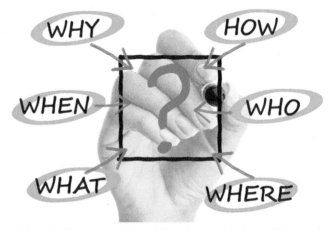

• **Fig. 10.2** Procedures Manual Questions to Address. (Source: © CanStock Photo Inc./adrian825.)

If you are employed in an office that does not have a procedures manual, or has a manual that needs updating, some topics for coverage are the following (listed alphabetically, not by order of importance):

- Accounting Procedures
- Appointments
- Banking
- Bill Collection (overdue)
- Billing Procedures and Systems
- Checklist for New Staff
- Clinical Skills and Responsibilities
- Daily Activity Routine
- Dress Code
- Medication Disposal
- Emergency and Referral Telephone Numbers
- Employee Benefits
- Electronic Medical Record (EMR) System and Functionality (screenshots of key processes)
- Equipment
- Fax Procedures (best practices and confidentiality)
- Filing Procedures, Manual and Digital Formats
- Hospital Records and Documents
- Infection Control
- Insurance—Claims and Policies
- Insurance Forms—Completion for Patients
- Inventory
- Job Description and Profile
- Medical Transcription Formats and Guidelines
- Office Policies
- Payroll
- Personnel
- Petty Cash
- Photocopier
- Records Management (regulations and standards)
- Staff Replacement (for holidays and emergency staffing)
- Supplies (ordering and storing)
- Telephone
- Travel Arrangements
- Work Schedule

DID YOU KNOW?

It is helpful to show information about procedures visually. Common belief is that we remember only 10% of what we hear, 20% of what we read, and 80% of what we see and do. That's why it's better to see something in a visual format once than to read it several times.

Specific procedures are unique to each organization. You would add to or delete from the above list as required—this is a starting point.

The chronological order or time sequence (daily, weekly, or monthly) in which jobs should be completed should also be recorded in the manual, so that no job is left undone. By looking through the manual, the new administrative assistant can verify whether any vital duties have been overlooked.

Uses

When detailed instructions are documented for all health care team roles, a temporary employee can effectively handle any emergency tasks. A procedures manual is also helpful for new employees. After reading the manual, the new employee has a general overview of the job requirements of the organization.

Of course, to be effective, the manual must have detailed information, such as EMR host information; photocopier, fax, and phone system contacts; the location of the petty cash box; where the list of medical supply companies and their addresses can be found; what time the mail and laboratory specimens are collected; and where important phone numbers are listed.

Preparing a procedures manual can sometimes reveal operational concerns related to a particular job or function. If you are involved in writing a comprehensive description of how to handle a job, you may discover that you are duplicating a process or performing a facet of the job that is unnecessary. From time to time, you should review your manual so that any changes can be incorporated. Think of continual quality and process improvement.

Cost savings and time management are important to the success of any business. As a responsible medical administrative assistant, you should take a personal interest in minimizing waste of both time and material. If you see others being inefficient and feel you can bring it to their attention diplomatically, you should do so.

CRITICAL THINKING

You recently developed a procedures manual for your medical office, and now three months have passed since its implementation. What steps could you take to evaluate the effectiveness of this tool?

Format

A paper-based binder for a procedures manual is typically considered an outdated format (see Fig. 10.3). A

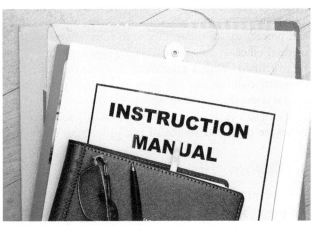

• **Fig. 10.3** Paper-Based Procedures Manual. (Source: © CanStock Photo Inc./ragsac.)

paper-based format may make sense in smaller organizations; however, in most organizations, moving to an online composition is more attractive for a number of reasons, such as:

- Ease of use
- Access, available 24/7
- Updated frequently
- Password protected
- Visually appealing because screenshots of systems processes can be demonstrated more easily
- Videos can be created and included
- Continual process improvement

DID YOU KNOW?

Physicians don't recite everything about a patient's medical history from memory; this is what a medical chart is designed to capture. The knowledge management team at the Mayo Clinic employs a sophisticated system that captures what everyone knows and archives it using computer informatics aligned with its EMR system.

Investigate a variety of digital platforms prior to arranging your procedures manual. Consider how the health care team will be able to access it while restricting access to outsiders. Security is a key attribute. Many platforms have material creation tools that can enable the development of your procedures manual. When creating shared digital resources, consider selecting software that is available to employees and a format that integrates into a variety of software packages. File names should be short and descriptive. Finally, plan for transition from one platform to another.

Documenting a Procedure

To write good procedures, you have to put yourself in the mind-set of someone who does not know how to do a task, and it should be detailed enough to walk that person through

it. This can be difficult when writing about something you are familiar with because it seems logical to you. When writing any procedure, walk yourself through it first, identify the steps, and capture them as you go. Document the steps in a checklist, and once you have a procedure described, go back and reread it to see whether it makes sense, or ask someone unfamiliar with the task to try it based on your written instructions.

Creating Checklists and Templates

The goal of your checklist(s) is to provide a tool to express detailed reminders and instructions, while not adding unnecessary complexity to a task or function. Start a checklist with time-sensitive tasks outlined first, for instance, turning on the computer and checking the daily appointment schedule. Then outline the operational tasks, which might include checking the examination rooms to make sure they are ready. Include reminders on the checklist, such as restocking materials. Include easily forgotten best practices.

For templates, consider their usage and design them in a format and application easily accessible by team members. A template is a sample document with specific components already completed. Building blocks are helpful if using a word processing software. Building blocks include features such as standard headers, footers, text boxes, page numbering, and tables. Assuming that most users are not design- or tech-savvy when it comes to using templates is a safer bet, but do not produce overly sophisticated templates. Basic is the best approach here.

CRITICAL THINKING

What changes do you see for the procedures manual of the future? In your estimation, will these changes be better, or will they create other challenges?

Summary

Task plans eliminate confusion. Clearly defined office policy and procedures are the requirements for a smooth-running medical office. A policy often directs how a procedure will be structured. With a procedures manual, your office can eliminate dull, routine questions and ensure that valuable time is spent where it matters.

As a goal, each employee in a medical facility should be aware of the existence of the procedures manual as

part of the onboarding orientation stage. As the institutional knowledge of the medical administrative assistant grows, they can contribute to the procedures manual's content development.

Use the recommendations and tactics presented in this chapter as a launching point to strive for greater efficiency in how you approach processes.

Assignments

Assignment 10.1

When you begin your duties for Drs. Plunkett and Pelham, assume that the office does not have a procedures manual. Using your imagination, prepare a section for the manual describing appointment scheduling. The description should

include such things as type of appointment scheduling used, what appointments are considered emergency bookings, amount of time to book for physicals, and so on. Design an SOP for several common reasons for appointments. Present the details to your instructor for discussion or evaluation.

Assignment 10.2

Devise a checklist to put in your procedures manual covering what information to source for a new patient on his or her first visit to the office.

Cover every aspect from greeting the patient to taking them into the examination room to meet Dr. Plunkett.

It will be necessary to use your imagination and previous knowledge to fill in missing information and clarify the information provided.

Assignment 10.3

Prepare a page for a medical office procedures manual entitled "Daily Activity Routine." You will have to imagine what duties you would perform and in which order they would be done. Also, decide whether the doctor has office hours all day or just in the morning or afternoon. Choose the type of medical office (private practice, hospital admitting, clinic reception, or other) in which you hope to find employment when you graduate. Insert this assignment in your portfolio.

Assignment 10.4

Research online office procedures manual platforms you may adopt. Find two you like and list the key features of each platform; based on the features, make a recommendation as to which one your office should adopt. Prepare a checklist comparing both platforms to present in your recommendation to your instructor or to present in front of your class for discussion.

Topics for Discussion

1. You have been asked on short notice to fill in at a general practitioner's office where you have never worked before. The only employee there is ill, and there is no one to show you what to do. What information would help you to get through your first day?
2. Do you feel that procedures manuals are helpful, or not? If not, what would be more helpful to you?
3. Consider how a medical administrative assistant would be sure to keep the procedures manual updated for accuracy and consistency.
4. Have you ever used a procedures manual in the past? Did you find it effective? Why or why not?
5. Suggest how a procedures manual supports succession planning in a health care facility.

11

Meeting Organization

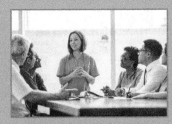

Source: istockphoto.com/FatCamera

Meetings in the medical environment can be effective when utilized in an efficient and productive manner. Finding the balance between meeting too much and too little is achieved through knowledge gained by experience and professional practice. This chapter will engage you in developing a working understanding of all aspects of meeting requirements, including preparing an agenda and planning for various events.

CHAPTER OUTLINE

Introduction

Notice of Meeting

Meeting Agenda

Events

Minutes

LEARNING OBJECTIVES

After reading this chapter, you will be able to:

1. Identify meeting structures and types
2. Describe the steps required in the preparation of a notice of meeting
3. Identify the requirements for preparing an agenda, and its purpose
4. Distinguish between various events
5. Write and prepare minutes for a meeting

KEY TERMS

Ad hoc: A committee formed for the purpose of achieving a specific goal; the group dissolves after the goal is met.

Chair/Chairperson: The individual who presides over or leads an event or meeting.

Committee: A group of people elected or appointed for a specific function and comprised of members of a larger group.

Conference: An event involving large groups of people with a specific focus; it usually involves several meetings and/or workshops throughout a day or over a period of several days.

Constitution: A set of rules that imposes a minimum standard regarding the activities of an association.

Convention: A type of conference usually hosted by an association with its members as participants.

Facilitator: The leader of the meeting, also referred to as a *chair* or *chairperson*.

Formal meeting: A pre-planned gathering of people with the intent of achieving shared goals and objectives.

Informal meeting: A meeting that is often not pre-planned and has less structure and documentation to record the meeting event compared with a formal meeting.

Proxy: When a vote is scheduled and a voting member cannot be present, he or she can give written permission to another member to vote for him or her on a specific issue.

Quorum: When a vote or action is recommended, the majority of members must be present to approve or disapprove it. The number needed is referred to as a *quorum*.

Resolution: A means of making formal decisions at meetings; a request is written and presented by the involved members, and the other members vote on the request.

Robert's Rules of Order: The recognized published guide to running meetings and conferences effectively and fairly. Covers parliamentary procedures.

Symposium: A small-scale conference that usually has an academic focus.

Webinar: A seminar hosted online; it usually involves a presenter sharing information with a group of participants. Two-way sharing is not the focus of a webinar.

Introduction

A meeting consists of two or more people gathered together. Meetings, when strategically planned, can be an excellent form of communication. Usually, this gathering of people is designed to deliver new knowledge and information and to discuss important issues such as upcoming projects. Holding meetings on a consistent basis creates a forum to manage matters affecting daily operation.

More medical administrative professionals are involved in meeting planning and development than ever before. Effective meeting planning comes down to three tenets: attention to detail, organization, and working within the boundaries of a budget.

The topics covered in this chapter are designed to facilitate the development of your meeting and planning skill set.

Meeting Structure

Usually meetings follow a structure type, either formal or informal. Formal meetings are pre-planned gatherings of people with the intent of achieving shared goals and objectives. Additionally, formal meetings involve the creation of a variety of documents, such as notice of a meeting, agenda, and minutes recorded from the process of the meeting. Formal meetings are governed by a set procedures and follow recognized guidelines, such as those presented in Robert's Rules of Order. The purpose of utilizing this publication is to clearly define processes for conducting meetings and making decisions as a group. The terms *motion, mover, and seconder* are discussed. A motion is the formal introduction of a matter at a meeting, a mover is the person who brings the motion forward, and the seconder is the person who supports the motion brought. For more information, see https://robertsrules.org. Associations hold formal meetings. An association develops a constitution, which is a set of rules that impose minimum standards regarding activities, including the frequency and structure of meetings.

Informal meetings are not as pre-planned as are formal meetings and have less structure and documentation to record the meeting event. Goals and objectives are not clearly defined in this structure. An informal meeting could involve a couple of team members quickly meeting to resolve a patient concern and reporting back to the rest of the team.

Types of Meetings

Meetings in the medical work environment support the culture and are essential for management of the office. Meeting types can consist of the following:

1. **Team/Staff.** By design, this type of meeting is intended to provide a forum for the entire health care team (HCT) to gather and discuss matters directly affecting the flow of work. This is usually the most common type of meeting in a medical office. With advances in technology available, e-meetings (electronic meetings) are gaining in popularity. Offices use a specialized phone system called a *polycom* for staff to call from another location to participate in the meeting, whereas others use a video streaming system so staff can participate remotely. The meeting should create a supportive, respectful environment for the team. It helps to establish ground rules from the beginning. Creating a set of ground rules together and agreeing on them as a team will create buy-in concerning team meetings and strengthened teamwork.

2. **Information Sharing.** These meetings are usually formalized in structure, with information shared through presentations, panel discussions, and guest lectures, for example. The purpose of these meetings is for attendees to learn new information.

3. **Committee Meetings.** A committee is a group of people elected or appointed for a specific function; it comprises members of a larger group. A committee is required to investigate or act on a specific subject matter. Examples of topics addressed in committee meetings in the medical environment include advisory, infection control, quality assurance, medical records, and safety. In larger health care settings such as hospitals, standing regulatory committees are required to ensure compliance and policy consistency. They have a continuum of existence, meet regularly, and have prescribed bylaws, which are the set of rules guiding the committee's operation and activities. An ad hoc committee is formed to achieve a specific goal and is dissolved afterward. An ad hoc committee could be formed in an office to review and select a new financial records system.

4. **Decision/Problem Solving.** This type of meeting is focused on a decision-making process that can include information gathering, sharing, and brainstorming as a group to guide next steps or formulate a plan.

A medical administrative assistant may be responsible for arranging meetings as well as for recording and producing minutes. To set an office meeting date and time, calendaring the meeting is essential to ensure that several people are available to attend the meeting. If electronic calendar systems are used, placeholders for new meetings, also known as *meeting ghosts,* are grayed out on team members' calendars to make sure that they are available to attend. The administrative assistant may also be responsible for sending out notices of the meeting, reserving an appropriate meeting place, deciding on and supervising table placement, ordering beverages (coffee, tea, water, juice) for participants, compiling an agenda, recording the minutes, and producing and distributing printed copies of the minutes. A meeting facilitator is considered the leader of the meeting. The meeting facilitator is responsible for making sure that the meeting runs smoothly and achieves its objectives.

DID YOU KNOW?

It is recommended that a meeting agenda be kept to three or four key items. An agenda of more than four items typically overwhelms the attendees, and the meeting can lose its momentum quickly.

A meeting of the Medical Aid Association will be held at 5 p.m. on December 15, 20__, in the Blue Room at the Fairmont Winnipeg, 2 Lombard Place, Winnipeg, Manitoba.

All committee heads are required to have their annual reports completed for presentation. Please confirm your attendance by (insert required date).

DATE: December 15, 20__
TIME: 5 p.m.
PLACE: Fairmont Winnipeg, Blue Room
2 Lombard Place
Winnipeg, Manitoba

(All committee heads are required to have their annual reports completed for presentation.)

Please confirm your attendance by (insert required date).

Notice of Meeting

When the date, time, list of participants, and purpose of the meeting have been established, the first responsibility of the administrative assistant is to find an appropriate physical space in which to hold the meeting. The meeting space helps to set the tone. If you want a small, intimate meeting, set up the chairs in a circle. Many offices have included a meeting space in the physical office setup. The number of participants will determine the size of the room; consider whether participants will be taking notes to ensure that the physical space setup will accommodate this requirement. Once an appropriate area has been reserved, the administrative assistant must inform the participants of the details in a notice of meeting. A notice of meeting should be written in a clear and professional manner (see Box 11.1).

Notices can be simply stated, as shown in Box 11.1, and sent to the attendees by email. The notice can also be in a poster format and sent to the attendees as an email attachment (see Box 11.2).

Attendees should be requested to confirm their attendance when the notice has been received. Some meetings will require a vote to take place. It is important to know the number of attendees because a quorum may be needed for the meeting to be held and for a vote to pass. The number that determines a quorum is normally outlined in the committee's bylaws or terms of reference. If no quorum is noted there, a quorum is usually understood as being the majority of members—half plus one or more. If the required number of members will not be present, the meeting may need to be moved to another date, the agenda item may have to be put on hold, or the vote may need to be achieved by proxy.

This notice should be distributed approximately 10 to 15 days before the meeting. Timing of notices is crucial: If sent too early, they may be forgotten; if sent too late, members may have made other commitments for the date you have arranged.

Meeting Agenda

An agenda is a document that itemizes activities in the order in which they are to be addressed in the meeting, often with a time allowance noted. The agenda begins with the call to order and ends with the closure. The agenda usually includes discussion items, information sharing, or matters to be actioned. Discuss with the facilitator/chairperson of the meeting the topics to be covered. A planned order for the meeting will avoid confusion, wasted time, and missed items. To counteract going off track and wasting time during a meeting, many utilize a parking lot technique. A parking lot is a productivity tool for managing items not part of the formal agenda; however, they become part of the meeting discussion. The items are noted during the process of the meeting; an attempt is made to address them later or at the end of the meeting, if time remains.

Some groups have an agenda committee as part of their team. In this case, the administrative assistant would attend an agenda meeting approximately two weeks prior to the meeting; an appropriate agenda would be discussed, and the administrative assistant would distribute the details. A computerized template would be developed in a style that suits the meeting and/or organization. Fig. 11.1 is an example of an agenda.

Effective Agenda Preparation

When preparing an agenda, whether using a template or creating your own format, remember it is a tool for keeping the meeting organized and structured. Follow these five steps for effective preparation:
1. Start early because it allows for adjustments based on feedback from participants.
2. Objectives should be defined so participants know how to prepare for the meeting.
3. Outline key topics to facilitate a focused discussion.
4. Show a time frame allowance for each item to ensure that the meeting flow is established.
5. Identify who is responsible for and leading each agenda item.

Ground Rules for Meetings

A workplace meeting is designed to achieve a goal or objective; however, recent studies show that 50% of meeting time is wasted for various reasons. To avoid this dysfunction, consider utilizing a best practice of establishing ground rules for meetings. Here are nine tips for ground-rule creation:
1. Arrive and start on time.
2. Participants should be encouraged to come prepared for the meeting.

Medical Aid Association

Meeting Agenda

December 15, 20___
Time: 17:00-19:00

Quarterly Meeting

Meeting Facilitator: _____

Location: Blue Room, Fairmont Winnipeg	Presenter	Time
I. Call to Order	Facilitator/Chair	17:00
II. Roll call	Members	17:05
III. Approval of minutes from last meeting	Members	17:10
IV. Business Arising		
a) Correspondence	A. Allister	17:30
b) Financial report	Treasurer	17:50
c) Revision of constitution	D. Martinez	18:00
V. New business		
a) Charity project	Nominating	18:10
b) Election of officers	Members	18:25
c) Guest speaker "Substance Misuse"	J.O. Scott, MD	18:45
VI. Adjournment	Chair	19:00
VII. Parking Lot Items		

    1. _____

    2. _____

    3. _____

• **Fig. 11.1** Meeting agenda.

AGENDA

Friday, June 2, 20___

2:00 - 6:00   Registration

6:30   Barbecue

8:30   Travelling Theme Party

Saturday, June 3, 20___

7:30 - 9:00   Breakfast
(8:00 President's Round Table)

9:00 - 9:30   Opening Ceremonies and Welcome

9:30 - 10:00   Annual Meeting

10:00 - 10:15   Coffee

10:15 - 11:00   "Rules My Grammar Never Taught Me"
- Sylvia Smith

11:00 - 12:00   "M.O.R.E." (Multiple Organ and Retrieval Exchange)
- L. Lars, Representative
• Heart Transplant Recipient
• Lung Transplant Recipient
• Mother of a young donor

12:00 - 1:00   Lunch

1:00 - 2:00   "Emergency Medicine"
- Dr. A. Vince
Emergency Department
Peterborough Civic Hospital

2:00 - 2:45   "What's Happening in Health Care ... What's Coming Up"
- D. Jones
Health Policies O.M.A.

2:45 - 3:00   Coffee

3:00 - 4:00   "Laughter is the Best Medicine"
- Tom White, Humorist

5:30   President's and International Reception

6:30   Social Time (Cash Bar)

7:00 - 9:00   Banquet
Awards/Presentations

9:30   Academy Awards

Sunday, June 4, 20___

8:00 - 9:00   Continental Breakfast
(Delivered personally to your cottage)

9:30 - 11:30   Country Store & Craft Sale

11:30 - 1:00   Buffet Brunch
Fashion Show

Visit the displays
on Saturday
in the Whistle Stop Room

Elmhirst Resort Total Convention Package is $242.94 per person

Includes: All Taxes and Gratuities
2 Nights Accommodation/
Fully Equipped Cottages
All Meals/Entertainment
Use of All Facilities/
Pool/Hot Tub/Sauna
Nature Trails

To reserve your accommodations or meal packages, please see enclosed flyer.

Convention Registration

Registration Fee:

Members	$30.00
Non-Members	$75.00
Retirees	$30.00

Please complete the reverse side, tear off this portion and return to OMSA by April 27, 20___.

To be eligible for an **Early Bird Draw**, registrations must be received at Head Office by May 1, 20___.

• **Fig. 11.2** Conference/convention agenda. From *Plunkett's Procedures for the Medical Administrative Assistant*.

3. Contribute to the meeting goals.
4. Encourage full participation.
5. Be open-minded.
6. Stay on point.
7. Never attack a person; instead address the issue.
8. Identify action items and follow up.
9. Utilize a parking lot technique.

DID YOU KNOW?

On average, 37% of staff time is spent in meetings, yet 47% of employees find meetings a waste of time. The key strategy is to make them memorable.

Events

Conferences, conventions, symposiums, and webinars are events that include meeting components. A conference is an event involving large groups of people with a specific focus; it usually consists of several meetings and/or workshops over the course of a day or several days. Increasingly, organizations are offering web-based conferences to bring people together from various locations remotely, harvesting the benefits available through technology tools such as online audio and video streaming. Platforms such as Skype for Business, GoToMeeting, and join.me provide an environment for web conferences. Your employer could attend a conference for primary care physicians covering a variety of health topics, such as cardiology, endocrinology, and gastroenterology, without ever leaving the office. A convention is a type of conference usually hosted by an association with its members as participants. A symposium typically has an academic focus and is a conference on a smaller scale in terms of participant numbers. Finally, a webinar is described as a seminar hosted online. A webinar usually involves a presenter sharing information with a group of participants. Two-way sharing is not the focus of a webinar.

Preparation for any of these events begins several months in advance. A planning committee is responsible for all facets of the event planning, including engaging speakers, setting the agenda, and marketing and promotion. As a medical administrative assistant, you may be a member of a planning committee responsible for selecting a venue, organizing food and beverages, arranging travel and accommodations, and securing multimedia platforms. Once details are finalized, the administrative assistant composes the agenda (see Fig. 11.2) and ensures that all those registered

Minutes

Meeting	Medical Aid Association Meeting	Date	December 15, 20___	Time	17:00	Location	Blue Room, Holiday Inn

Members present:

J. Hayes (President)	R. Mastrianni	T. Intersoll	A. Mosta	C. Fortran
M. Zincovich	T. Cavanagh	D. Moore	G. Farley	T. Fergus
D. Fergus	D. Dudley	J. Bluett	E. Chambers (Treasurer)	

Members absent:

Nil

Items for agenda	Presenter	Discussion/decision (Who do we need to consult prior to and inform after?)	Who is responsible for follow-up? Timeframe/deadline
1. Call to order	J. Hayes	The meeting was called to order at 17:15	
2. Review of ground rules			
3. Approval of agenda		The agenda was approved as distributed	
4. Approval of minutes (date)	T. Cavanagh	T. Cavanagh noted that Paragraph 2, section 5.2 of the November 14, 20___ minutes should read '…At a purchase price of $218.28.' Moved by D. Moore, seconded by T. Fergus that the minutes be accepted and amended. MOTION CARRIED	D. Moore/T. Fergus
5. Business arising			
5.1 Correspondence	Secretary	Letters were received from the Homecare Workers requesting a donation of baked goods for their Christmas Tea and Bazaar to be held on	

• **Fig. 11.3** Meeting minutes. From *Plunkett's Procedures for the Medical Administrative Assistant*

Item	Presenter	Notes	Action
		Wednesday, December 3, 20____, and from the Heavenly Home for the Aged inviting our association to attend their Christmas party on December 10, 20____, tickets are $8.00.	C. Fortran/M. Zincovich
5.2 Financial report	E. Chambers	Treasurer Eleanor Chambers reviewed the financial statement (copy distributed) Moved by C. Fortran and seconded by M. Zincovich that the financial report be adopted as read and that all accounts be paid when properly vouched. MOTION CARRIED	
5.3 Resuscitating equipment	G. Farley	G. Farley reported on his investigation into the cost or purchasing resuscitating equipment for use by the fire department. The TX60 equipment discussed at the November meeting can be acquired for $4,926.50. Mr. Farley has discussed the purchase with the fire chief and he feels the TX60 would improve their efficiency 100 percent when dealing with cardiac and drowning victims. A. Mosta moved that we purchase the TX60 package at a cost of $4,926.50. D. Dudley seconded the motion. MOTION CARRIED	A. Mosta/D. Dudley
		D. Moore reported that the constitution committee is still meeting twice a month and they will be ready to present a draft revision at the January meeting.	D. Moore
6. New business			
6.1 Charity project for 20____	T. Intersoll	T. Intersoll recommended that our charity project for 20____ be directed toward providing tables, chairs, cards, and trays for the Senior Citizens' Bridge Club. A brief discussion ensued. No other suggestions were brought forward. I. Bluett moved that we defer this topic to the next meeting and hopefully more suggestions will be made at that time. R. Mastrianni seconded the motion.	I. Bluett/R. Mastrianne
6.2 Election of officers	Nominating committee	The nominating committee presented a slate of officers for 20____ and an election was held. The new executives are: President: R. Mastrianni Vice-president: J. Bluett Secretary: T. Intersoll Treasurer: E. Chambers	
6.3 Guest speaker, 'Crib Death'	J.A. Coons, MD	Dr. J.A. Coons was introduced by A. Mosta. His presentation on crib deaths was both interesting and informative. G. Farley thanked Dr. Coons on behalf of the membership.	G. Farley
7. Attachment – FYI-Treasurers report			
8. Vision statement/committee effectiveness			

• **Fig. 11.3, cont'd**

9. Round table/information sharing			
10. Next meeting			
11. Adjournment	D. Moore	The meeting was adjourned at 19:15 p.m.	
Parking lot items		Constitution committee Charity project	

• Fig. 11.3, cont'd

to attend the event receive a copy. The agenda may be sent out electronically prior to the event or used as a handout on the day of the event.

Minutes

You may be required to attend the meeting and record the minutes of the meeting (MoM), or your employer may record the minutes and ask you to prepare them from handwritten notes. Alternatively, a recording device may be used, and you would produce the minutes from the recording device. Regardless of the method used to record the minutes, they must be prepared and distributed to the participants in an acceptable format. A general guideline for producing minutes is as follows:

1. Pre-plan meeting minutes. A well-planned meeting helps ensure effective meeting minutes. If the chairperson and the minute taker work together to ensure that the agenda and meeting are well thought out, taking minutes is much easier. The minute taker should work with the chairperson to create a document format that meets the organization's standards.
2. Identify the type, the location, and the time of the meeting.
3. Identify those in attendance, those who have sent regrets, and those who are absent.
4. Identify the chairperson and the minutes-taker.
5. Use the prepared agenda as a guideline for recording the minutes. It should be noted if a deviation from the agenda order occurs.
6. Place subject captions such that they can easily be located and such that the subject number corresponds to the agenda number (see Fig. 11.1).
7. Some minutes are produced with "motion" captions formatted in the same manner as the subject captions.
8. The words "motion carried" or "motion defeated" should be in all capitals, underlined, and should follow each motion. The minute taker might also wish to note the number of "for," "against," and "abstaining."
9. Do not record personal comments or opinions such as, "John Smith thought it would be wise if . . ." Only business matters are recorded.
10. Try to summarize discussions; motions should be recorded exactly as presented.
11. If a thank-you letter is requested, or if an expression of gratitude is recommended, it should take the form of a **resolution**.
12. Attach any pertinent reports to the minutes.
13. All motions must be seconded and voted on by the membership (a motion of adjournment is an exception). Be sure to include both the "mover" and "seconder" when recording the minutes.

    For an example of completed minutes, refer to Fig. 11.3.

Summary

Whether you love meetings or feel somewhat indifferent to them, they are a necessary aspect of your working world. It's important to make them as useful as possible. Be sure to follow up after a meeting, because each person's takeaway will vary, plus action items frequently are assigned during a meeting.

A meeting or event is a collaborative effort for all involved. Meetings can define the who, what, where, and when of an objective. Remember, if you are responsible for planning a meeting or an event, start with understanding and stating the purpose. Finally, be sure to employ the strategies, recommendations, and proven tactics outlined in this chapter.

Assignments

Assignment 11.1

Assume that Dr. Plunkett has just informed you that the meeting outlined in Box 11.1 will be held. You are responsible for making all physical arrangements for this meeting. Dr. Plunkett is also the treasurer/secretary of this society and has asked you to take care of all the administrative duties surrounding this meeting.

First, consider what this duty involves, and then prepare a simple checklist of all items that need to be completed, such as tasks related to documents and meeting space. After you have completed your first list, determine the approximate date on which each task should be completed, and then prepare a chronological list of these tasks. Hand in your checklist to your instructor for evaluation and feedback.

Assignment 11.2

Assume that you are employed as the administrative assistant of the physician responsible for organizing a conference for a local medical association. Prepare a printed copy of the conference schedule (see Fig. 11.2) using an appropriate and attractive format (use your creativity). Computer application programs have many formats, symbols, and pictures to choose from. A copy of the schedule is sent to each participant electronically.

The schedule for the conference is the same each day, except for the registration beginning at 10 a.m. on May 14 and the dinner at 6 p.m. on May 18.

On May 14, the conference meetings begin at 1 p.m. and conclude at 4 p.m. On May 15, 16, and 17, morning sessions begin at 9 a.m. and conclude at 11:30 a.m.; afternoon sessions are from 2 p.m. to 4 p.m. On May 18, sessions conclude at 11:30 a.m., and the afternoon is free.

The afternoon sessions are lecture meetings, and the morning sessions are workshops. The speakers are Dr. Janette McGilvray, anaesthetist, on "Advances in Administering Techniques"; Dr. Meera Sharma, pediatrician, on "Learning Disabilities"; Dr. Fraser McGee, heart specialist, on "The Killer Disease"; and Dr. Terry Fisher, neurologist, on "The Human Mind."

The workshops are discussions pertaining to the previous afternoon's lecture.

Assignment 11.3

Research online and locate three videos providing information on how to master taking minutes of a meeting. Prepare a numerated list of 10 best practices you have learned from viewing the media. Discuss your findings and present them to your class, or present the list to your instructor for review and feedback.

Assignment 11.4

You are the administrative assistant to Dr. Janice Lawson, chairperson of the medical records committee. Using the following minutes as a guide, produce a notice of meeting and agenda that would be sent to the committee members prior to the meeting.

Reproduce the minutes and agenda using the format provided on the Evolve website.

Minutes

Minutes of a meeting of the Medical Records Committee held on May 20, 20__, at 1215 hours in Conference Room A, Peterborough Regional Health Centre (PRHC).

PRESENT: Dr. J. Lawson, Dr. S. Kapoor, R. Smith, Dr. Trims, D. Stanley, R. Sevich, L. Bazio, N. Taylor, A. Rawlins, P. Clark, Z. Copping, T. Kezia, H. Bragg, Dr. A.T. Khan.

MINUTES: The minutes of the previous meeting were approved on a motion by Dr. A.T. Khan, seconded by N. Taylor.

Business Arising from the Minutes

1. New Medical Records Policy for Incomplete Records

Dr. Kapoor noted that the policy recommended by this committee has now been passed by the Medical Advisory Committee and the Board of Governors. It is now up to the Medical Records Committee to decide when and how the new policy should be implemented. It was agreed that a notice should be sent to all medical staff members explaining the policy and including a copy of the policy. R. Smith noted that the next count would be taken on Friday, May 21. It was agreed that overdue records would be ignored for this one week. The notice to physicians would be distributed electronically as quickly as possible, and implementation of the new policy would begin the week of May 25.

2. Patient Profile Form

There is nothing to report on this form at the present time. Dr. Kapoor noted that she suggested to A. Rawlins that she obtain suggestions for the Patient Profile Form from all medical departments before updating the design in the health records system. Committee members agreed that medical staff input is necessary.

3. Obstetrical Form

H. Bragg noted that the Obstetrical Form, which includes intrapartum risk factors, was used on a trial basis for several months. At the end of this time, its use was reviewed by the department of obstetrics, which has recommended discontinuing use of the form.

Dr. Trims drew the attention of committee members to the vast amount of duplication from physicians completing medical records. He asked that the committee be aware of this when new forms are being considered, and that all possible attempts be made to avoid duplication wherever possible.

4. Diet Order Form

R. Sevich reported that the new Diet Order Forms have been implemented electronically and are now in use.

5. Staff Electronic Patient Records Systems Training

L. Bazio reported that the training guidelines have been updated for all new staff.

New Business

1. Letter from Wellesley Hospital re Transfer of Information

A request was received from Wellesley Hospital asking to set up a formal transfer procedure between our hospitals. Wellesley Hospital is gathering this information from a number of hospitals in an effort to determine a systematic approach.

A. Rawlins noted that the process right now depends on what procedures are to be performed. A. Rawlins noted that it is one process for a patient being transferred to Princess Margaret, but that it is quite a different situation if a patient is being transferred to Sunnybrook Medical Centre.

Dr. Kapoor noted that it is difficult for one hospital to know what will be useful in another hospital.

R. Smith noted that nursing staff find it very helpful to receive the nursing notes with the patient and not at a later date.

R. Sevich will respond to the Wellesley Hospital request, noting that it would be helpful to establish a formal transfer process at this time.

2. Availability of Old Charts

T. Kezia noted that the physicians like to have old charts scanned and added to their patients' current charts. The anaesthetists in particular find this most desirable, and it has been recommended that the old record be added to the current record. L. Bazio outlined the procedure used for surgical patients. He is attempting to organize the logistical problems to reach the goal of having all old charts attached in the current record.

R. Sevich noted that the department is looking at ways to increase the storage potential in her department; however, noted records of 20 years and older cannot be restored to their previous form.

3. Record Review

This item was tabled because of lack of time to deal with it adequately.

4. Problem Charts

P. Clark noted that there were two patient records flagged in the system for which she was unable to determine which physician should complete the record. Committee members reviewed this situation and assigned the records to physicians for completion.

Topics for Discussion

1. You know that there is a major vote issue on the agenda for the upcoming meeting. You are not sure whether there will be a quorum at the meeting. What will you do before you consult the chairperson?

2. You are coordinating a conference, and you have several speakers coming. What information will you need from each speaker to arrange the conference?

Adjournment

Dr. Kapoor moved that the meeting be adjourned at 1530.

Next Meeting

June 21, 20__, 1215, Conference Room A, PRHC
Janice Lawson, M.D., Chairperson
Medical Records Committee

Assignment 11.5

Divide the class into several teams depending on class size. Aim for six to eight members per team. Each team will conduct a formal meeting. In each team, appoint one student as the chairperson. The team will decide the topic for the meeting. Decide on names, titles, and active roles for the remaining team members as meeting participants. Each team will produce a notice of meeting and an agenda using an appropriate format, and will distribute them to the attending members and the rest of the students. A copy could be posted in the Learning Management System used by the class. Develop a script for each team member's role during the meeting. Consult the *Robert's Rules of Order* website, located at https://robertsrules.org, for formal meeting rules. Host the meeting as a presentation in front of the rest of the class. The meeting could also be pre-recorded and shown in class. The other teams will observe, record, and prepare MoM. Each team will present its own meeting and will have meeting minutes captured from observing the other teams' meetings. As a class, debrief with a discussion about how the meeting ran. Was it on time? What were the challenges you found during the meeting? Was the discussion captured in the minutes? Your instructor will act as an observer.

3. What types of distractions might affect the progress of a meeting? How would you address this up front?

4. You want your meetings to be successful; how would you build rapport in a meeting?

5. What video streaming systems have you used? How does this technology benefit and enhance a meeting?

12

Hospital Records, Requisitions, and Reports

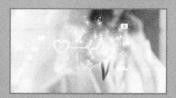

Hospital health records are the most important database for the care and treatment of patients. These records are utilized by physicians, nurses, and other staff to ensure appropriate monitoring of a patient's health status and quality and care, and to ensure continuity. These records also serve as a legal document. This chapter will provide an overview of hospital records from admission or first point of contact to discharge.

CHAPTER OUTLINE

Introduction

Hospital Records

Hospital Admissions

Hospital Notes

Unit Clerk/Ward Clerk/Hospital Unit Coordinator

Processing the Physician's Orders

Confidentiality

Discharge of a Patient

LEARNING OBJECTIVES

After reading this chapter, you will be able to:

1. Identify hospital record composition
2. Understand the advancements in health records
3. Identify hospital departments
4. Describe the responsibilities and roles of the medical administrative assistant in the hospital setting
5. Describe the types of patient reports
6. Recognize diagnostic and laboratory testing
7. Describe the importance of confidentiality concerning health records
8. Identify appropriate formats for history and physical reports
9. Identify appropriate formats for admission/consult notes
10. Identify appropriate formats for discharge summaries/final notes

KEY TERMS

Computerized physician order entry (CPOE): In this process, a medical professional such as a physician provides instructions electronically instead of on paper charts.

Elective: Elective means that the admission or procedure is not considered urgent or an emergency and can be pre-booked.

Health Information Management (HIM): Relates to certified experts in health information performing analyses of the health record to support patient care and safety.

Hospitalist: This physician works either full time or part time in the hospital to provide in-hospital medical services to patients who do not have a family physician or whose family physician has permanently or temporarily given up his or her admitting privileges. In some areas, these physicians provide short-term medical support for the patient on discharge.

Most responsible physician (MRP): Refers to the physician who has overall responsibility for the patient in the hospital.

Point-of-care testing (POCT): This involves the ability in a hospital to bring the test to the bedside using point-of-care devices offering immediate results.

Provisional diagnosis: This is the original diagnosis made by the physician based on the patient's presenting symptoms.

Stat: In the medical environment, stat means "immediately." The action(s) should be completed right away.

In addition to discussing hospital records, this chapter will explore standard procedures surrounding orders and requisitions and will explore the medical administrative assistant's roles and responsibilities in a hospital setting versus an office setting.

Introduction

A hospital record is documentation that details a medical history, treatment, and care over a period of time. Health professionals make entries in the hospital record detailing everything from illnesses, symptoms, testing, results, and physicians orders, to the types of medication that have been prescribed.

It is important to remember with hospital admissions that some are planned and some are not. Going to the hospital is stressful for most patients. The medical administrative staff should remain thoughtful regarding these stressors during their contact with patients in this setting.

In your role in a hospital environment, you will be accessing medical records as well as handling sensitive patient information. The topics covered in this chapter will provide a framework to prepare you to work in a hospital setting in an administrative capacity.

Hospital Records

Most hospitals in Canada maintain and navigate an electronic health record (EHR) system. The system maintains a collection of electronic medical records for every patient who visits or is admitted to the hospital for care. This approach has greatly reduced the need for paper-based charts because almost all information related to the patient is accessible and inputted electronically. Additionally, hospitals are integrating more advanced digital health strategies that allow hospitals to share information with each other. Patients have complex health needs, and hospital services do vary. Therefore a patient may have treatment at more than one hospital, and the availability of these records at all institutions involved significantly improves the quality of care offered.

A hospital records system will consist of several components; of course, information will vary depending on the patient and treatment received. Here is a list of typical information found within a patient record:

- Patient information including admission notes
- Medical history (Hx)
- Physical examination (PE)
- Physician's orders (CPOE)
- Clinical progress notes
- Diagnostic imaging
- Medication orders and records
- Reports (operative, consultative, procedures)
- Nursing care plan (NCP)
- Laboratory results
- Discharge summary
  A patient seen as an outpatient may also have:
- Emergency note
- Medical outpatient notes
- Diagnostic imaging

- Physiotherapy
- Surgical outpatient report

A hospital patient record can be as simple as an outpatient emergency visit consisting of a few documents containing information, or multiple pages as an inpatient admission.

The inpatient hospital record can be initiated in several ways:

1. A patient may be assessed in the Emergency Department (ED) and subsequently admitted.
2. The patient may enter the hospital for an outpatient procedure and subsequently require admission.
3. The patient may be pre-booked for an admission for a surgical procedure in a non-urgent manner.
4. A patient who is in labour.

Advancements in Patient Hospital Records

Hospitals are utilizing a personal health record (PHR) portal for patients to access components of their electronic patient record; an example of this is a portal known as *MyChart*®. See the sample patient record from MyChart® in Fig. 12.1. A patient portal is designed to have patients actively engaged in their health management. Not all information contained in the EHR transfers to the PHR. Data privacy and security are maintained through encryption technology protection. Canada Health Infoway, a self-governing, federally funded organization responsible for integrated digital solutions such as EHRs, provides privacy and security standards across Canada. In its publication guidebook *Privacy and Security Requirements and Considerations for Digital Health Solutions* (2014), security and emerging technologies are addressed as they affect EHRs. The guide can be downloaded at https://www.infoway-inforoute.ca.

Hospitals typically have medical advisory and operation committees whereby policy is outlined in terms of electronic documentation process requirements specific to the institution. There are several (EHR) platforms in use in Canada, and one such system is known as *MEDITECH*. The MEDITECH platform is used in approximately 40% of acute care facilities Canada-wide. See Fig. 12.2 showing a MEDITECH screen of a critical care patient record. You will notice that the patient identifying data as recorded in the EHR is located in the upper portion of the screen, whereas the main window lists the treatment plan.

DID YOU KNOW?

According to Canada Health Infoway, 76% of patients who have accessed and reviewed their laboratory results online were certain that they understood the results posted.

Source: https://www.infoway-inforoute.ca/en/myths

Hospital Departments

There are many departments and units within a hospital, which are staffed by a variety of health care professionals, including medical administrative assistants. These departments and units can include:

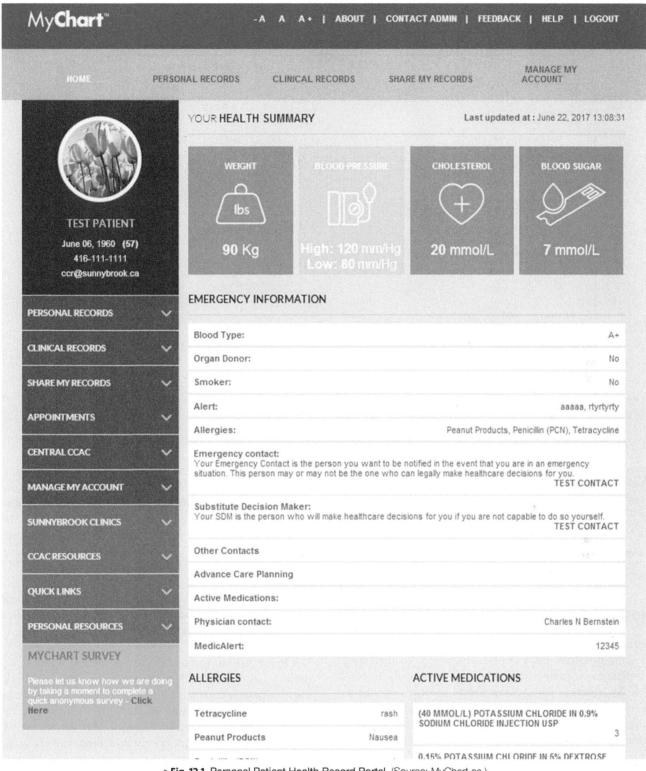

• **Fig. 12.1** Personal Patient Health Record Portal. (Source: MyChart.ca.)

- Admission/registration
- Emergency
- Administrative/business
- Pediatric
- Intensive care
- Acute medical care unit
- Diagnostic imaging

- Gynecology/obstetrics
- Laboratory medicine
- Nuclear medicine
- Neonatal unit
- Logistics
- Pharmacy
- Surgical pre-operative and post-operative

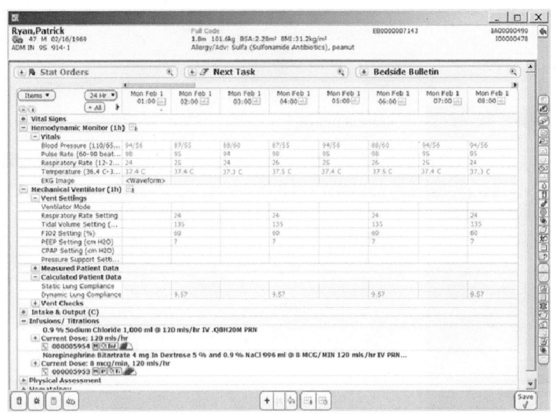

• **Fig. 12.2** MEDITECH Hospital electronic medical record. (Source: 2019 Medical Information Technology, Inc.)

Hospital Admissions

Admissions are processed in the admitting department. In some hospitals, the ED or nursing units do their own admissions. Administrative personnel are usually responsible for entering patient data for all inpatient as well as all outpatient visits. This information is entered into the hospital EHR system. Because some hospitals are linked to other facilities, it is extremely important that this information is accurate and up to date. Departments and physicians depend on this information to access patient records. Hospital billing to the provincial or territorial health insurances is also generated from this patient information.

The admitting physician will provide the provisional diagnosis (reason for admission), which is recorded on the admission portions of the electronic patient record under Reason (see Fig. 12.3 showing an admission screen). The provisional diagnosis cannot appear in abbreviated form. For example, U/A must appear as unstable angina. The original diagnosis stays the same on the Admission/Discharge Record even though the patient's diagnosis may change during the hospital stay. See Table 12.1 for an example of a drop-down menu choice for a hospital unit as determined through the admissions process. Fig. 12.4 shows an admissions patient registration as an EHR entry.

When a patient is being admitted on a pre-arranged (elective) basis, the patient's demographics and medical information are provided to the admitting department prior to the admission date.

On admission, the sociological or demographic information (see Chapter 3) is secured. This includes checking the patient's name, address, telephone number, and so on for accuracy as well as scanning or keying in the patient's health card for verification. This information is very important for future reference, billing, and statistical purposes. The admitting facility is responsible for informing the patient how this information will be used by the hospital. All of Canada's provinces and territories have laws guiding health information privacy as well as e-health laws designed to protect personal health information. Refer to Chapter 7 concerning provincial and territorial privacy legislation. This privacy information is conveyed to patients through various communication channels, such as notices posted and documents shown in the admitting

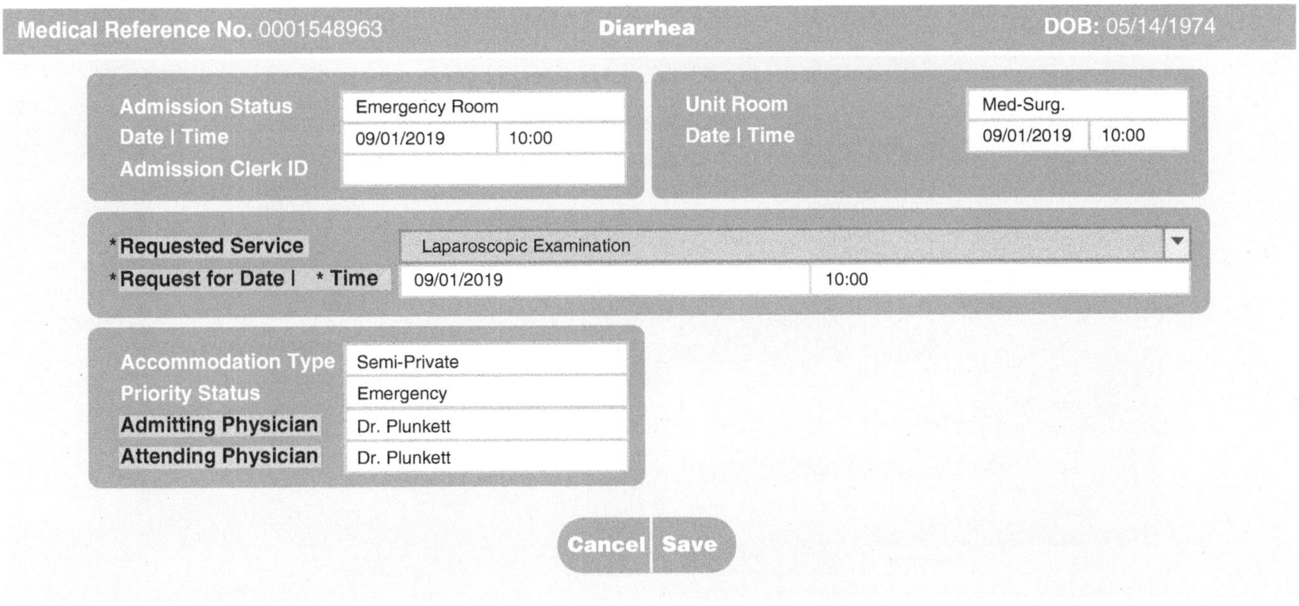

Medical Reference No. 0001548963		Diarrhea	DOB: 05/14/1974

Admission Status	Emergency Room		Unit Room	Med-Surg.	
Date	Time	09/01/2019	10:00	Date	Time	09/01/2019	10:00
Admission Clerk ID					

*Requested Service	Laparoscopic Examination	
*Request for Date	* Time	09/01/2019	10:00

Accommodation Type	Semi-Private
Priority Status	Emergency
Admitting Physician	Dr. Plunkett
Attending Physician	Dr. Plunkett

Cancel Save

• **Fig. 12.3** Patient Admission Screen View. (Source: Alberta Health Services. https://www.albe-tahealthservices.ca/assets/info/hp/edu/if-hp-edu-meditech-edm-filing-admissions-request.pd4.)

Table 12.1 Standard Admission Departments

Dept Code	Department Name
ALC	Alternative Level Care Chargeable
CLS	Clinical Specialty
CON	Convalescence
GER	Geriatrics
GYN	Gynecology
ICU	Intensive Care
MED	General Internal Medicine
NB	Newborn
OBS	Obstetrics
PAL	Palliative Care
PED	Pediatric
PSY	Psychiatry
REH	Rehabilitation in Acute Care
RES	Respite
SB	Stillborn
SDC	Surgical Daycare
SUB	Sub Acute
SUR	General Surgery

department and on care units. If the patient has concerns, the staff members are aware of the appropriate steps to take to ensure that the patient's requests are met. This disclosure is required under privacy legislation.

At the time of admission, the patient will be asked to identify which accommodation he or she is requesting or which accommodation he or she is covered for by third-party insurance. Typically, there are three types of hospital accommodation: standard, four beds per room; semi-private, two beds per room; private, one bed per room. Canada's provincial and federal health insurance covers standard ward accommodation. If the request is for private or semi-private and the patient has no additional insurance (most provincial health care insurances cover ward accommodation only), the patient will be responsible for paying the difference in cost.

Patients are provided with an ID band that is created on admission and placed on the patient's wrist. For years, hospitals have used a variety of colour-coded bracelets to also identify allergies, fall risk, do-not-resuscitate orders, and various other special precautions. A patient could be wearing up to four bracelets at a time so that hospital personnel could easily recognize these warnings. Recent changes in wristband technology have seen the movement to a single band embedded with a bar code that is easily scanned by hospital staff, providing critical patient information in seconds. Each time the patient has laboratory work done or has a treatment, the wristband is checked to verify the patient's identity.

If the patient is not being admitted from outpatient or emergency status, the Admission/Discharge report will be the first of several documents that will make up the patient's record. Fig. 12.5 is an example of an emergency admissions report.

In most hospitals, all entries and ordering (Order Entry) of tests, procedures, care routines, and medications are accessed through the EHR network. With this system, the patient's record can be accessed by authorized personnel

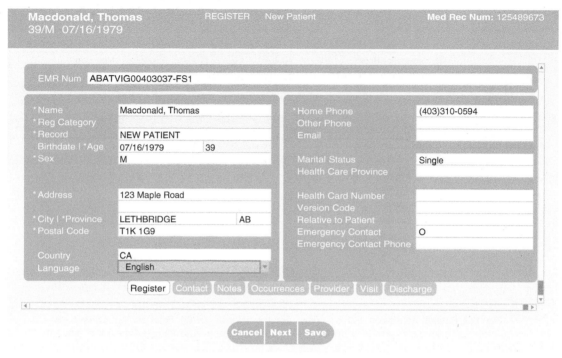

• **Fig. 12.4** Patient Registration Screen. (Source: https://www.albertahealthservices.ca/assets/info/hp/ed u/if-hp-edu-meditech-adm-user-manual.pdf.)

throughout the hospital involved in the patient's circle of care. To maintain security of data, each user of the EHR is restricted to only the components used in his or her department. The most accurate way to verify a patient is by entering his or her medical record number (MRN) for a search. The MRN is also known as the *health record number* (HRN), the unique number, or the patient ID number. This number is assigned to the patient on his or her first visit to that hospital and remains a unique number to that patient for any other visit. This number electronically files the health record and all the associated information, including diagnostic imaging files. The account number or visit number will change with each separate visit, but the MRN remains the same. In some systems, the patient status screen will be shown in different colours. For example, outpatient visits may be in red, current inpatient visits may be in bright green, and discharged patients may be in black.

A medical admission is facilitated by a physician. All physicians have admitting privileges at the facility where they want to admit a patient. If they do not have admitting privileges, they must arrange for a physician to assume care for the patient while in the hospital. The role of the hospitalist will be discussed later in this chapter. The traditional components of the hospital medical record for an admitted patient can include admission notes, physician and nursing progress notes, physician orders, and operative, treatment, procedure, and discharge notes. Remember, the medical record is a legal document and should be managed with significant care and accuracy.

When the patient is admitted for surgery, or if surgery is required during the patient's hospital stay, surgical information is added to the EHR. For a surgical admission,

the most responsible physician (MRP), also known as the *Most Responsible Practitioner*, would be the surgeon. According to the Canadian Medical Protective Association (CMPA), the MRP refers to the physician who has overall responsibility for directing and coordinating the care and management of an individual patient at a specific point in time (CMPA, n.d.a.).

DID YOU KNOW?

According to a 1993 Supreme Court ruling from the landmark case McInerney v. MacDonald, the information contained in a patient record belongs to the patient, but the physical record belongs to the person or organization, such as a hospital, responsible for its creation.

Hospital Notes

In a hospital environment, all investigations must be documented. When a patient is admitted, the attending or admitting physician will prepare an Admission or Consult Note (it may read Admission/Consult note). This may also be entitled History and Physical (see Fig. 12.6). History of the present illness, past illnesses, family's health, and the patient's lifestyle are reported because they may play a part in diagnosing the illness. The physician will then proceed with a physical examination and, subsequently, prepare a report on the findings. The information contained is generally included in a specific order, as follows:

Demographic/Sociological Information—The patient's name, address, date of birth, and so on are recorded. If the

EMERGENCY ADMISSION REPORT
HISTORY & PHYSICAL

Patient Name: Steve Moore

Health Record ID: 112592   **DOB:** 11/05/---   **Sex:** Male

Date of Admission: 12/05/20xx

Emergency Room Physician: Daniel Thompson, MD

Admitting Diagnosis: Acute onset, severe chest pain, and indigestion.

HISTORY OF PRESENT ILLNESS: This 52-year-old man has had severe bouts of heaviness across his chest, which was eventually relieved by nitroglycerin. He has also complained of increased shortness of breath for 8 days. He has had no fainting episodes. His bowels seem to be moving all right.

PAST HISTORY: He has tendinitis of the right leg.

GENERAL: The patient is an alert cooperative male, clutching at his chest at times during the interview. He states he is still uncomfortable at times. Pulse 95 and irregular. Temperature 36.7.

SOCIAL HISTORY: Patient admits to alcohol ingestion on weekends. Denies tobacco use, denies illicit drug use. He is married.

FAMILY HISTORY: There is no history of cardiac disease in his family.

HEENT: PERRLA. Ears are normal. Pharynx normal. No thyroid enlargement.

CHEST: Decreased air entry, but no crackles or wheezes appreciated. Normal S1 and S2 with faint heart sounds.

ABDOMEN: Soft with no hepatomegaly or tenderness.

RECTAL: Deferred

ANALYSIS/PLAN: It would appear this man is having prolonged bouts of angina. He may also have COPD. He will be admitted to hospital, some basic tests will be done, and he will be observed.

_____
Daniel Thompson, MD
Emergency Department Physician

AM:xx

D: 12/05/----
T: 12/06/----

• **Fig. 12.5** Emergency Admission Report

HISTORY AND PHYSICAL EXAMINATION

Patient Name: Marianne Ramos

Health Record No.: 678956

Date of Admission: 08/20/20xx

Admitting Physician: Candace Miller, MD

Admitting Diagnosis: Rule out adenomyosis of uterus.

CHIEF COMPLAINT: Heavy and painful menses.

PRESENT ILLNESS: Patient is a 35-year-old, mildly obese Hispanic female, gravida 4, para 3 whose youngest child is 9 years old. Patient states that over the past year or so she has had increasing difficulty with moodiness, depression, generalized fatigue, weight gain, and bloating premenstrually. The symptoms described precede her menses by about a week. She was seen by another physician and diagnosed as having menstrual endometrium.

PAST SURGICAL HISTORY: She has had D&Cs on two occasions four or five years ago for what sounds like menorrhagia/metrorrhagia. A sterilization procedure was done after the birth of her last child.

ALLERGIES, PAST HISTORY, AND MEDICATIONS: The patient is allergic to Penicillin and Iodine especially in the form of IVP dye. Her only medication at present is Advil used prn menstrual cramps.

PHYSICAL EXAMINATION: VITAL SIGNS: Completely within normal limits. HEENT: Normocephalic. PERRLA. NECK: No crepitus. Trachea is midline. BREASTS are pendulous No masses, tenderness, or discharge. ABDOMEN: Fatty abdominal apron with a well-healed scar at the site of her sterilization procedure. No hepatosplenomegaly. Positive bowel sounds. PELVIC/RECTAL: Introduction of speculum reveals the cervix multiparous and clean. No vaginal wall lesions are noted. On bimanual exam, uterus is tender to compression and is retroverted in position. Adnexa are negative for masses but are moderately tender. SKIN: Patient has had some itching between her breasts and on her inner thighs. NEUROLOGIC: No focal deficits.

IMPRESSION
1. Cyclic edema inadequately compensated.
2. Probable adenomyosis of the uterus.

_____

Candace Miller, MD

HS:xx
D:10/20/20xx
T:10/21/20xx

• **Fig. 12.6** History and Physical Report

patient is seen in the hospital, information such as date of admission is included.

Chief Complaint—This refers to the reason the patient has engaged the physician.

Present Illness—The patient is asked to give a detailed outline of the chief complaint, for example, when the discomfort first began and the severity of the discomfort. If the patient has been referred by another physician, details of previous tests and treatments should be available. The Present Illness section is sometimes referred to as *History of Present Illness* or *History of Chief Complaint.*

Past History—Reference to previous surgeries, illnesses, and diseases is added here. This section may be broken down into specific areas with appropriate subheadings such as Surgeries and Diseases.

Family History—This section comprises documentation of the medical history of the patient's parents, brothers and sisters, grandparents, and so on. Other details, such as age and cause of death of any of the individuals mentioned previously, may be significant.

Personal History—This includes such things as hobbies, alcohol or drug use or abuse, use of tobacco, socio-economic and marital status, and type of employment. (This section may be included with Past History and entitled Past and Personal History.)

After the above details are recorded, the physician will undertake the physical examination. This section of the report may be entitled Physical Examination, or it may be referred to as a *Systemic Review, Review of Systems, Functional Inquiry,* or *Inventory of Systems.*

The examination usually begins with the head area and contains the following subheadings:

Integumentary (skin and hair)—An examination of the appearance of the skin including rashes, discolouration, and so on.

HEENT—Pertains to the head, eyes, ears, nose, and throat and includes such things as use of glasses, blurred vision, loss of hearing, dizziness, pain, discharges, ability to smell, colds, condition of teeth, taste, dentures, gums, swallowing, neck movement, and so on.

Cardiorespiratory (CR)—Refers to the patient's heart and respiratory system.

Gastrointestinal (GI)—This is an examination of the digestive system and may include questions about appetite, indigestion, change in weight, and diet or bowel habits.

Genitourinary (GU)—Refers to the urinary organs and genitals and may include urgency, frequency, sexually transmitted infection, incontinence, hesitancy, and pain.

Neuropsychiatric (NP)—Refers to headaches, pains, paralysis, emotional state, convulsions, and so on.

Musculoskeletal (MS)—Discusses such things as pain, stiffness, movement ability, and fractures.

The physician does not necessarily cover all of the previous details. The examination varies depending on the reason for the assessment and the physician's preferences. If the patient's history or any other aspect of the examination has been covered previously, the report will state, for example, "Past Illness: as outlined in the patient medical record." A physician's personal preference of terms will also determine the subheading titles; for example, "Gastrointestinal" may be broken down into "Abdominal" and "Rectal."

If the examination of a system does not reveal any problems, the physician may record "unremarkable" or "nothing of note" beside the subheading. If an examination of a system is not performed, the record may state "deferred" or "not done."

Usually, the report will conclude with a diagnosis of the complaint and the physician's recommendations, and plan, for the patient. The subheading may be "Impression," "Admission Diagnosis," "Clinical Impression," or perhaps "Analysis and Plan."

With the increased use of the EHR, the need for traditional dictation and paper-based transcription has decreased substantially. Many hospital settings use an integrated voice recognition platform through the EHR system for physicians to dictate extensive notes, consultations, and procedures. The software captures the information by text and then converts and filters it through a pre-set hospital template. The Health Records (transcription) Department often reviews the completed document and edits text that was not transcribed correctly through the software platform. Once completed, the reports will be available in the patient record.

The format for these report templates will vary depending on the integration being used by the facility. The basic information, however, is as follows:

- Patient's name
- Medical/Health record number (MRN/HRN)
- Patient's Health Card number
- Patient location (i.e., room number, Medical Outpatient, Surgical Outpatient, Emergency)
- Admission date or date of visit
- Dictating physician
- Where copies are to be sent
- Date of creation

DID YOU KNOW?

According to Canada Health Infoway, 69% of patients who don't have access (online) to their records would like to have access. Furthermore, 94% of patients who use portals say they find it valuable; 74% of those with access find that it provides for a more targeted discussion with their primary care providers.

Source: https://www.infoway-inforoute.ca/en/myths

Progress Notes

These notes, which are entered into the patient record during a hospital visit or stay, outline a patient's care, status and communicate findings, opinions, and plans between physicians and other members of the medical care team. When a patient is cared for in a health unit, nurses involved in patient care will complete nursing progress notes in the EHR over the duration of the hospital stay, besides preparing a nursing care plan NCP. An example of the NCP is shown in Fig. 12.7.

A SOAP note is a documentation method employed by health care providers in a variety of health care settings to create a patient's entry. Notes in the EHR are somewhat based on this methodology. There are four parts of a SOAP note: Subjective, Objective, Assessment, and Plan. Subjective indicates the narrative form of the patient complaint in his or her own words. Objective refers to the objective, repeatable facts about the patient's status, which could involve vital signs, physical examination, and laboratory results. Assessment consists of the physician's medical diagnoses for the medical visit on the given date of a note written. Plan reflects what the physician or provider will do to treat the patient.

Physician Order

For a patient to receive care and or treatment in a hospital environment, a physician's order is required. When orders are created, they are routinely revised and updated through the duration of patient hospital stay. Traditionally, in paper-based charting these orders would be handwritten or keyed on a form as shown in Fig. 12.8. EHRs utilize a computerized physician order entry (CPOE), which is the process of a medical professional or physician providing instructions electronically instead of on paper charts. A primary benefit of CPOE is that it can help reduce errors related to poor handwriting or transcription of orders. The CPOE outlines medications (dosage and times to administer), tests to be done, appropriate diet, physical activity, and general instructions for the patient's initial admission and ongoing care.

The MRP will update the physician's orders as needed during the patient's hospital stay. At times, a consultant may be requested to see the patient. The consultant's orders will be added to the CPOE. The consultant will also dictate a note with regard to his or her findings on this patient.

Many locations in Canada have a shortage of family physicians, and many family physicians have given up their admitting privileges, which leaves patients without a primary health care provider. Some hospitals have physicians called "hospitalists." Hospitalists care for patients who require hospitalization but do not have a physician able to look after them while they are in hospital for a medical admission. The role of the hospitalist varies in hospitals throughout Canada. In some parts of Canada, a hospitalist is a family physician who may have additional training in internal medicine or in another area, or they could be physicians who have focused their professional practice in a hospital. Patients admitted for surgery have the surgeon as the MRP. The hospitalists care for the patient while in hospital and, in some areas, also provide short-term support when the patient is discharged.

Unit Clerk/Ward Clerk/Hospital Unit Coordinator

Commonly, medical administrative assistants are assigned to a unit in the hospital setting, and this role is referred to as a *ward secretary, unit clerk,* or *hospital unit coordinator.* As in a physician's office, a significant amount of time is focused on patient records and supporting the health care team. See Box 12.1 for a unit clerk responsibilities description.

This can be a very fast-paced and ever-changing environment. The same skills that were discussed in Chapter 1 also apply to this position. Unit clerks play a vital role in managing the flow of information on a hospital unit. The responsibilities of the unit clerk differ from those of a position in a physician's office. The unit clerk does not conduct health card or third-party insurance billing, perform medical transcription, or have as much phone contact with patients. The phone calls received are usually internal calls—physicians or, occasionally, a patient's family. The position requires awareness of appropriate communication channels throughout the hospital.

Hospitals also have codes for emergency response and an extension to call to expedite awareness throughout the facility. Review Box 12.2 for a list of sample codes a hospital may utilize. It is important to remember that each hospital has its own unique code setup, and all staff are provided knowledge-based training for the codes utilized by the institution. Codes are often printed on the back of ID badges issued by the hospital.

Most hospitals have outpatient specialty clinics and these clinics are supported in function by a medical assistant. Even though these clinics are in a hospital setting, the clinic secretary's responsibilities can mirror those of a medical administrative assistant in a physician's office. The responsibilities could include scheduling appointments, records management, contacting patients, ordering supplies, and some billing activities.

In the Admissions/Registration department, clerks are responsible for entering patient data for *all* inpatient visits as well as *all* outpatient visits. This information is entered into the hospital EHR system. Because some hospitals are linked to other facilities, it is extremely important that this information be accurate and up to date. Departments and physicians depend on this information to access patients and patient records. Hospital billing to the provincial or territorial health insurances is also generated from this patient information.

As mentioned earlier, a sound knowledge of terminology and anatomy is needed for any of these positions.

CONTACT PERSON: _____

DIAGNOSIS _____

TRANSFER PLAN: _____

SPECIAL OBSERVATIONS/1:1 CARE REQUIRED: ☐

DPO _____

| RESUSCITATION STATUS |
DATE:
ADVANCED DIRECTIVE: Yes ☐ No ☐

| SURGERY & DATE |

DISCHARGE: INITIATED: _____

DISCHARGE PLANS

| PERTINENT HISTORY |
Any Previous hospitalization in past 3 months Yes ☐ No ☐
ALLERGIES
DRUG
FOOD
OTHER

CARE PROGRAM _____

HOME CARE REFERRAL: ☐ NEEDED ☐ COMPLETED ☐ SIGNED

| HYGIENE |
BATHES SELF ☐
BATHES SELF WITH HELP ☐
COMPLETE BATH ☐
PM CARE/POST - OP BATH ☐
MOUTH CARE Q1 - 2 HRS ☐

| MOBILITY |
WALKING WITH ASSISTANCE/UP IN CHAIR ☐
POST-OP MOBILITY ☐
TWO PERSON TRANSFER ☐
BEDREST WITH ASSISTANCE ☐
BEDREST WITH TURNING ☐
MECHANICAL LIFT ☐
TRANSFER TECHNIQUES ☐

| NUTRITION |
DIET
FEEDS SELF/NPO/FAMILY FEEDS ☐
FEEDS WITH ASSISTANCE ☐
TOTAL FEED ☐
TUBE/GASTRIC FEED ☐

| ELIMINATION |
TOILETS WITH HELP/BEDPAN/CATHETER/COMMODE/ ☐
OCCASIONAL INCONTINENCE ☐
TOILETS WITH SUPERVISION ☐
INCONTENENT CARE ☐
CATHETER SIZE _____
INSERTED _____ REMOVED _____
OSTOMY BAG CHANGE ☐
OSTOMY CARE ☐

| VITAL SIGNS ROUTINE |
ROUTINE VS ☐
V.S. UP TO Q 4 H/CLOSE OBS. ☐
VASCULAR/NEURO V.S. ☐
OTHER _____

| SAFETY |
SPECIAL PRECAUTIONS

| PLANNED TEACHING EMOTIONAL SUPPORT |
TIME: 15 MINUTES ☐ 20 MINUTES ☐ 30 MINUTES ☐
PATIENT CONFERENCE ☐

MOST RESPONSIBLE PHYSICIAN:

NAME: _____ ROOM: _____

• **Fig. 12.7** Nursing Care Plan. From *Plunkett's Procedures for the Medical Administrative Assistant*.

DIAGNOSTIC TESTS

DATE	FREQ		CULTURE COLLECTIONS		
			DATE	SITE	RESULTS
		CBC, DIFF, PLTS, PTT, INR		BLOOD	
		GLUC, LYTES, BUN, CR			
		CK q 8H X3, AST, CK.ECG DAILY X3		URINE	
		RESTART WITH ANY EPISODE > 20 MIN.			
		ECG STAT WITH CHEST PAIN			
		CHEST X-RAY		SPUTUM	
	DAILY	APTT			
				WOUND	

TREATMENTS

DATE		
	ECG ON DAY OF DISCHARGE - COPY TO E.P. & ATTENDING M.D.	
	OXYGEN THERAPY	

I.V. THERAPY

DATE	☐ CV LINE	☐ P.I.V
☐	MAINTENANCE	
☐	TITRATED INFUSIONS	
☐	TPN	

PAIN MANAGEMENT

☐	PAIN MANAGEMENT
☐	IV PCA ☐ MORPHINE ☐ FENTANYL ☐ MEPERDINE
☐	EPIDURAL
	EPIMORPHINE _____ mg q _____ h prm
	BUP/FENT@ _____ ml/hr

• Fig. 12.7, cont'd

MEDICATIONS

PERSONAL MEDICATIONS TO PHARMACY ☐ YES ☐ NO

DATE (mm/dd/yy)	MEDICATION	ROUTE	FREQ	07 - 19	19 - 07	STOP	DATE	PRN MEDICATION	STOP

REFERRALS & CONSULTS

DEPARTMENT/SERVICE	NOTIFIED	COMMENTS

PHYSIOTHERAPY ☐   OCCUPATIONAL THERAPY ☐

NUTRITION ☐   SPEECH THERAPY ☐

SOCIAL WORK ☐   RESPIRATORY ☐

ISOLATION ☐

NAME: ROOM:

LINE INSERTION & REMOVAL

LINE/ DRAIN	INSERTION DATE (mm/dd/yy)	DRESSING CHANGE	SOLUTION CHANGE	TUBING CHANGE	REMOVAL DATE (mm/dd/yy)

VENTILATOR PHYSICIAN:

FAMILY PHYSICIAN:

CONSULTANT:

MOST RESPONSIBLE PHYSICIAN:

• Fig. 12.7, cont'd

PETERBOROUGH REGIONAL HEALTH CENTRE PATIENT CARE PLAN

DATE	NURSING ORDERS	NURSING ORDERS	DATE	EXPECTED OUTCOMES
	ALTERATIONS IN CARDIOVASCULAR	BP _____ HR _____ RR _____ NEURO V/S		READY FOR TRANSFER WHEN:
	FUNCTION RELATED TO:	CVP _____ PAPS _____ PAWP _____ CO _____		1. VS & HEMODYNAMIC PARAMETERS WITHIN
		TEMP. _____ PULSES _____		NORMAL RANGE FOR PATIENT
		PA CATCHER LENGTH AT INTRODUCER _____ CM		
		☐ TTVP MA _____ RATE _____		2. ABSENCE OF ARRHYTHMIAS
		☐ CHECK THRESHOLD q SHIFT		
	ALTERATION IN RESPIRATORY	CHECK AUSCULATION q _____ h		READY FOR TRANSFER WHEN:
	FUNCTION:	F1O2 _____ RATE _____		
	1. IMPAIRED GAS EXCHANGE	VENTILATOR MODE: SIMV AC PC CPAP		1. PATIENT'S RESPIRATORY FUNCTION IS ADEQUATE
	RELATED TO:	RATE _____ VT _____ CPAP/PEEP _____ PS _____		
		☐ BIPAP IPAP _____ EPAP _____		
	2. INEFFECTIVE BREATHING	ETT SIZE _____ @lip _____ cm		2. PATIENT IS MAINTAINING AN ADEQUATE AIRWAY
	PATTERNS RELATED TO:	☐ WEANING AS PER PROTOCOL		
		SUCTION PRN		
	3. INEFFECTIVE AIRWAY	CHEST PHYSIO q _____ h		
	CLEARANCE RELATED TO:	INCENTIVE SPIROMETRY q _____ h		
		SP02 MONITOR q _____ h		
		ETC02 MONITOR q _____ h		
		TRACH CARE q _____ h		
	ALTERATION IN COMFORT/PAIN/			READY FOR TRANSFER WHEN:
	SLEEP			1. PATIENT'S PAIN IS CONTROLLED
	RELATED TO:			2. PATIENT'S NORMAL SLEEP PATTERN IS RE-ESTABLISHED

• Fig. 12.7, cont'd

DATE ORDERED	TIME ORDERED	PHYSICIAN'S ORDER
May 1	08:15	1. CBC & ESR
		2. Weight please
		3. Dietician to see
		4. 1200 cal. DD NAS
		5. Urine bid ac & hs for sugar
		6. Daily FBS
		7. 2 hour pc lunch BS
		8. Tylenol # 2 tabs 1 q8h prn
		9. Halcion 0.25 mg. hs prn
		10. BRP
		11. LES prn
		12. CXR
		13. ECG
		14. BUN
		15. Lytes
		16. Proteins

Erika Shultz

Erika Shultz

• **Fig. 12.8** Physician's Order Sheet

CRITICAL THINKING

You are working as a Unit Clerk on a medical/surgical unit of a hospital. One day, you notice two physicians, Dr. Ronn and Dr. Sims, entering notes into the electronic records system while seated side by side at workstations. One of the physicians, Dr. Ronn, asks Dr. Sims how a patient is doing and then says, "Never mind. I will just look up the patient's record." Dr. Sims reminds Dr. Ronn that the patient is not in Dr. Ronn's care. Then Dr. Ronn says, "It's OK. The patient is my wife's close friend, and we want to know." You then notice that Dr. Ronn accesses the patient's record. What would you do?

Processing the Physician's Orders

The physician's orders are processed as soon as possible after a patient is admitted as well as when the orders are updated after a physician's hospital rounds. The physician and a multi-disciplinary health care team assess the status of patients under their care during rounds. The orders are transferred to the appropriate documents and requisitions line by line. unit clerks are generally responsible for transferring information. It is helpful to process orders by following these general guidelines:

1. Scan the previously documented orders:
   - Ensure that no prior orders have been missed.
   - Orders may appear on several lines.
   - Ensure that the previous order has all been actioned and signed off.
2. Read/scan the entire set of orders to prioritize tasks:
   - Determine priorities.
   - Prepare yourself for necessary steps.

- Each word/abbreviated symbol carries a special meaning.
3. Process STAT/NOW (urgent) orders first:
   - It may be a matter of life or death.
   - This order must be completed first, before the next decision is made.
   - Staff may require additional resources, such as medications from the hospital pharmacy.
   - Staff may need to be notified to carry out this order immediately.
4. Process orders one at a time. Starting from the top of the set:
   - Be methodical (always start at the beginning of the electronic or paper record).
   - You will know where you have stopped and need to start if interrupted.
5. Record action
   - This ensures that the health care team knows that the order is transcribed.
   - The action is updated immediately in the records system.

The unit clerk should check for any stat (urgent) orders and process them first. Notify the appropriate personnel or department (e.g., the nurse, laboratory, or diagnostic imaging department). When an order is completed, the unit clerk should record this information to show the order status.

Because nursing units are extremely busy, it is unreasonable to expect the unit clerk to process *all* of the orders. Registered nurses (RN), registered practical nurses, or both, will often share this task. It is good practice to have the charge RN check the orders to ensure that they are completed correctly. If some orders are unclear, it may be necessary to clarify them with the ordering physician.

Medication Orders

Medications are included in a physician's orders. It is imperative that an accurate record of all medication orders be maintained for each patient. The electronic medical patient record will have a section to record medication orders for the nurse to review and administer on a unit. See Fig. 12.9 for a sample medication record. Three divisions identify medication orders. These divisions are explained in Box 12.3.

Diagnostic and Laboratory Orders

Diagnostic tests, such as echocardiography and colonoscopy, are also part of physician orders (see Fig. 12.10 showing common diagnostic tests). Complete blood count (CBC) and prothrombin time (PT) are common blood tests that are included as diagnostic laboratory tests. For more information regarding diagnostic tests and normal values, refer to Appendix B.

Each test requires the unit clerk to initiate an electronic requisition through the EHR of the hospital. According to the CMPA article *Safety of Care,* in a hospital setting,

MEDICATION RECORD   DATE: _____

PATIENT NAME: _____ Health #: _____

DRUG ALLERGIES: _____

MEDICATION	ROUTE	DOSE	FREQ.	REMARKS

• **Fig. 12.9** Medication Record

ROUTINE medications: Must be taken at a specific time, either daily or on a regular basis (i.e., every other day or once a week).

PRN medications: Must be administered as needed. The frequency will be identified so the patient does not receive too much (e.g., Tylenol No. 2 tabs 1 q8h prn).

STAT medications: Must be administered immediately. These medications are ordered by the physician to get results and improve the patient's condition as soon as possible. These medications are usually single-dose medications, meaning that they are given only one time.

Test	Type
Mammography	Imaging
Echocardiography	Ultrasonography
Complete Blood Count (CBC)	Blood test
Colonoscopy	Endoscopy
Prothrombin Time (PT)	Blood test
Bone Density Study	Imaging
Magnetic Resonance Imaging (MRI)	Imaging
Computer Axial Tomography (CT or CAT)	Imaging
Electrocardiogram	Laboratory
Prostate Specific Antigen	Blood test

• **Fig. 12.10** Diagnostic Tests

managing test results is not the sole responsibility of the physician who orders the test. The hospital, laboratories, and other health care professionals also play a role in communicating on test results or following up. All members of the team are accountable for their respective role, whether it is ordering a test, conducting it, communicating results, or ensuring clinical follow-up (CMPA, 2018).

Review of a Physician's Order

For clarity of the order process, we will review a handwritten manual physician order sheet. Review Fig. 12.8. It is an example of a physician's order for Erika Shultz. Ms. Shultz has been admitted to the hospital by Dr. Plunkett after complaining of severe thirst, headaches, and dizziness. The provisional diagnosis is diabetes mellitus/obesity as indicated at the top of the order sheet. Steps 1 to 16 will explain the process line by line. Examples of the appropriate requisitions will follow.

1. CBC and ESR mean that a complete blood count and erythrocyte sedimentation rate are required. On a blood testing requisition (Hematology and Biochemistry combined), the boxes beside "CBC" and "ESR" would be checked. See Fig. 12.11

2. Weight please: the patient's weight would be recorded by the nurse on the Nursing History record.

3. Dietitian to see: the dietitian would be contacted and a consultation/appointment arranged.

4. 1200 Cal. DD, NAS means a diabetic diet of 1200 calories with no added salt. The information would be recorded on the diet record under "Nutrition: diet" as well as on the Nursing History record. The dietary department would also need to be notified to ensure that the proper meals are prepared.

5. Urine bid ac & hs for sugar: The ward nurse is required to check the patient's urine twice a day, before breakfast and at night, to determine whether there is glucose in the urine. This would be done by using chemistry sticks and recording the results of the tests on the Nursing History record under section reminders.

6. Daily FBS means that a fasting blood sugar test is to be done daily. The request for this test would be recorded on the biochemistry laboratory requisition section by placing a check mark beside "glucose fasting."

7. Two hours ac lunch BS means that a blood sugar is to be done two hours before lunch, requiring another blood testing requisition to be completed, but this time a check is placed beside "glucose random." A separate requisition is completed because this test is to be done at a different time.

8. Tylenol No. 2 tabs 1 q8h prn gives permission to administer one Tylenol No. 2 tablet every 8 hours as needed. This would be charted on a Medication Administration record.

9. Halcion 0.25 mg hs prn gives permission to administer 0.25 mg of Halcion at night as needed. This would be charted on the Medication Administration record.

10. BRP means that the patient is allowed bathroom privileges and would be so recorded on the Nursing History record beside "BRP."

11. LES prn gives permission to administer, when necessary, a laxative, enema, or suppository. Laxatives and suppositories are treated as prn medications. The enema order would be recorded on the Nursing History record under "Treatments."

12. CXR is a request for a routine chest x-ray. This would include a PA (posterior/anterior) and lateral view. The information would be recorded on the Diagnostic Imaging requisition in the EHR.

13. ECG means that an electrocardiogram is to be given and that the appropriate laboratory requisitions must be completed.

14. BUN stands for blood, urea, and nitrogen, and a check mark would be placed beside "urea" on the Biochemistry requisition to order the test.

15. Lytes means a testing of sodium, potassium, and chloride is requested. This test would also be ordered on the blood testing or Biochemistry requisition by placing a check mark beside "Lytes." Some requisitions will require that "sodium," "potassium," and "chloride" be checked individually. This can be included on the requisition ordering CBC, ESR, and glucose fasting.

16. Proteins are checked through urinalysis, and the order would be processed by completing a Urinalysis requisition and placing a check mark beside "protein."

| *Physician Request | Plunkett | Plunkett, John | Source | Electronic |
| Patient Name | Olivia Taucher | | | |

Biochemistry	Hemotology	Microbiology
☐ Electrolytes	☐ White Blood Count	☐ Urine Analysis
☑ Creatinine	☐ Red Blood Count	☐ Urine C&S
	☑ Complete Blood Count	

• **Fig. 12.11** Laboratory Order Entry. (Source: https://www.albertahealthservices.ca/assets/info/hp/edu/if-hp-edu-meditech-oe-user-manual.pdf.)

NOTE: The same requisition can be used for numerous tests if they are to be completed at the same time.

Advances in medicine have led to point-of-care testing (POCT). This involves the ability in a hospital to bring the test to the bedside using point-of-care devices offering immediate results. POCT is often conducted through the use of transportable, portable, and handheld instruments, such as blood glucose meters, nerve conduction study devices, and test kits such as hemoglobin A1C blood testing.

During the patient's stay, new orders will be created. The EHR system will flag this as uncompleted orders to identify that a new order has been created. It is understandable that in a busy environment, this can be forgotten or overlooked. The unit clerk or ward clerk should check the charts at the beginning of the shift and then periodically during the shift.

Confidentiality

As mentioned throughout this text, all areas of health care give personnel access to highly confidential information. In the hospital setting, personnel who are not involved in the direct care of a patient should not access patient records without being part of the circle of care. Even checking the computer to see whether someone is in the hospital or coming into the hospital is a data breach of confidentiality if the information is not required for their role. This policy applies to all personnel, including physicians.

If the unit clerk has concerns that a confidentiality or a data breach has occurred and is not comfortable confronting the individual, concerns should be reported to the unit charge nurse or unit director.

Discharge of a Patient

Discharge planning begins as soon as the patient arrives in the hospital. The unit clerk responsible will check to ensure that the discharge order is completed. Often the MRP will prepare a Discharge Summary or Final Note (see Fig. 12.12). The Admission/Discharge record will identify the discharge date and the discharge diagnosis. The discharge diagnosis may be different from the provisional diagnosis.

If the patient has been to the hospital for an outpatient procedure, there will be a clinical note or an outpatient operative note prepared by the attending physician.

In the Health Records department, the scanning, indexing, and quality assurance standards are evaluated relative to the patient record. Hospitals have bylaws, rules, regulations, accreditation standards, and legislation that govern the content as well as the completion of records. If physicians do not comply with the regulations, various penalties may result, including loss of admitting privileges and a request to appear before the Medical Advisory Committee (Administrative Committee of Medical Staff); sometimes a report on the infraction may be sent to the College of Physicians and Surgeons.

DID YOU KNOW?

Informed discharge is telling patients at discharge about the signs and symptoms to look for that may indicate the need for additional care. The patient is also informed as to who the most responsible physician is for follow-up care. Health care providers should be alerted of the need for follow-up care.

Source: https://www.cmpa-acpm.ca (CMPA)

Additionally, in the Health Records department, the **health information management** (HIM) professional is responsible for the coding and abstracting of records of personal health information in accordance with Canadian Institute for Health Information (CIHI) guidelines. CIHI was established in 1994 and has a 16-member board of directors that links federal, provincial, and territorial governments with health groups.

A position in the Health Records department would most likely require a medical administrative graduate to earn an additional certification for a HIM designation. Another role a graduate may acquire in the hospital is that of a medical transcriptionist or speech recognition editor. In these roles, the medical administrative assistant listens to and transcribes the recorded dictation of a physician or other health care professional; he or she also reviews and edits drafts prepared by speech recognition software, making sure that the transcription is correct, complete, and has a consistent style.

As discussed in Chapter 1, other employment areas of interest in a hospital setting include a variety of clerk positions including, but not limited to, patient registration, inpatient services, dietary, communications, booking an finance.

DISCHARGE SUMMARY

Patient Name: Thomas Lee

Health Record No.: 78540

Admitted: 01/04/20xx

Discharged: 01/18/20xx

Consultations: Ruthanne Ellis, MD, Surgeon

Procedures: Appendectomy

Complications: None

Admitting diagnosis: Rule out acute appendicitis.

This is a 45-year-old Asian male seen in my office on January 14 with the onset of acute abdominal pain at 10 a.m. that day. He was admitted directly to the hospital with a diagnosis of probable acute appendicitis.

DIAGNOSTIC DATA: Serum amylase was normal at 64. Cultures of peritoneal fluid at the time of discharge showed no growth. CBC performed as a follow-up on January 16 showed a white count of 12,400 (decreased from 21,000 on January 14). Hemoglobin today is 12 (decreased from 15.5 on January 14). Pre-op laboratory data were performed in the office prior to admission. The remainder of the values were within the reference range for our facility.

HOSPITAL COURSE: The patient was admitted and surgical consultation was obtained from Dr. Medina. The patient was taken to surgery the evening of admission where acute appendicitis with a small perforation was found. Pathology confirmed acute appendicitis. The patient convalesced without difficulties, although he did have a low-grade fever of 37.8°C until January 17. He was discharged on the following medication: Darvocet-N 100 one q6h prn for pain and Keflex 500 mg po q6h for three days. Diet and activities at the time of discharge are as tolerated.

DISCHARGE DIAGNOSIS: Acute suppurated appendicitis.

DISPOSITION: Dr. Medina will see him in five days. He will be seen in my office in six weeks to be evaluated for possible hypercholesterolemia and possible hypothyroidism.

_____

Ruth Ellis, MD

RE:xx

D:01/20/20xx
T:01/22/20xx

• **Fig. 12.12** Discharge Summary/Final Note

Summary

The appropriate structure for hospital records is a professional standard guided by rules and regulations. A number of forms must be completed depending on the level of care a patient requires, and the hospital record will vary from patient to patient, but all records will contain many of the same basic components.

Accurate, up-to-date records are a key piece of the health care puzzle. It is important to recognize that although gathering this information can be time-consuming, the outcome of this process can be lifesaving. With the use of technology, records can be more easily updated, and the records are more readily accessible.

This chapter presented an opportunity for you to develop knowledge and understanding of the various components of the hospital record and of your role in the creation, management, and protection of hospital records.

Assignments

Assignment 12.1

Your instructor will provide you with a Physician's Orders record (Assignment 12.1A) for Erika Shultz. Ms. Shultz was admitted to the hospital last July 1. Requisitions were completed on July 2, 20__, Health record no. 56762, Room 2. You are the unit clerk responsible for manually transferring the doctor's orders onto the appropriate requisitions. (You will find the necessary forms on the Evolve site.) After completing the requisitions, translate the orders on Physician Order Translation Form. For example, FBS would be fasting blood sugar; tid, three times in a day.

Assignment 12.2

Consider that you have employment as a medical transcriptionist in a hospital setting. Locate on the Evolve site the History and Physical document dictated into the EHR from the admitting physician in the emergency room. Review it and correct any errors the voice recognition software may have made in the creation. Present the corrected version to your instructor for evaluation.

Assignment 12.3

An Autopsy Report (located on the Evolve site) will be given to you by your instructor as a production assignment. You will be informed of the time allowed to produce the report. The student is responsible for making all necessary corrections to produce an acceptable document.

Topics for Discussion

1. As a medical administrative assistant, the position of unit clerk or ward clerk is one that you would be qualified to apply for. What other positions within the hospital setting do you feel you would be qualified for?

2. What challenges do you believe exist working in a hospital compared with an office setting?
3. What are the benefits of working in a hospital?
4. Considering the differing roles, which one interests you? Why?

References

Canadian Medical Protective Association. (n.d.a).. *Navigating legal or regulatory processes*. Retrieved from https://www.cmpa-acpm.ca/en/advice-publications/browse-articles/2012/the-most-responsible-physician-a-key-link-in-the-coordination-of-care.

Canadian Medical Protective Association. (n.d.b). *Safety of care*. Retrieved from https://www.cmpa-acpm.ca/en/advice-publications/browse-articles/2012/effectively-managing-hospital-test-results-key-to-timely-diagnosis-and-patient-safety.

13

Your Job Search

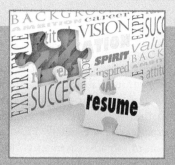

The chapter will assist you in identifying entry-level job opportunities for medical administrative assistants. You will be encouraged to explore your expectations and abilities and to consider these against the available employment. You will be introduced to employment documents, including résumé-writing options, cover letters, and reference sheets. Tips for completing applications and attending interviews are offered.

CHAPTER OUTLINE

Introduction

Entry-Level Positions

Where to Find Job Opportunities

What to Consider

Your Employment Documents

Interview Skills

Career Advancement

LEARNING OBJECTIVES

After reading this chapter, you will be able to:

1. Identify entry-level positions
2. Identify considerations for your job search
3. Recognize the importance of résumés and cover letters
4. Recognize appropriate formats to fit your résumé style
5. Plan carefully for your interview

KEY TERMS

Networking: The term *networking* means a netlike combination or system of lines or channels (*Canadian Intermediate Dictionary*). Your personal network can consist of relatives, friends, professional associations, or acquaintances who may have information or contacts to assist you. Networking is information sharing; it is not one-sided.

Résumé: The term *résumé* simply means a summary. Also spelled resumé (one accent), and resume (no accents), this summary of education and work experiences is used for most job applications. The exception is for career paths such as academics and medicine. These professions use a similar document called a "curriculum vitae," or CV, which is longer in length and more comprehensive than a résumé.

Introduction

Your medical administrative assistant program has taken you through all the basic requirements for a position in a medical office or a medical environment. The next step is to find the "right" job. In today's society, education and experience are generally listed as requirements of the position in job advertisements. You have the education and, if your program offered a practicum experience, you have had the opportunity to explore one or more work environments firsthand. Now you need to gain an entry-level position to launch your health care career. The following paragraphs will assist you in identifying opportunities for new graduates and in preparing your job search documents.

Entry-Level Positions

Most entry-level positions, such as file clerk and receptionist, do not require the same level of experience that would be required for, say, a medical administrative assistant in a physician's office or for a ward secretary in a hospital emergency department. It may be necessary for you to begin your career as a file clerk or a receptionist to gain the experience that will allow you to advance to a higher-level job.

Entry-level positions allow you to gain valuable knowledge and experience without having the responsibilities of a more senior job. Entry-level jobs also provide the opportunity to observe and learn the activities in your environment. You will receive ideas and constructive criticisms from your administrators and peers that will help you increase your knowledge of the requirements of your chosen career.

It is essential that you always heed the pointers covered in Chapter 1 concerning personal qualities and appearance, customer service, and skills.

Where to Find Job Opportunities

Several months before graduation, you should begin thinking about sources of information for your job search. Start working on your employment documents (résumés, cover letters, and applications), and speak with your instructors about job search resources. Remember, many of your instructors have worked in the health care industry and have contacts and resources that are valuable to you as a student. Many colleges also have a placement office that publishes notices on its website or in-house bulletin boards. Staff members will advise program instructors of employment opportunities that come through their offices.

As mentioned in Chapter 1, common areas of employment for medical administrative assistants include the federal government, provincial governments, and private offices. Many of these organizations and institutions now require applications to be submitted online or by e-mail. Some smaller offices may still rely on faxes or paper copies of your employment documents. Almost all employment competitions will be found on company or agency websites, job search websites, social media, or through career development agencies or networking sites, such as LinkedIn. Face-to-face and online networking remains an excellent way to obtain job leads and to let others know you are seeking employment.

Federal Government Opportunities

Federal government job opportunities are located on the website for the Public Service Commission of Canada at GC Jobs. The Public Service Commission of Canada is responsible for advertising, recruiting, screening, interviewing, and referencing for all federal government jobs in Canada. You will find listings for the creation of "pools" or "lists" of administrative candidates for future positions, along with the regular positions it is seeking to fill. To apply for positions, you will need to create an account. You can use this account to sign up for e-mail alerts to be sent to you when jobs matching your education, experience, and interests are posted. The advertisements and application processes are quite long and detailed; you will need to be mindful of competition closing dates and application instructions on this site. You run the risk of being screened out of competitions if you do not follow the instructions carefully. If you successfully pass the initial screening—your application was completed properly, and you have met the minimum requirements for education and experience—you may be invited for further screening through an assessment process. Any assessment or testing required will be noted on the job advertisement; it may include typing timings; testing of language, general knowledge, grammar, writing, filing, or medical terminology; or some combination of these evaluations and others, depending on the position. If you are successful in your testing, you may be invited for an interview or placed on a list for future openings. Before offering employment, the commission will perform reference checks and may request that you submit a criminal record check or take part in a credit check. Box 13.1 lists some of the government agencies that hire administrative assistants.

Provincial Government Job Opportunities

Provincial and territorial governments advertise job opportunities on their individual Public Service Commission websites. Jobs in hospitals, government-run clinics, and government-run long-term care facilities fall under their jurisdictions. As with the federal government, many of the positions posted will require you to complete some entrance testing, despite your having a diploma. The testing may be mandated by a union associated with the position, by the individual institution, or as a general Public Service Commission screening requirement. The

---

• BOX 13.1 **Federal Government Areas of Employment**

- Veterans Affairs Canada
- Health Canada
- Royal Canadian Mounted Police
- Defense Construction Canada
- Correctional Services of Canada
- National Research Council of Canada
- Immigration, Refugees and Citizenship Canada

TABLE 13.1 Public Service Commissions

Alberta	Public Service Commission	https://www.alberta.ca/public-service-commission.aspx
British Columbia	Public Service Agency	https://www2.gov.bc.ca/gov/content/governments/organizational-structure/ministries-organizations/central-government-agencies/bc-public-service-agency
Manitoba	Civil Service Commission	http://www.gov.mb.ca/csc/index.html
New Brunswick	Public Service (NBJobs)	http://www2.gnb.ca/content/gnb/en/gateways/employment.html
Newfoundland and Labrador	Public Service Commission	https://www.psc.gov.nl.ca/psc/
Northwest Territories	Government of the Northwest Territories	https://www.gov.nt.ca/careers/en/search/job
Nova Scotia	Public Service Commission	https://novascotia.ca/psc/
Nunavut	Government of Nunavut	https://www.gov.nu.ca/public-jobs
Ontario	Ontario Public Service	https://www.gojobs.gov.on.ca/jobs.aspx
Prince Edward Island	Public Service Commission	https://psc.gpei.ca/
Quebec	Commission de la function publique	https://www.carrieres.gouv.qc.ca/accueil/?no_cache=1
Saskatchewan	Public Service Commission	https://www.saskatchewan.ca/government/government-structure/boards-commissions-and-agencies/public-service-commission
Yukon	Public Service Commission	http://www.psc.gov.yk.ca/

position you are applying for at the provincial level will likely be through your department of health, and any testing will be more specific to your medical knowledge and administrative skills related to the job. Tests in the areas of keyboarding speed and accuracy, medical terminology (word parts, abbreviations, spelling), medical transcription, word processing, spreadsheet creation and manipulation, grammar, and general knowledge (foundational math skills, filing, punctuation, English spelling) can be expected for some medical administrative positions. Applications will be submitted online in many cases; be sure to read the advertisement carefully and to follow the submission instructions exactly. You do not want to get screened out by giving a first impression that includes an inability to follow instructions. See Table 13.1 for a list of provincial Public Service Commissions or the equivalent provincial government employer.

Private Office Opportunities

Smaller private offices may not have their own websites or dedicated human resources professionals. In these cases, job advertisements may be posted on popular local, regional, or international job search sites (see Box 13.2).

DID YOU KNOW?

Single-practitioner offices may not advertise at all—they may use their contacts in industry or with the public to identify potential applicants. For this reason, letting others know that you are seeking employment is essential.

BOX 13.2 Job Search Sites

Canada Job Bank (https://www.jobbank.gc.ca/home)
Indeed (https://www.indeed.ca/)
Monster (https://www.monster.ca/)
Workopolis (https://www.workopolis.com/en/)
LinkedIn (https://ca.linkedin.com/jobs)
Eluta (https://www.eluta.ca/)
Jobboom (https://www.jobboom.com/en)
Indigenous Link (https://careers.indigenous.link/)
Jobpostings (https://www.jobpostings.ca/)
Career Beacon (https://www.careerbeacon.com/)

Physician employers may be dealing directly with the applications, or they may have their senior office staff person handling the candidate search. Either way, following the instructions on the advertisement will assist them in processing your application and will allow you to make a great first impression. The screening process is likely to be less stringent than with government jobs; however, this may mean also that you do not get as many chances to prove your worth to the employer and organization. Take some extra steps to demonstrate to your potential employer your interest in the opportunity. Follow up on any fax applications with a phone call, and accept any invitation to drop off your application in person (dress professionally and introduce yourself); if you mail your employment documents, call to see whether they were received, and ask questions about the remainder of the process—when interviews will be held, whether there will be testing, whether the employer will require a copy of your diploma, and so on. All of these efforts will give you a chance to display your professionalism, interest, and dedication to working in health care. If the employer is unable to offer you a position, taking these steps will help them remember you, and they may recommend you to a colleague or for future positions.

Networking Opportunities

Networking is an excellent way to secure a job. Inform your primary care doctor or his or her staff members that you will soon be graduating. They may hear of job opportunities through their medical network. It is unlikely that your primary care physician will hire you to work in his or her office if family members also attend the same physician, due to access to confidential information.

Take advantage of any practicum, on-the-job training, or internship opportunities offered through your college or by industry. Not only will you gain valuable work experience, but you will also connect with other medical professionals and expand your network. You may have an opportunity to speak with human resources representatives, who can provide insight into upcoming opportunities within the organization.

Join professional associations; speak to members of the local chapter, attend meetings, or visit their websites for job listings and other networking ideas. Associations offer professional development opportunities, conferences, and online discussion forums—all opportunities for networking.

Social media sites such as LinkedIn, Facebook, and Twitter have become popular networking spaces. You can enhance your networking opportunities by connecting with others in health care, following professional associations and organizations, and letting others know that you are seeking employment by posting your résumé and accomplishments. However, it is important to keep in mind that social media platforms, and what you post to them, can negatively affect your job search. Make sure your online campaign is a positive one. This may mean removing past information that no longer reflects your values or attitudes; it may mean making a switch to posting, liking, and sharing information that is related to, and positively impacts, your chosen career area. For instance, post your professional development achievements, "like" appropriate industry-related content, and "share" job search information. Avoid posting negative information about former co-workers, past employers, or potential employers—you need to use social media in a positive manner to get positive results.

Career development services offices are available to residents across the country. They assist people with career inventories, retraining, job readiness, and employment searches. If you have worked with a career development representative during the course of your program, continue to touch base about potential opportunities. If you have not consulted with a career development agency, seek out a local office and speak to a case worker about how he or she can assist you. Staff members may be organizing a job fair you can attend, they may know of upcoming opportunities, and they may be able to help you with your employment documents.

What to Consider

When beginning your job search, it is important to consider your expectations, needs, and abilities. For example, if you had difficulty with medical transcription, it would be unwise to seek a job as a transcriptionist. If you have a pleasing personality, a pleasant smile, and enjoy meeting people, a job in the admitting office in your local hospital or a position as a receptionist in a complementary care setting might be of interest to you.

Another important point to consider is whether it may be necessary for you to relocate to get a job. Administrative skills are very portable. Can you think of any business that does not require some type of office skills? Providing there is no language barrier, your skills are required in all parts of the world. Of course, you may not have to move to another city, region, or country to get a job. Currently, many companies hire telecommuters or virtual assistants for administrative and specialty work, such as medical transcription. Online transcription companies such as M*Modal, Terra Nova, and Nuance contract remote medical transcriptionists for most of their work.

Investigate the salary level, skill requirements, location, benefits, and working hours of the position you want. Are the services provided by the organization in your area of interest? Is there room for advancement in the organization? Will the salary level allow you to reach a goal you have set, such as to buy a car or move into your own apartment? All of these things must be considered, because if you accept a position and you are not happy, you will not work to your fullest potential. The Canada Job Bank is an excellent source of labor market information, including salary ranges and job outlook data from across the country. Knowledge of this information may be helpful when negotiating wages and benefits.

At the beginning of your career, it may be necessary to accept a job that is not exactly what you want; however, work with the idea that you are gaining valuable experience and qualifications for when the right job comes along. For instance, many hospitals hire new employees on a casual or part-time basis. Casual employees are called in to work when regular employees are absent. Some casual opportunities offer substantial weekly hours. Many workers prove their abilities while performing casual work. This helps them move into part-time positions and, eventually, full-time positions. Consider a casual opportunity as a great starting point in your career.

When you are invited for an interview, be prepared. Learn as much as you can about the employer and the position. If the employer has a human resources department, call them prior to the interview and ask for the job fact sheet. Having this information can provide additional information that was not in the job advertisement—you can use this information to enhance your interview answers. During the interview, you will be assessed on your ability to communicate (i.e., maintain eye contact, use appropriate grammar, and provide descriptive answers to questions, rather than a simple "yes" or "no"), on your appearance (dress in appropriate business attire), and on your attitude (be courteous and positive). Ask a peer or instructor to conduct a mock interview for practice. The person may point out mannerisms or nervous habits that are distracting, for example, finger tapping, voice inflections, or constant throat clearing. Be ready to sell yourself. Tell the interviewer about your achievements. Following the interview, send a thank-you letter.

Your Employment Documents

A résumé, cover letter, reference sheet, and application form may all be required when applying for employment. These documents are the employer's first impression of you and should be prepared in a manner that best represents you. In addition to these employment documents, be prepared to supply a copy of your academic transcripts and a criminal records or vulnerable sector check. Read the job advertisement carefully to ensure that you are submitting the correct documents.

Résumés

In developing your résumé, you should use a format that best reflects your knowledge, skills, and abilities and emphasizes the particular requirements of the position you are seeking. Chronological and functional résumés meet the needs of most applicants; however, a combination or hybrid of these two styles is also a common choice.

Chronological

Chronological is the most common résumé style. This format allows the reader to see your career progress in a straightforward time line. Its use of concise bulleted lists makes it visually attractive and easy to read. Your experiences are listed in order, with the most recent experience being at the top. For this reason, it is sometimes called a "reverse-chronological" résumé. Your primary job duties and responsibilities for each work experience are noted; any supporting information can be included in your cover letter or discussed at your interview. See Fig. 13.1 for an example of a chronological résumé. For a beginner résumé writer, this format is the easiest to modify. Once you have a good working copy, you can simply add your new experience to the top of your list of experiences.

Functional

Functional résumés take the focus off your time line. Unlike the chronological approach, the functional approach focuses on skills and experiences and does not group responsibilities with specific job headings (see Fig. 13.2 for a functional résumé example). These résumés work well for those who have left the work force for a period of time, have no work experience, or are self-employed. If you are a new graduate who does not have any work experience, the functional résumé may be a good choice. Or, maybe you have employment gaps due to parental leaves or other familial obligations—again, the functional résumé may best reflect your skills and experiences.

Chronological-Functional Combination

The chronological-functional combination, or hybrid résumé, draws on the skills focus of the functional résumé while retaining the dates and lists of duties and responsibilities for relevant employment experiences, as in the chronological (see Fig. 13.3). This style draws attention to a strong skill set required by a specific job and away from limited work experience, career change, or re-entry into the job market.

Considerations

Résumé writing is not an exact science. When you put all of the facts and ideas together, make certain that the finished product projects *you*. The person reading the application wants to know about you, not a textbook character you copied. Your résumé is also a demonstration of your word processing skills and knowledge. As a graduate of an administrative program, you are expected to have good word processing skills and abilities. Consider the following tips, guidelines, and suggestions to improve your résumé writing.

Headings

The first item on your résumé is your personalized "letterhead." This letterhead should contain your first and last name (in a larger font than the body of your résumé), your permanent address (do not use your school address if you will be moving after graduation), your contact numbers, and your personal email address (be sure it is appropriate for professional use; do not use your school address if it will expire). You will use this letterhead on the first page of your résumé (not the second), on your cover letter, and on your reference sheet. Be sure it is exactly the same on all three documents—simply copy and paste it from document to document when you have a format you like. This will give your employment documents a professional appearance.

As a new college graduate, you may want to place the *Education* section at the beginning of the résumé, and you may want to list your courses so that the potential employer can clearly see your accomplishments and better understand the focus of your program (see Fig. 13.1). Once you have secured your first position, you can move the *Education* section below the *Experience* section. At this point, you can also remove your courses if you need the space.

Other examples of headings that you can organize in various ways are *Objective, Volunteer Experience, Certifications, Interests,* and *Memberships.* Although you will not normally add your specific reference information to your résumé, you do acknowledge that it will be attached (if sending electronically), enclosed (if sending paper copies), or available upon

DAPHNE R. SMITH

1356 Gloucester Drive, Ottawa, ON Z8X 1X9

daphrsmith@gmail.com

613-742-9856

Education

Medical Office Administration Diploma   September 2016 to June 2018
Anytown Business College   Anytown, XX

- Medical Terminology I & II
- Medical Transcription I & II
- Grammar for MOAs
- Health Unit Coordinating I & II
- Keyboarding: Advanced
- Medical Office Procedures I & II

- Document Management
- Computer Applications
- Pharmacology for MOAs
- Professionalism in Healthcare
- Medical Office Billing
- Practicum (On-the-Job) Placement

Relevant Experience

Office Assistant (Two-week practicum)   May 2018 to June 2018
Dr. J.E. Plunkett's Medical Office   Ottawa, ON

- Performed medical transcription and speech-recognition editing
- Answered telephones and scheduled appointments
- Prepared and transmitted computerized billing
- Prepared consultations and medical correspondence
- Monitored patient flow and ensured records management
- Assisted physician with medical tests
- Practiced confidentiality and adhered to office policies

Office Worker (Part-time)   May 2017 to September 2017
Anytown Medical Centre   Anytown, XX

- Handled high volume of bookings
- Performed all routine filing, reception, and telephone duties
- Prepared and handled billing documentation for computer input
- Accurately transcribed medical dictation
- Organized and maintained filing system of over 400 patient files
- Assisted nurses with routine medical procedures
- Handled high-pressure situations and deadlines

Teen Volunteer   July 2015 to September 2016
Anytown Hospital   Anytown, XX

References

- Available upon request

• **Fig. 13.1** Chronological Résumé

DAPHNE R. SMITH

1356 Gloucester Drive, Ottawa, ON Z8X 1X9

daphrsmith@gmail.com

613-742-9856

Education

Medical Office Administration Diploma
Anytown Business College

September 2016 to June 2018
Anytown, XX

- Recipient of Medical Secretarial Association Outstanding Graduate Award for academic excellence

Highlights of Qualifications

- Work effectively in a busy medical office environment
- Knowledge of medical procedures, terminology, and anatomy
- Familiar with computers
- Effective communication skills
- Ability to recognize and solve problems
- Effective time management

Medical Administrative Experience

- Performed reception duties and secretarial functions: medical machine transcription, filing medical documents, answering telephones and scheduling appointments
- Effectively monitored patient flow and ensured records management
- Knowledge of medical terminology, anatomy and physiology, and paramedical studies
- Exceptional keyboarding and office skills
- Organized and maintained a workable filing system of over 400 medical files respecting patient confidentiality
- Assisted physician with medical tests and nurses with routine medical procedures and errand service
- Transported newly admitted patients to rooms and patients for tests

Computer Knowledge

- Computer software applications: Microsoft Word, Excel, and PowerPoint
- Prepared computerized billing and transmitted electronically
- Entered all patient records and retrieved data from the electronic medical record (EMR)
- Composed correspondence, prepared reports, completed hospital requisitions, merged letters with labels for mailing of 500

• **Fig. 13.2** Functional Résumé

Daphne R. Smith

Page 2

Management and Problem Solving

- As receptionist, answered and redirect heavy load of incoming calls and relayed messages to staff
- Handled high volume of patients while meeting appointment book schedule
- Effectively handled high-pressure situations and office procedures; met all billing deadlines
- Greeted patients and suppliers in a friendly and courteous manner

Relevant Experience

Office Assistant (Two-week practicum)   May 2018 to June 2018
Dr. J.E. Plunkett's Medical Office   Ottawa, ON

Office Worker (Part-time)   May 2017 to September 2017
Anytown Medical Centre   Anytown, XX

Teen Volunteer   July 2015 to September 2016
Anytown Hospital   Anytown, XX

Memberships and Certifications

CPR with AED, Standard Care First Aid, and WHMIS   December 2017
- St. John Ambulance

Medical Secretaries Association, Student Member   October 2016 to Present
- Assisted with organizing 2018 Clinic Day

Anytown Curling Club, President (Junior Section)   December 2015 to Present
- Certified Curl Canada Instructor

References

Available upon request

• **Fig. 13.2, cont'd**

DAPHNE R. SMITH
1356 Gloucester Drive, Ottawa, ON Z8X 1X9
daphrsmith@gmail.com
613-742-9856

Highlights of Qualifications

- Work effectively in a busy medical office environment
- Knowledge of medical procedures, terminology, and anatomy
- Familiar with computers
- Effective communication skills
- Ability to recognize and solve problems
- Effective time management

Medical Administrative Experience

- Performed reception duties and secretarial functions: medical machine transcription, filing medical documents, answering telephones and scheduling appointments
- Effectively monitored patient flow and ensured records management
- Knowledge of medical terminology, anatomy and physiology, and paramedical studies
- Exceptional keyboarding and office skills
- Assisted physician with medical tests and nurses with routine medical procedures and errand service
- Transported newly admitted patients to rooms and patients for tests
- Organized and maintained a workable filing system of over 400 medical files respecting patient confidentiality

Computer Knowledge

- Computer software applications: Microsoft Word, Excel, and PowerPoint
- Prepared computerized billing and transmitted electronically
- Entered all patient records and retrieved data from the electronic medical record (EMR)
- Composed correspondence, prepared reports, completed hospital requisitions, merged letters with labels for mailing of 500

Time Management and Problem Solving

- As receptionist, answered and redirect heavy load of incoming calls and relayed messages to staff
- Handled high volume of patients while meeting appointment book schedule
- Effectively handled high-pressure situations and office procedures; met all billing deadlines
- Greeted patients and suppliers in a friendly and courteous manner

• **Fig. 13.3** Chronological-Functional Combination

Daphne R. Smith

Relevant Experience

Office Assistant (two-week practicum)
Dr. J.E. Plunkett's Medical Office

May 2018 to June 2018
Ottawa, ON

- Performed medical transcription and speech-recognition editing
- Answered telephones and scheduled appointments
- Prepared and transmitted computerized billing
- Prepared consultations and medical correspondence
- Monitored patient flow and ensured records management
- Assisted physician with medical tests
- Practiced confidentiality and adhered to office policies

Office Worker (part-time)
Anytown Medical Centre

May 2017 to September 2017
Anytown, XX

- Handled high volume of bookings
- Performed all routine filing, reception, and telephone duties
- Prepared and handled billing documentation for computer input
- Accurately transcribed medical dictation
- Organized and maintained filing system of over 400 patient files
- Assisted nurses with routine medical procedures
- Handled high-pressure situations and deadlines

Teen Volunteer
Anytown Hospital

July 2015 to September 2016
Anytown, XX

Education

Medical Office Administration Diploma
Anytown Business College

September 2016 to June 2018
Anytown, XX

- Recipient of Medical Secretarial Association Outstanding Graduate Award for academic excellence

Memberships and Certifications

- CPR with AED, Standard Care First Aid, and WHMIS
- Medical Secretaries Association, Student Member
- Anytown Curling Club, President (Junior Section)

December 2017
October 2016 to Present
December 2015 to Present

References

- Available upon request

• **Fig. 13.3,** cont'd

request. The notes are made under the final résumé heading of *References*.

Style and Format

Sometimes very small touches can give you an advantage. Human resources staff members may be sifting through dozens of résumés from qualified applicants, and a little extra effort may help you stand out.

One way to demonstrate your word processing skills is by avoiding pre-formatted templates. Your advanced word processing skills will shine if you can create your résumé from scratch. Templates can be attractive and seem like a simple solution; however, they can be difficult to modify. They sometimes have standardized font types, font sizes, text boxes, and tabs that may not allow you to achieve the result you are looking for. Even if a résumé is submitted in print form, most experienced administrative professionals can spot a template. They may wonder why you did not attempt to create a résumé style yourself.

You should keep your résumé length to no more than two pages; you will occasionally have to remove or modify older experiences to accomplish this. When you do remove entries, be sure that you are keeping information that is most relevant to the position you are applying to. For instance, if you worked as a volunteer at the hospital where you are applying to work, do not remove this volunteer experience. Instead, choose something unrelated to that work, like a part-time position you held during high school. You may need some guidance on these decisions in the beginning. College employment officers and instructors can provide some advice. In addition, you can research trends and formats in textbooks and online.

Using non-proportional or varying-width fonts is a good choice for résumé writing. These fonts tend to be easier to read and are the most common for published materials; they will give your résumé a professional look. Examples of non-proportional fonts are Times New Roman, Arial, and Verdana. Your font size should be in the 11 to 12 range, with the exception of headings. Headings within the body of the résumé can be up to 14, and your personalized letterhead can be in the range of 14 to 16. The size you use will be determined by font style, the length of your résumé, and overall appearance.

If you are sending a paper copy of your résumé, invest in a heavier paper (24 to 32 lb or 90 to 120 g/m^2) with some texture (woven or linen) and discreet colouring (ivory, almond, light grey).

Storage

It is good practice to review and revise your résumé as necessary for each job you apply to. Keep an electronic master copy that contains all your work experiences, old and current, with a list of all your duties and accomplishments. When you need a new résumé, you can draw from this master file. Give all your new résumés unique file names that reflect the positions you are applying for. Create a résumé folder in your word processing software, and store all of the individual résumé files in this folder for easy access. Back up your files periodically—copy them to a USB drive, email them to yourself, or use a cloud-based program for easy access. Because you will be modifying your files regularly, there is not much need to store paper copies of your résumé.

Sending Your Résumé

When sending your résumé by email, be sure that you have created it in a format that the receiver can download and open. Do not type your résumé into the body of the email; send it as an attachment, and be sure to fill in the subject line of your email to indicate its contents. Also write a brief note in the body of the email (see Fig. 13.4).

If sending your application by mail, package your employment documents flat, in a letter-sized envelope, with an address label that you have created. If you do not have address labels, you can run the envelope through your printer using the envelope function. Be sure you have the proper postage—larger envelopes should be weighed and measured by post office staff. If you wish to send your documents by courier, have all of the receiver's information ready to transfer to the waybill if you do not have one in advance.

Some offices will request employment documents by fax. Be sure that you have the correct fax number, be sure to create a fax cover sheet with your return information, make sure that your documents are in the right order and that you orient them properly on the fax machine. Place a follow-up call to the receiver of your documents to confirm their arrival. If you do not have access to a personal fax machine or software, you can use the faxing services offered at many business centres and office supply stores.

Cover Letters

Your cover letter should begin with your established letterhead. Choose the same fonts and font sizes that you used in your résumé (or copy and paste it from your résumé), and stick with a simple letter format, such as the popular full-block letter with mixed punctuation. Make sure the spacing is correct between all letter elements, and proofread for spelling and format errors. You should have someone else proofread your electronic copy to be sure that you are not overlooking

---

SUBJECT: Resume for Competition No. 654321

TO: lplunkett@drplunkettsoffice.com

SUBJECT: Resume for Competition No. 654321

Dear Lorna:

As discussed, I am attaching my resume in Word format for Competition No. 654321.

Regards,

Daphne R. Smith

Office Assistant Position_Dr. Plunkett.docx (12k) ✕

• **Fig. 13.4** Sample Email Note with Attachment

any errors. Do not forget to sign your name in the signature block. Once you have your format and spacing perfect, save a master cover letter file that you can work from in the future.

The cover letter is most effective when it is brief. Focus on creating three to four brief paragraphs. The first paragraph should include a note on why you are writing to the person or company. Mention the job advertisement, where and when you saw the advertisement, and note any competition numbers associated with it (you can also use a *Subject* or *Reference* line for this). State that you wish to be considered for the opportunity. The next paragraph(s) should connect your hard skills and abilities to those outlined in the advertisement. For instance, if the employer says that they need someone with excellent transcription and time management skills, explain how you can meet these needs specifically. This section of the cover letter will be the most difficult and require you to reflect on your abilities and think critically about how you will deliver your message. Your closing paragraph should thank the advertiser and express your interest in meeting with them to discuss the opportunity. See Fig. 13.5 for a sample cover letter.

Reference Sheets

Most employers will request two to three work references (also call referees). New graduates may be encouraged to use an instructor as a reference. You should always speak to people you are choosing before you offer their name as a referee. Be clear that they are offering a "good" reference. Have a conversation, or send them information, about the job opportunity and your recent experiences. This will give them a chance to imagine how your skills will match the position and how your strengths can help the employer. A referee who is informed and confident in their reference will make a better impression on the employer than one who is surprised by a call.

Your reference sheet should be a document that is separate from your résumé and cover letter. It should begin with your personalized letterhead—matching your résumé and cover letter exactly (see Fig. 13.6). The fonts, font sizes, spacing style, and paper weight and colour (if applicable) should match those of your résumé and cover letter. As discussed above, include a *References* heading in your résumé, and use a notation appropriate for the situation. If you want to submit your application but have not been able to reach your references, add the notation "references available upon request" and keep working on contacting your supporters. If you are sending your application by email, use the notation "attached," and if you are sending by regular mail, use the notation "enclosed."

Application Forms

Many public service commissions and other large employers request the completion of an application form to gather information not normally provided in your other employment documents. The application forms help human resources staff members screen for location preferences,

DAPHNE R. SMITH
1356 Gloucester Drive, Ottawa, ON Z8X 1X9
daphrsmith@gmail.com
613-742-9856

February 25, 20XX

Dr. Jasbir Sandhu
310 O'Connor Street
Ottawa, ON J5Z 2X8

Dear Dr. Sandhu:

Subject: Application for a Medical Assistant Position

Please accept my application for your Medical Administrative Assistant position as listed on the Canada Job Bank web site on January 8, 20XX. I have attached my résumé and references for your consideration.

As a recent graduate of a medical office administration program, I am prepared to begin my career as a medical administrative assistant. In addition to my education, I have knowledge of the hospital atmosphere through volunteer work, and I have learned much about medical office dynamics, transcription, billing, records management, and patient care through related part-time and practicum experiences. My excellent administrative skills, sound knowledge of medical terminology and anatomy, and demonstrated computer skills will positively influence your practice.

I believe my combination of education and experience would be an asset to your team, and I look forward to speaking with you further about this exciting opportunity.

Sincerely,

Daphne Smith

Daphne R. Smith

Attachments: Résumé
                References

• **Fig. 13.5** Cover Letter in Full-Block Style with Mixed Punctuation

DAPHNE R. SMITH

1356 Gloucester Drive, Ottawa, ON Z8X 1X9

daphrsmith@gmail.com

613-742-9856

References

Dr. J. E. Plunkett   **Relationship: Practicum Supervisor**
278 O'Connor Street
Ottawa, ON K2P 1V4
Phone: 613-212-1212
Fax 613-212-2121
www.drplunkettsoffice.com
jeplunkett@dr.plunkettsoffice.com

Rachel Keenan   **Relationship: Administrative Supervisor**
Anytown Medical
22512 Jackson Street
Anytown, XX X0X 0X0
Phone: 902-303-2727, Ext: 12
Fax: 902-303-7272
www.anytownmedical.com
rhkeenan@anytownmed.com

Alexandra DuPont   **Relationship: College Instructor**
Anytown College
0927 College Drive
Anytown, XX X0X 0X0
Phone: 902-303-1010 Ext: 10
Fax: 902-303-0101
www.anytowncollege.com
aldupont@anytowncollege.com

• **Fig. 13.6** Reference Sheet

language abilities, licensed drivers, skill levels (keyboarding speed), and other factors related to the Canadian *Employment Equity* and *Human Rights Acts*.

Many application forms are available in electronic fillable format; however, if you find that you are required to fill in a paper form, print clearly and carefully. A very small error may be corrected by drawing a line through the error and adding your initials. If you make more substantial errors, you should obtain a new form and start the process again. If you cannot download copies of the form, be sure to make copies before you start writing on the original. Submit the form in the manner indicated and by the date requested.

Interview Skills

Plan carefully for your interview, and remember that the interview begins the moment you arrive in the building. Treat everyone you encounter, not just the interviewers, with courtesy. All employees will notice how you present yourself. The following factors will be evaluated by the interviewer:

- Punctuality
- Appearance
- Posture
- Mannerisms
- Courtesy
- Attitude

Arrive 10 to 15 minutes before your appointment. If you are going to be late due to transportation or other unavoidable circumstances, call as soon as you can and explain the situation. If you are not sure where the exact location of the interview is, scout it out in advance.

Your appearance should be professional. You should appear well groomed and in business-style dress. Clothes should be pressed and clean and should fit well. Much of health care remains quite conservative in its policies on dress and personal hygiene because of patient and employee safety concerns; this fact should be kept in mind as you prepare your professional image.

If you are attending more than one interview, be sure that you bring the correct information to the correct interview. Make a file for each competition that includes the job advertisement, the job fact sheet (if available), any questions you may have, and a copy of your application, résumé, cover letter, and references. If you did not provide your reference sheet at the time of your application submission, be sure to bring it to the interview.

Before the interview, network with people in the industry who can give you some advice on what to expect. Human resources professionals can also be contacted for more information about the interview process. If there is no dedicated human resources professional available, research interview question types and practice answers to some possible questions. Visit the institution's website, and gather some facts

---

• BOX 13.3   What Not to Do During an Interview

Do not chew gum or candy.
Do not display nervous gestures such as fidgeting, stroking your face, or tugging at your clothes.
Do not interrupt.
Do not argue, brag, or criticize.

• BOX 13.4   What Does the Employer Want?

A person with both the hard and soft skills to do the job
A person who has a professional appearance that complements the employer's image
A person who is dependable and can prove that he or she is a reliable team member

---

about the employer. All of these steps will make you more confident and comfortable on interview day.

Box 13.3 and Box 13.4 provide additional interview and employment tips.

Career Advancement

Although we have been discussing how to obtain your first job in health care, it is never too early to think about what might come next. As mentioned previously, the job outlook for medical administrative assistants in Canada is healthy. In addition to the 19,000 new positions estimated by Canada Job Bank, many existing positions held by senior administrative assistants will open up as employees retire or change positions. You may want to consider how to move into more responsible positions once you have gained some experience. Even if you are not interested in moving into leadership roles, additional training will bring many advantages; security in your role, potential wage increase, and a higher level of competence and confidence in your abilities are just a few.

Take advantage of any professional development opportunities or funding that your employer offers. You can also consider continuing your formal education by enrolling in a post diploma bachelor's degree, such as a bachelor of health administration. These degrees can expand your knowledge in the areas of accounting, health care law, writing for health care organizations, and others. Some colleges offer articulation agreements that allow your college credits to be transferred for credit toward a bachelor's degree, allowing you to finish your degree in less than the traditional time frame. These opportunities have the potential to open you up to a future that you may not even be able to imagine currently. Would you like to be a supervisor? Perhaps a medical office manager? What about an instructor in a medical administrative assistant program?

Summary

This chapter has provided valuable information that will assist you in future job searches. You know where to seek employment and how to prepare yourself for the opportunities that are coming your way. You have the knowledge and the skills to create professional-looking employment documents that highlight your education, employment, and skills in a logical way. The factors that interviewers will assess during the interview process have been outlined; attending to these factors will positively influence the interview experience for you and the interviewer. Your dedicated attention to all of the details that go into a job search will help you stand out from the crowd, and making a commitment to life-long learning will prepare you to leap forward in your career. You are well on your way to enjoying an exciting future in the Canadian health care industry.

Assignments

Assignment 13.1

Select an advertisement for a medical or general administrative assistant from one of the job search sites discussed in the chapter. Prepare a cover letter, résumé, and reference sheet. Save these documents in a dedicated résumé folder for future use.

Assignment 13.2

Extract from your portfolio the rating sheet you completed in Assignment 1.3. Would your ratings in any of the categories change?

Assignment 13.3

Research types of interview questions. Try to create five questions (a combination of the styles you find) that you think may be asked by the interviewer for the job advertisement you choose. Have a classmate ask you the questions and provide you some feedback on your mannerisms, posture, courtesy, and attitude.

Assignment 13.4

Extract from your portfolio the skills and personal qualities inventory sheet completed in Assignment 1.4. Reassess your skill levels. Have you acquired any new skills? How would you rate those skills? Have any of your skills improved; if so, how much?

Reassess your personal qualities. Would you rate any of your personal qualities as being stronger than in your original rating?

Assignment 13.5

With your instructor's assistance, search local or online universities for post diploma programs that may complement your college credential. Find out whether your current program of study offers an articulation agreement with another academic institution.

Topics for Discussion

1. What are some examples of positive body language during an interview? What are some examples of negative body language?

2. Discuss appropriate attire and hygiene considerations for an interview. Also discuss inappropriate attire.

Appendix A

Common Abbreviations Used in the Health Care Field

The following is a list of common abbreviations and short forms used in the medical profession. Some abbreviations should never be used in medical documentation. A list of these "dangerous" abbreviations is provided at the end of the common abbreviations.

Even when abbreviations are not considered "dangerous," caution must be used when applying them to any medical documentation. The same combination of letters with different letter casing and punctuation may have a different meaning. Many abbreviations also have more than one meaning, so the context in which an abbreviation is being applied must be considered.

The terms of use for abbreviations and short forms may vary depending on the workplace setting, the purpose, or your area of specialization (medical transcriptionist versus a health unit coordinator) be sure to consult the appropriate style guide or policy for each situation.

A

ABGs	arterial blood gases
a.c.	before eating; before meals (L. ante cibum)
ad lib.	as desired; at pleasure (L. ad libitum)
adhib.	to be administered (L. abhibendus)
ADL (or ADLs)	activities of daily living
ADT	admission, discharge, transfer
AED	automated external defibrillator
afeb (or abs. feb.)	without fever (L. absente febre)
Afib	atrial fibrillation
AHDI	Association for Healthcare Documentation Integrity
alt. dieb.	every other day (L. alternis diebus)
alt. hor.	every other hour (L. alternis horis)
alt. noc.	every other night (L. alternis nocte)
a.m.	before noon; morning (L. ante meridiem)
AMA	against medical advice
ANA	antinuclear antibodies
aq.	water (L. aqua)
ARDS	acute (adult) respiratory distress syndrome
as tol	as tolerated
ASA	acetylsalicylic acid

B

b.i.d.	twice daily (L. bis in die)
bili (or Bil)	bilirubin
b.i.n.	twice a night (L. bis in nocte)
bis in 7d.	twice a week
BMI	body mass index
bol.	bolus
BP	blood pressure
BRAT	bananas, rice cereal, applesauce, toast
BRP	bathroom privileges
BUN	blood urea nitrogen
Bx (or bx)	biopsy

C

c̄	with (L. cum)
C	Celsius
C&S	culture and sensitivity
Ca	cancer
ca.	about (L. circa)
CABG	coronary artery bypass graft
cal	calorie
cap (or cap.)	capsule (L. capsula)
CAT	computerized axial tomography
cath	catheter/catheterize/catheterization
CBC	complete blood count
CC	chief complaint
cc	cubic centimetre
cm	centimetre
c.m.	tomorrow morning (L. cras mane)
CMA	Canadian Medical Association
CMPA	Canadian Medical Protective Association
c.m.s.	to be taken tomorrow morning (L. cras mane sumendus)
c.n.	tomorrow night (L. cras note)
CNS	central nervous system
CO_2	carbon dioxide

compd (or Comp.)	compound (L. compositus)
COPD	chronic obstructive pulmonary disease
CPAP	continuous positive airway pressure
CPOE	computerized physician order entry
CPR	cardiopulmonary resuscitation
CTS	carpal tunnel syndrome
CV	cardiovascular
CXR	chest x-ray

D

d	day
/d	per day
D	dose
D&C	dilation and curettage
DAT	diet as tolerated
diff	differential
DIN	drug identification number
D/LR	dextrose in lactated Ringer's
DM	diabetes mellitus
DNR	do not resuscitate
DOB	date of birth
dr	dram
DVT	deep vein thrombosis
Dx (or dx)	diagnosis

E

ECG	electrocardiogram; electrocardiography
ECT	electroconvulsive therapy
EEG	electroencephalogram; electroencephalography
e.g.	example (L. exempli gratia)
EHR	electronic health record
EKG	electrocardiogram; electrocardiography
EMG	electromyogram; electromyography
e.m.p.	in the manner prescribed (L. ex modo praescripto)
EMR	electronic medical record
ENT	ears, nose, and throat
ESR	erythrocyte sedimentation rate
etc.	and so forth (L. et cetera)

F

FBS	fasting blood sugar
FCFP	Fellow of the College of Family Physicians
FF	forced fluids

fl oz	fluid ounce; fluidounce
FRCP	Fellow of the Royal College of Physicians
FRCP(C)	Fellow of the Royal College of Physicians of Canada
FRCS(C)	Fellow of the Royal College of Surgeons of Canada
FROM	full range of motion
FSH	follicle-stimulating hormone
FU (or F/U)	follow-up (adj.); follow up (v.); followup (n.)
Fx	fracture

G

g	gram
GERD	gastroesophageal reflux disease
GH	growth hormone
GI	gastrointestinal
GP	general practitioner
gr	grain
Grad.	by degrees (L. gradatim)
gt.	drop (L. gutta)
gtt.	drops (L. guttae)
GTT	glucose tolerance test
GU	genitourinary

H

h (or hr, hrs, h.)	hour (L. hora)
H&H	hemoglobin and hematocrit
H&P	history and physical
H/O	history of
H_2O	water
Hct	hematocrit
HDL	high-density lipoprotein
HEENT	head, eyes, ears, nose, throat
Hgb	hemoglobin
HIM	health information management/manager
h.n.	tonight (L. hora nocte)
HOB	head of bed
HRN	health record number
h.s.	at bedtime (L. hora somni)
HTN (or htn)	hypertension
HUC	health unit coordinator
Hx (or hx)	history

I

I&D	incision and drainage
I&O	intake and output
IBS	irritable bowel syndrome

IBW	ideal body weight
ICD	implantable cardioverter-defibrillator; international classification of diseases
ICU	intensive care unit
IM	intramuscular
IN	intranasal
IP	intraperitoneal
IUD	intrauterine (contraceptive) device
IV	intravenously
IVF	intravenous fluids
IVP	intravenous pyelogram
IVPB	intravenous piggyback

J

J	joule
Jt (or jnt)	joint
Jts	joints
JV	jugular vein/venous
JVD	jugular venous distention
JVP	jugular venous pulse

K

K	potassium (L. kalium)
kcal	kilocalorie
KCl	potassium chloride
Kg	kilogram
kHz	kilohertz
kj	knee jerk
KJ	kilojoule
kl	kilolitre
KO	keep open
KUB	kidneys, ureters, bladder
kV	kilovolt
kW	kilowatt

L

L	litre
L&R	left and right
L&U	lower and upper
L/min	litres per minute
LAD	left anterior descending (coronary artery)
Lat	lateral
LDL	low-density lipoprotein
LE	lower extremity/extremities
lig.	ligament (L. ligamentum)
ligg.	ligaments (L. ligamenta)
LLE	left lower extremity

LLL	left lower lobe
LLQ	left lower quadrant
LPN	licensed practical nurse
LTC	long-term care
LUE	left upper extremity
LUL	left upper lobe
LUQ	left upper quadrant
lytes	electrolytes

M

MD	medical doctor
MDI	metered-dose inhaler
mets	metastasis; metastases
mEq	milliequivalent
Mg	magnesium
mg	milligram
MI	myocardial infarction
min	minute
mL	millilitre
mm	millimetre
mm HG	millimetres of mercury
MOM	milk of magnesia
MRP	most responsible physician
MRI	magnetic resonance imaging
MRN	medical record number
MRSA	methicillin-resistant *Staphylococcus aureus*
MS	multiple sclerosis
MT	medical transcriptionist

N

N&V	nausea and vomiting
N/A	not applicable
N/S	normal saline
Na	sodium
NaCl	sodium chloride
NAS	no added salt
NCS	nerve conduction studies
NEC (or nec.)	not elsewhere classified
NG	nasogastric
noc	night
NOS	not otherwise specified
NP	nurse practitioner
NPO	nothing by mouth
NSA	no salt added
NSAID	non-steroidal anti-inflammatory drug
NTE	not to exceed
NYD	not yet diagnosed

O

O_2	oxygen
O&P	ova and parasite
OA	osteoarthritis
OB	obstetrics
OE	otitis externa
OM	otitis media
OOB	out of bed
OR	operating room
ORIF	open reduction internal fixation
OT	occupational therapy
oz	ounce

P

P	pulse
p.c.	after meals (L. post cibum)
p.m.	after noon; evening (L. post meridiem)
p.o.	by mouth (L. per os)
p.r.n.	as needed; as necessary (L. pro re nata)
PACS	picture archiving and communication system
PBI	protein-bound iodine
PCP	primary care physician
PE	physical examination
PERRLA	pupils equal, round, reactive to light and accommodation
PET	positron emission tomography
PHI	personal health information
PHR	personal health record
PICC	peripherally inserted central catheter
PID	pelvic inflammatory disease
PMH	past medical history
POCT	point-of-care testing
ppm	parts per million
PR	per (through the) rectum
PROM	passive range of motion
PSA	prostate-specific antigen
PT	physical therapy/therapist; pro-thrombin time
PTCA	percutaneous transluminal coronary angioplasty
PUD	peptic ulcer disease

Q

q.	each; every (L. quaque)
QA	quality assurance
QC	quality control
q.2 h.	every two hours (L. quaque seconda hora)
q.4 h.	every four hours (L. quaque quarta hora)
q.h.	every hour (L. quaque hora)
q.i.d.	four times a day (L. quater in die)
q.l.	as much as wanted (L. quantum libet)
q.s.	sufficient quantity (L. quantum satis)
qns (or QNS)	quantity not sufficient
qt	quart

R

R	respiration
R/O	rule out
RBC	red blood count; red blood cell
RLE	right lower extremity
RLL	right lower lobe
RLQ	right lower quadrant
RML	right middle lobe
RN	registered nurse
ROM	range of motion
RR	respiratory rate
RT	respiratory therapist
RUE	right upper extremity
RUL	right upper lobe
RUQ	right upper quadrant
Rx	prescription, treatment, or medication

S

$\bar{s}$	without (L. sine)
S&A	sugar and acetone
SARS	severe acute respiratory syndrome
SGOT	serum glutamic oxaloacetic trans-aminase
SGPT	serum glutamic pyruvic transaminase
SOB	shortness of breath
sol'n	solution
Staph	Staphylococcus
stat. (or STAT)	urgent; rush; immediately (L. statim)
stet.	let it stand (L. steti)
Strep	Streptococcus
sub-q (or SQ, sq)	subcutaneously
subling (or sl, sL)	sublingual
supp	suppository
syr.	syrup (L. syrupus)

T

T (or temp)	temperature
tab	tablet
tabs	tablets

TKO	to keep open
TENS	transcutaneous electrical nerve stimulation
T&C (or T&X-match)	type and crossmatch
T3, T4, T7	thyroid tests
TB	tuberculosis
T&S	type and screen
TIA	transient ischemic attack
TKR	total knee replacement
TKA	total knee arthroplasty
THR	total hip replacement
THA	total hip arthroplasty
TPAL	term, premature, abortions, living
TPR	temperature, pulse, respirations
TSH	thyroid-stimulating hormone
TURP	transurethral resection of the prostate
trig (or TG)	triglycerides
Tx	traction
top.	topically
TEE	transesophageal echocardiography
t.i.d.	three times daily (L. ter in die)
t.i.n.	three times a night (L. ter in nocte)
tinct.	tincture
TKVO	to keep vein open

U

ung.	ointment (L. unguentum)
ur (or UR)	urine
URI	upper respiratory infection
U&L	upper and lower
UA (or U/A)	urinalysis
UC	urine culture
UO (or U/O)	urine output
UTI	urinary tract infection
US	ultrasound
UV	ultraviolet

V

VDRL	Venereal Disease Research Laboratory (laboratory test)
Vfib	ventricular fibrillation
VRE	vancomycin-resistant Enterococcus
VS	vital signs
$\dot{V}/\dot{Q}$	ventilation/perfusion (quotient)

vol	volume; voluntary
vf	visual field
vent (or VENT)	ventral; ventricular
VAD	vascular access device

W

WBC (or wbc)	white blood count; white blood cell
WBAT	weight bearing as tolerated
WHO	World Health Organization
wt	weight
w/v	weight by volume
WOW	workstation on wheels
WNL	within normal limits
WA (or W/A)	while awake; while awake
wk	week
wc (or w/c)	wheelchair

X, Y, Z

XR	X-ray
XM	crossmatch
x	times
y.o. (or YO)	years old
yr (or y)	year
YOB	year of birth
yd	yard
Zn	zinc

The Institute for Safe Medication Practices (ISMP) Canada has compiled a list of abbreviations that are considered to be dangerous. The list identifies abbreviations that have been reported as causing actual or potential harm to patients due to misinterpretation. Abbreviations on this list should never be used to communicate medical information.

Do Not Use

Dangerous Abbreviations, Symbols and Dose Designations

The abbreviations, symbols, and dose designations found in this table have been reported as being frequently misinterpreted and involved in harmful medication errors. They should NEVER be used when communicating medication information.

Abbreviation	Intended Meaning	Problem	Correction
U	unit	Mistaken for "0" (zero), "4" (four), or cc.	Use "unit".
IU	international unit	Mistaken for "IV" (intravenous) or "10" (ten).	Use "unit".
Abbreviations for drug names		Misinterpreted because of similar abbreviations for multiple drugs; e.g., MS, MSO_4 (morphine sulphate), $MgSO_4$ (magnesium sulphate) may be confused for one another.	Do not abbreviate drug names.
QD QOD	Every day Every other day	QD and QOD have been mistaken for each other, or as 'qid'. The Q has also been misinterpreted as "2" (two).	Use "daily" and "every other day".
OD	Every day	Mistaken for "right eye" (OD = oculus dexter).	Use "daily".
OS, OD, OU	Left eye, right eye, both eyes	May be confused with one another.	Use "left eye", "right eye" or "both eyes".
D/C	Discharge	Interpreted as "discontinue whatever medications follow" (typically discharge medications).	Use "discharge".
cc	cubic centimetre	Mistaken for "u" (units).	Use "mL" or "millilitre".
µg	microgram	Mistaken for "mg" (milligram) resulting in one thousand-fold overdose.	Use "mcg".

Symbol	Intended Meaning	Potential Problem	Correction
@	at	Mistaken for "2" (two) or "5" (five).	Use "at".
> <	Greater than Less than	Mistaken for "7"(seven) or the letter "L". Confused with each other.	Use "greater than"/"more than" or "less than"/"lower than".

Dose Designation	Intended Meaning	Potential Problem	Correction
Trailing zero	$x.0$ mg	Decimal point is overlooked resulting in 10-fold dose error.	Never use a zero by itself after a decimal point. Use "x mg".
Lack of leading zero	$.x$ mg	Decimal point is overlooked resulting in 10-fold dose error.	Always use a zero before a decimal point. Use "$0.x$ mg".

Adapted from ISMP's List of *Error-Prone Abbreviations, Symbols,* and *Dose Designations 2006*

© 2006 ISMP Canada, reaffirmed 2018

Report actual and potential medication errors to ISMP Canada at https://www.ismp-canada.org/err_report.htm **or by calling** 1-866-54-ISMPC.

Institute for Safe Medication Practices Canada
Institut pour la sécurité des médicaments aux patients du Canada

Source: Institute for Safe Medication Practices (ISMP) Canada. (2018). Do not use: Dangerous abbreviations, symbols and dose designations. Retrieved from https://www.ismp-canada.org/dangerousabbreviations.htm

Laboratory Medicine

In the field of laboratory medicine, tests are conducted on specimens to assess an individual's health status. The results provide an avenue for diagnosis and treatment as well as for aid in the development of illness prevention strategies. Standard laboratory ranges will vary slightly from laboratory to laboratory depending on the type of tests conducted. Test results that fall outside the standard range will be flagged on the reports generated. Each reporting laboratory identifies the standard range for each test performed.

More recently, to promote the availability of test results, health care practices have encouraged patients to set up a user profile through the laboratory-hosted website; this enrollment enables the patient to view his or her own test results online as they become available. Patients may contact the office of their primary health care provider for a more robust explanation after self-reviewing their results. As an effective medical administrative assistant, you will benefit from developing an understanding of commonly ordered tests in laboratory medicine.

As a medical administrative assistant, you may be involved in collecting, handling, and storing specimens prior to distribution to the laboratory for analysis. Secure from your local laboratory its specimen management guidelines. Be mindful that inappropriate specimen management can compromise a result.

Several subdivisions or departments fit under the umbrella of laboratory medicine. The headings provided in this appendix outline common departments and tests performed.

Biochemistry

Biochemistry—is the analysis of testing performed on bodily fluids such as blood, urine, cerebrospinal fluid (CSF), and other fluids. Typically, biochemical blood tests are performed on the liquid portion of a blood specimen known as *serum* or *plasma*. The specimen is collected by a phlebotomist using a Vacutainer for collection, storage, and transportation to the lab.

Biochemical tests can determine the level of various drugs, hormones, and other substances in the body from the blood sample obtained. Remember, biological variants commonly exist from laboratory to laboratory due to homeostatic setting points.

Laboratory tests are ordered based on the critical need and the patient's condition. The physician, nurse practitioner, and other allied health professionals ordering the testing determine the critical need. Expected turnaround times for laboratory tests vary according to the urgency of the initial request. Test time lines fall into one of three categories: routine, urgent, and emergent, also known as *STAT testing*.

Routine tests are orders without any indication of priority need. Most results are available within 24 hours after the receipt of the specimen at the lab.

Urgent testing requires the laboratory to process the specimen as soon as possible after receipt of the specimen. In most cases, the patient's health status has been compromised, and the testing will help provide a greater insight. Usually, a three-hour window is standard for processing results for orders of the urgent category.

The term *STAT,* or emergent, is derived from the Latin word *statim,* meaning instant or immediately. The specimen is collected and processed immediately. Results are usually available within 60 minutes. STAT tests are ordered by a physician when a life-threatening medical emergency is occurring.

Following is a list of some laboratory tests and turnaround times for reference.

Test	Routine	Urgent	Emergent/STAT
Acetaminophen	24 hr	3 hr	90 min
Alkaline phos-phatase	8 hr	na	na
Amylase	8 hr	2 hr	na
Barbiturates	8 hr	3 hr	90 min
Bilirubin total	8 hr	na	na
Calcium	8 hr	2 hr	60 min
Chloride	24 hr	na	na
CK (total)	8 hr	2 hr	na
CK-2 (MB)	24 hr	na	na
Creatinine	8 hr	90 min	na
CSF—protein	na	3 hr	60 min
CSF—glucose	3 hr	90 min	na
Digoxin	24 hr	na	na
Dilantin	24 hr	na	na
Drug screen	10	na	na
Electrophoresis	72 hr	na	na
Glucose	8 hr	2 hr	60 min
HDL—C	5	na	na
Iron	4	na	na

Continued

Test	Routine	Urgent	Emergent/STAT
Lithium	2	na	na
Magnesium	8 hr	na	na
Occult blood	24 hr	na	na
Osmolality	8 hr	na	na
pH	hr	1 hr	20 min
Phosphates	8 hr	na	na
Potassium	8 hr	90 min	60 min
Pregnancy test	8 hr	2 hr	1 hr
Protein—CSF	na	3 hr	60 min
Protein—total	8 hr	na	na
SGOT (AST)	8 hr	na	na
Sodium	8 hr	2 hr	60 min
Triglycerides	8 hr	na	na
Urate	8 hr	na	na
Urea (BUN)	8 hr	2 hr	na
Urinalysis	8 hr	60 min	na

NOTE: The electrolytes—sodium, potassium, and chloride—are sometimes shown in short form on a requisition simply as *lytes*.

   Enzymes = SGOT, LDH, CK

   BUN = Blood, urea, and nitrogen

   The following information is included when completing a biochemistry requisition:

Patient's name

Patient's birth date

Patient's medical record number (if an inpatient)

Attending physician

Ordering physician

Tests required

Date and time of collection

Diagnosis or relevant clinical information

   See Fig. B.1 for an example of a Biochemistry/Blood Testing Requisition from Ontario.

Cytology

Cytology—is the examination under a microscope and study of cells from the body. Cytology tests commonly check for infection, inflammatory disease, cancer, or precancerous conditions. Cytology testing comprises gynecological cervical-vaginal specimens as well as a complete range of non-gynecological specimens.

   The following is a sample list of cytology tests for reference.

Bronchial washing

Broncho-alveolar lavage

CSF (for malignant cells)

Fine needle aspirates

Gynecological smears

Pericardial fluid (for malignant cells)

Peritoneal fluid (for malignant cells)

Pleural fluid (for malignant cells)

Sputum (for malignant cells)

Urine for cytology

The following information must be included when completing a cytology requisition:

a. Gynecological Requisition

   Patient's name

   Patient's birth date

   Ordering physician

   Type of specimen

   Date smear taken

   Date of last menstrual period (LMP)

   Relevant clinical information

b. Non-gynecological Requisition

   Patient's name

   Patient's birth date

   Ordering physician

   Type of specimen

   Date and time specimen taken

   Relevant clinical information

   See Fig. B.2 for an example of a Gynecological Cytology Requisition from Alberta. Note the selection of Pap smear on the requisition.

Hematology

Hematology—is the study of blood cells, bone marrow, and coagulation. Hematology contrasts biochemistry blood testing because the solids of blood are analyzed instead of the fluid-based components. The solids include erythrocytes, leukocytes, and thrombocytes (red, white, and clotting cells).

   The following is a list of some of the hematological laboratory tests and turnaround times for reference.

   Note: The most routine hematological test is known as a *complete blood count,* commonly referred to using the short form, CBC. A CBC is used to evaluate overall health and to detect a wide range of disorders, including anemia, infection, and leukemia. The components analyzed include erythrocytes, which are oxygen-carrying blood cells; leukocytes, which are infection-fighting cells; hemoglobin, a protein in red blood cells that carries oxygen; and thrombocytes, which assist with blood clotting.

a. Hematology

Test	Routine	Urgent	Emergent
Leukocytes	4 hr	90 min	10 min
Hemoglobin	4 hr	90 min	10 min
Hematocrit	4 hr	90 min	10 min
MCV	4 hr	90 min	10 min
Platelets	4 hr	90 min	10 min
ESR	6 hr	na	na
Reticulocytes	6 hr	na	na
Mono screen	4 hr	90 min	na
CSF count	2 hr	90 min	60 min
CSF diff.	3 hr	2 hr	90 min
Malarial parasites	3 hr	90 min	60 min
Sickle screen	3 hr	90 min	60 min
Bone marrow prep.	24 hr	2 hr	na

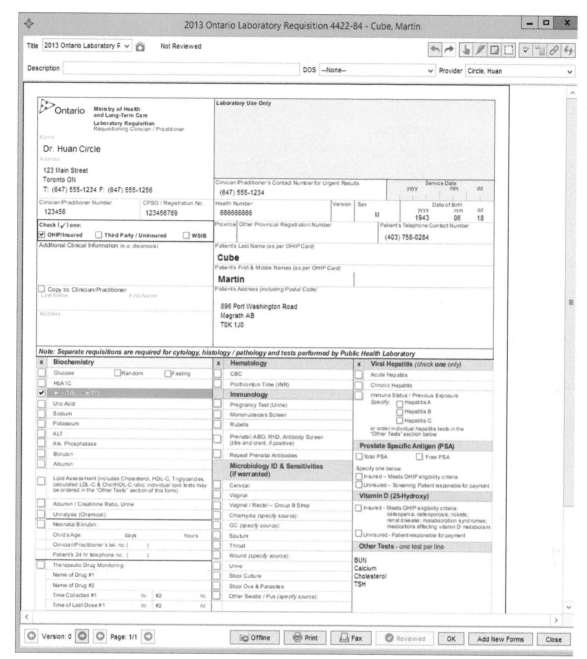

• **Fig. B.1** Combined Biochemistry/Blood Testing Requisition. (Source: EMR Accuro (Permissions: contact Lauren Romano, lauren.romano@QHRtech.com))

b. Hematology—Coagulation

Test	Routine	Urgent	Emergent
Prothrombin time	4 hr	90 min	30 min
Pro-time—anticoagulant	4 hr	90 min	na
Bleeding time	4 hr	na	na
Thrombin time	4 hr	2 hr	60 min
Lupus anticoagulant	4 hr	na	na
Protein C	10	na	na
Protein S	10	na	na
Platelet antibodies	10	na	na
Platelet count	4 hr	90 min	10 min

The following information, which is similar to that required on a biochemistry requisition, should be included when completing a hematology requisition:

Patient's name
Patient's birth date
Ordering physician
Tests required
Date specimen to be taken
Relevant clinical information

Refer to Fig B.1 and B.2 sample requisitions, and note the sections for selecting hematological testing.

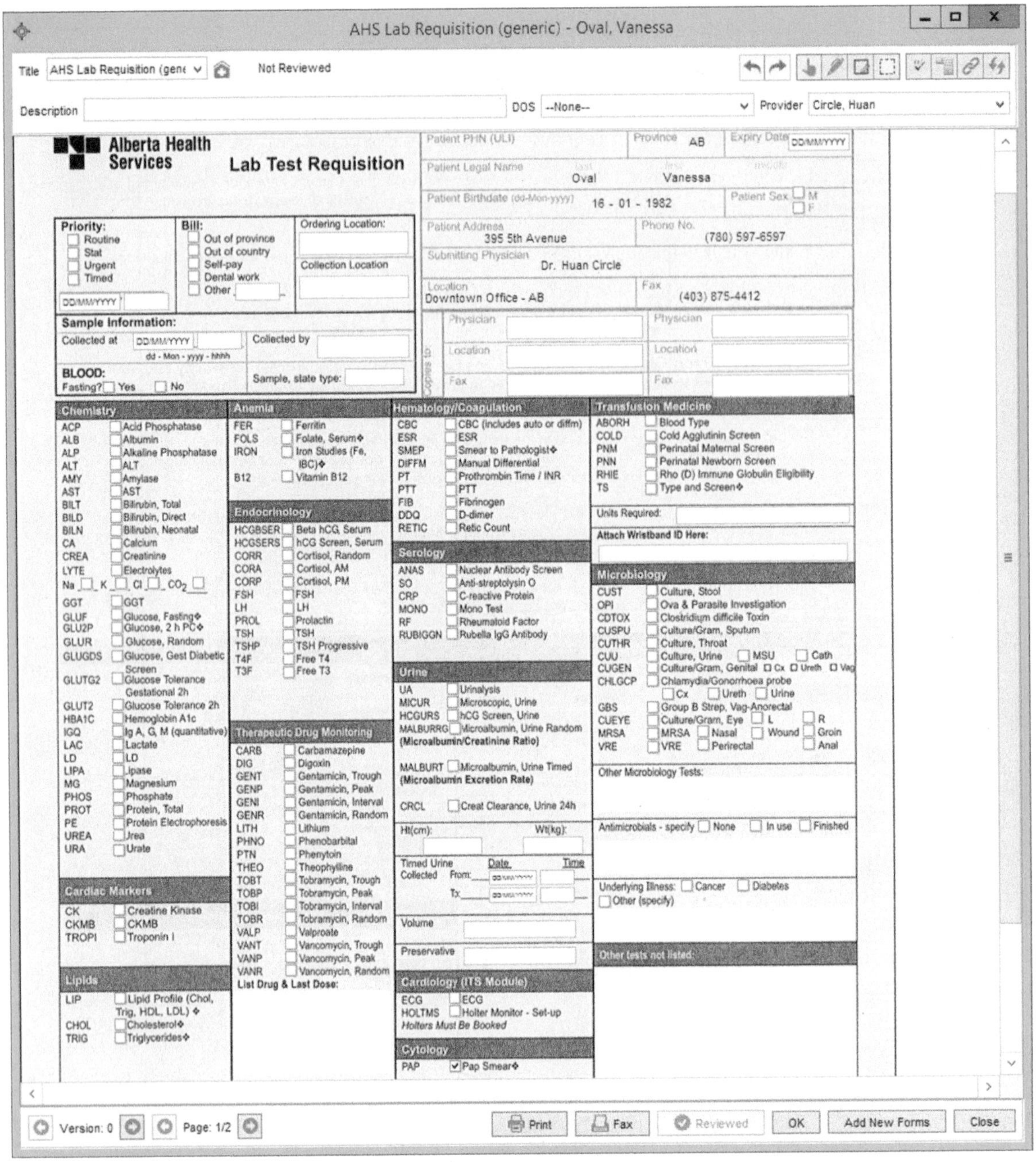

• **Fig. B.2** Gynecological Cytology Requisition. (Source: Accuro (see above permissions information))

Histology

Histology—is the study of tissues; it is used for routine pathology reporting. This medical application is referred to as *histopathology*, which means the study of diseased tissue. Tissue obtained for testing is usually prepared or treated in a specific way to maintain the integrity of the originating specimen. The three main types of tissue specimens analyzed through histopathology are identified as follows:

1. Whole specimens involve large sections or a complete organ after removal, such as a uterus after a hysterectomy.
2. Section specimens involve pieces of tissue, also known as a *biopsy;* examples include a biopsy of breast, liver, or lymph tissue.

3. Fluid specimens involve tissue gathered through a needle aspiration, such as a lung fluid tissue sample. It is a much finer sample than a section specimen.

The following is a list of some specimens that are analyzed in the histology division of a laboratory, along with turnaround times for your reference.

Test	Turnaround Time
Intra-operative consultations	15–20 min variable
Surgical pathology (without special stains, consultations, etc.)	24–36 hr

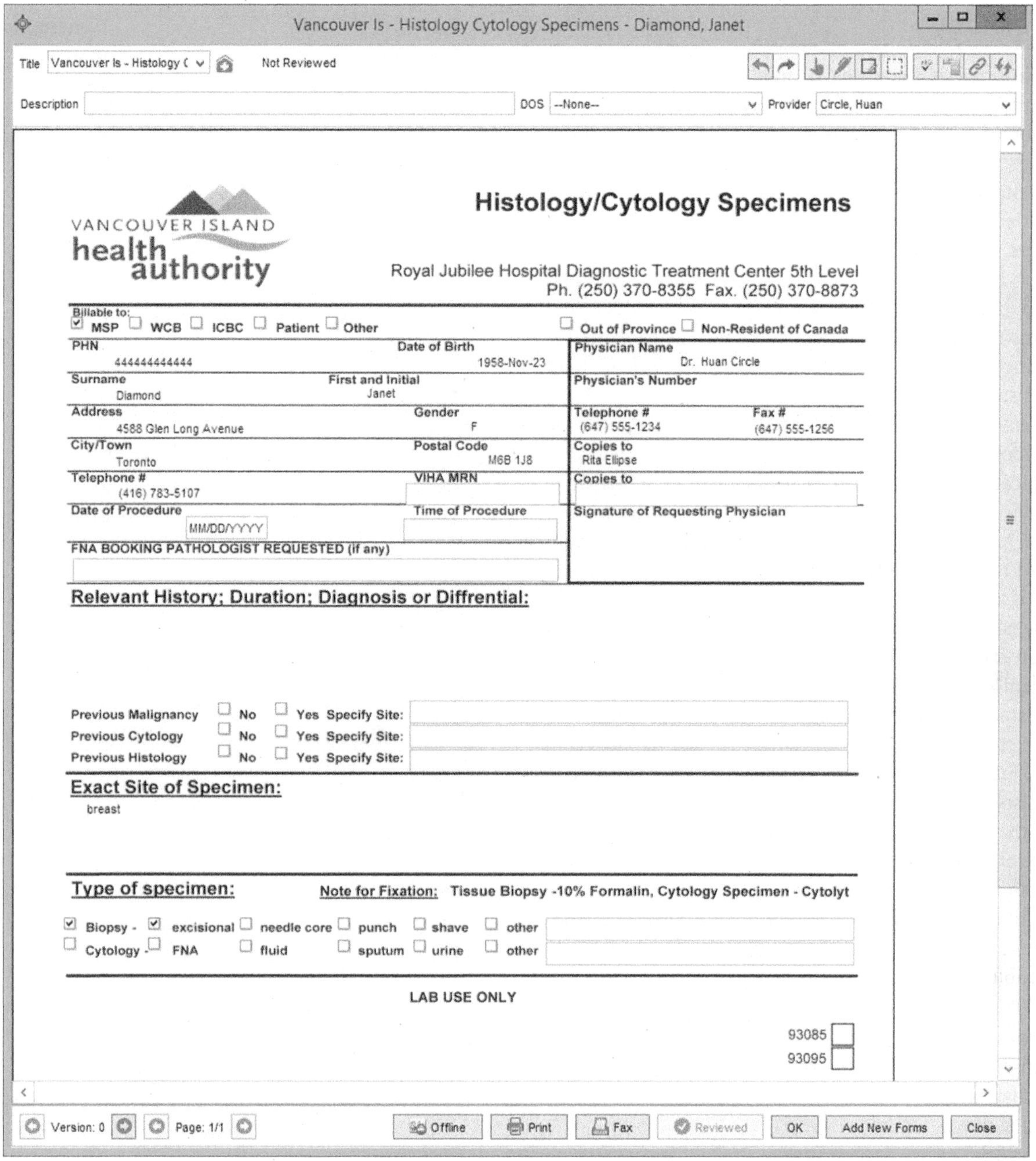

Fig. B.3 Histology Requisition. (Source: Accuro (see above permission and credit information))

Test	Turnaround Time
Fresh tissue for possible malignant lymphoma	24 hr 48 hr (depending on time received by laboratory)
Estrogen receptors	1–2 wk
Renal biopsies	May be sent to another facility
Muscle biopsies	May be sent to another facility
Unstained slides	1–3 wk
Mammographically directed biopsies	24–48 hr 48–72 hr (varies depending on time received by laboratory)

The following information is included when completing a histology requisition:

Patient's full name
Patient's birth date
Sex
Type of specimen
Anatomical location
Pertinent history, including where and when previous diagnosis was made
Date of surgery
Preoperative diagnosis
Postoperative diagnosis
Submitting physician or surgeon
See Fig. B.3 for a sample Histology Requisition from British Columbia.

Microbiology

Microbiology—is the study of microscopic living organisms. Laboratory microbiology involves testing and identifying bacteria, fungi, parasites, and viruses in patients' specimens. As a science, microbiology helps improve health for patients by identifying treatment methods to combat a wide variety of bacterial infections and disease-producing organisms.

Many microbiology tests require that the specimen obtained be placed through a culture process. A culture maintains the specimen in suitable conditions to allow for growth in an artificial environment. A medium, often a solid jelly-like substance known as an *agar*, is used to permit the growth environment. If growth occurs, the disease-producing microorganism is identified, which is the culture result, and typically a treatment is recommended. For instance, a microbiology test ordered for a nose C&S. The nose is swabbed for a suspected bacterial infection, and the swab is sent to the laboratory for analysis. With a test for C&S, the "C" is the culture component of the testing, and the "S" is the sensitivity. A report is generated detailing the nasal specimen results; if it is positive for an infection, the bacteria is identified and listed on the report. The sensitivity on the report identifies which antibiotic will treat the infection. Antibiotics that will not work against the bacterial infection cultured are listed as resistant or simply denoted with an *r*. This assists the physician in ordering the correct medication to treat the infectious condition. Table B.1 shows an example of a Urine for C&S report, detailing the bacterial growth and antibiotic sensitivity.

The following is a list of some of the microbiology laboratory tests and turnaround times for your reference.

a. Microbiology (Routine)

Test	Turnaround Time
Abscess for C&S (culture & sensitivity)	48 hr
Acid fast bacilli	24 hr
Auger suction—C&S	48 hr
Bile—C&S	48 hr
Blood culture—C&S	72 hr
Blood culture—mycobacteria	8 hr
Bronchial washing—C&S	48 hr
Bronchial washing—fungus	4 wk
Bronchial washing—T.B.	8 wk
Catheter tip—C&S	48 hr
Chlamydia	3–6 d
Corneal scrapings	48 hr
CSF—C&S	72 hr
CSF—routine Gram stain	24 hr
Fluid (body)—C&S	48 hr
Genital swab—C&S	48 hr
Genital swab—GC culture	72 hr
Genital swab—gonorrhea	72 hr
Gram stain—routine	24 hr
Lung washing—fungus	4 wk
Lung washing—G&S	48 hr

Test	Turnaround Time
Lung washing—T.B.	8 wk
Mouth and gums	48 hr
Mycology (skin scraping/hair)	4 wk
Mycoplasma	10–14 d
Nails—fungus culture	4 wk
Nose—C&S	48 hr
Parasitology	7 d
Pinworm	1 d
Rectal culture	72 hr
Rectal culture—gonorrhea	72 hr
Skin—C&S	48 hr
Skin scrapings (fungus culture)	4 wk
Stool—C&S	72 hr
Stool—O&P	7 d
Stool—RSV	24 hr
Stool—*Clostridium difficile*	48 hr
Throat	48 hr
Throat washing—(virus)	7–10 d
Tissue	72 hr
Tuberculosis—respiratory	8 wk
Tuberculosis—urine	8 wk
Urine—culture and colony count	48 hr

TABLE B.1 **Microbiology Urine for Culture and Sensitivity**

Urine Culture: *Klebsiella Oxytoca*	
Antibiotic	**Sensitivity**
Ampicillin	Resistant
Cefotetan	Sensitive
Ciprofloxacin	Resistant
Gentamicin	Resistant
Levofloxacin	Sensitive
Tobramycin	Resistant

b. Microbiology (Medical Emergency Requests)

Test	Turnaround Time
Blood Gram stain	<30 min
CSF and body fluid—Gram stain	<30 min
Lower respiratory Gram stain	<30 min
Wound Gram stain	<30 min

The following information should be included when completing a microbiology requisition:

Patient's name
Patient's birth date
Patient's medical record number (if an inpatient)
Attending physician
Ordering physician
Tests required
Date and time of collection

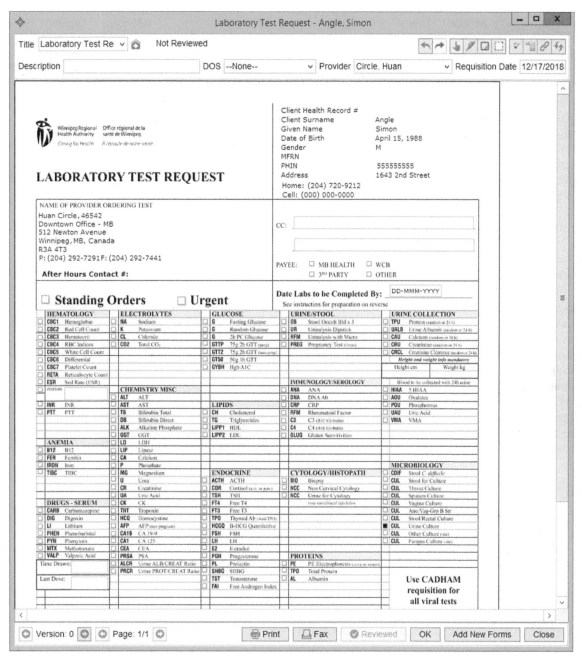

• **Fig. B.4** Microbiology Test Requisition. (Source: Accuro (see above permission and credit information))

Diagnosis or relevant clinical information
Antibiotics currently being given or preferred by physician

See Fig. B.4 for an example of a Microbiology Test Requisition from Manitoba.

Blood Bank

Blood Bank—Performs pre-transfusion compatibility testing before blood is issued. Administering incompatible blood can result in serious complications. The compatibility blood testing is often referred to as a *cross and type*. The typing of blood indicates a test to determine a patient's main blood grouping from either A, B, AB, or O. The cross represents the presence of the Rhesus (rh) factor on the surface of red blood cells; blood that has the rh factor is considered positive, whereas blood that does not have it is considered negative.

Serological testing is also performed to predict obstetrical sensitization and to aid in the diagnosis of certain immune disorders.

Following is a list of some laboratory tests and turnaround times for your reference.

Test	Routine	Urgent	Emergent
Blood Grouping—ABO	24 hr	10 min	10 min
—Rh	24 hr	10 min	10 min
—Other phenotypes	24 hr	30 min	30 min
Antibody investigation—screen	24 hr	60 min	60 min

Continued

Test	Routine	Urgent	Emergent
—Identification	24 hr	60 min	60 min
Complex antibody identification	4 d	na	na
Blood group & anti-body screen	24 hr	60 min	60 min
T&S (type & screen) (pre-op, prenatal, & poss. transfusion)			
Investigation of autoimmune hemolytic anemia	24 hr	2 hr	20 min
Direct antiglobulin test	24 hr	2 hr	20 min
Neonatal testing (D.A.T., ABO, & Rh)	24 hr	2 hr	60 min
Compatibility testing (ind. T&S)	24 hr	90 min	60 min
Investigation of transfusion reaction (non-hemolytic)	24 hr	na	na
Immediate spin crossmatch after type & screen	na	10 min	5 min
Issue uncross-matched group O blood (trauma)	na	na	5 min
Group patient and issue	na	na	10 min

Test	Routine	Urgent	Emergent
uncrossmatched group compatible blood			
Investigation of suspected hemolytic transfusion reaction	na	2 hr	20 min

The following information must be included when completing a blood bank requisition:

Patient's surname and given name (no abbreviation)

Medical record number for inpatients and birth date for outpatients

Location

Sex

Ordering physician

Priority of red cell transfusion

Clinical information or surgical procedure "type and screen"—check this area except when there is an order to transfuse the products, when the MSBOS (maximum surgical blood order schedule) calls for a crossmatch, or when it is an emergency situation.

Electronic Reports

Many laboratory facilities process their reports electronically. The requisitions have bar codes that can be scanned when ordering and processing. Figure B.1 is an example of a combined blood testing and biochemistry requisition.

Appendix C

Pharmacology

The following is a list of commonly prescribed drugs that shows their generic names and brand names (where available) for your reference.

Many drugs are used to treat more than one type of illness, or they are used in combination with other drugs to treat illnesses; therefore, drug names may be included in more than one category.

When referencing brand name drugs in written communication, medical administrative assistants should capitalize the first letter of the drug. For generic drugs, all letters should be lowercased unless the drug name begins a sentence or immediately follows a period or other terminal punctuation. Some health care facilities have additional rules for communicating drug names. Always consult your institution's chosen style guide for rules related to transcribing or writing drug names.

Because drugs are marketed, approved, and cancelled regularly, Health Canada's Drug Product Database and Drug and Health Products Register should be consulted for the most up-to-date information. Other important drug references include the *Compendium of Pharmaceuticals and Specialties* (CPS) and the National Association of Pharmacy Regulatory Authorities (NAPRA).

Health Canada's Drug Product Database (https://www.canada.ca/en/health-canada/services/drugs-health-products/drug-products/drug-product-database.html)

Health Canada's Drug and Health Product Register (https://hpr-rps.hres.ca/index.php)

Compendium of Pharmaceuticals and Specialties (https://www.pharmacists.ca/products-services/)

National Association of Pharmacy Regulatory Authorities (https://napra.ca/national-drug-schedules?keywords=&schedule)

Analgesics

Agents that relieve pain. These include narcotics and nonsteroidal anti-inflammatory drugs (NSAIDs).

Generic Name	Trade Name
acetaminophen	Tylenol
buprenorphine	BuTrans, Belbuca
celecoxib	Celebrex
codeine phosphate	Tylenol with Codeine No. 2, 3, and 4

Generic Name	Trade Name
diclofenac sodium	Voltaren
fentanyl citrate	Fentora
hydrocodone bitartrate	PDP-Hydrocodone
hydromorphone	Dilaudid
ibuprofen	Motrin, Advil
ketorolac tromethamine	Toradol, Acuvail
ketoprofen	Ketoprofen-E
meperidine	Demerol
methadone	Methadose, Metadol
morphine	Doloral, Statex, MS Contin, Zomorph
naproxen	Naprosyn, Vimovo
naproxen sodium	Anaprox, Aleve
oxycodone	OxyNeo, Rivacocet
sumatriptan succinate	Imitrex
tapentadol	Nucynta
tramadol hydrochloride	Durela, Ralivia, Ultram, Tridural

Antianxiety Agents

Agents that relieve feelings of apprehension, uncertainty, and fear; they treat the psychological and physical symptoms of anxiety disorders.

Generic Name	Trade Name
alprazolam	Xanax
chlordiazepoxide	Chlorax, Librax
citalopram	Celexa
clomipramine	Anafranil
clonazepam	Rivotril
diazepam	Valium, Diastat
duloxetine	Cymbalta
escitalopram	Cipralex
fluoxetine	Prozac
lorazepam	Ativan
oxazepam	Apo-Oxazepam

Antibacterials

Agents that have properties to destroy or suppress growth or reproduction of bacteria.

Generic Name	Trade Name
amoxicillin	Clavulin
azithromycin	Zithromax
cefixime	Suprax
cefuroxime	Ceftin
cephalexin	Apo-Cephalex
ciprofloxacin	Cipro
clarithromycin	Biaxin
doxycycline	Teva-Doxycycline; Apo-Doxy
erythromycin	Eryc Delayed-Release Capsules
metronidazole	Flagyl
moxifloxacin	Avelox
norfloxacin	Norfloxacin
trimethoprim-sulfamethoxazole	Septra
vancomycin	Vancocin

Anticholinergics and Antispasmodics

Agents that block the passage of impulses through the parasympathetic nervous system.

Generic Name	Trade Name
clomipramine	Anafranil
ipratropium bromide	Atrovent
meclizine	Bonamine
oxybutynin chloride	Ditropan XL; Oxytrol
phenobarbital	Phenobarb
quetiapine	Seroquel; Seroquel XR
olanzapine	Zyprexa

Anticoagulants

Agents that act to prevent clotting of blood.

Generic Name	Trade Name
acetylsalicylic acid (A.S.A.)	Entrophen, Aspirin
apixaban	Eliquis
dabigatran	Pradaxa
rivaroxaban	Xarelto
warfarin sodium	Coumadin

Anticonvulsants

Agents that control seizures.

Generic Name	Trade Name
carbamazepine	Tegretol
clonazepam	Rivotril
diazepam	Valium, Diastat
divalproex sodium	Epival
ethosuximide	Zarontin
gabapentin	Neurontin
lamotrigine	Lamictal

Generic Name	Trade Name
lorazepam	Ativan
nitrazepam	Mogadon
phenytoin	Dilantin
valproic acid	Depakene
vigabatrin	Sabril

Antidepressants

Agents that prevent or relieve depression.

Generic Name	Trade Name
amitriptyline	Elavil
citalopram	Celexa
bupropion	Wellbutrin SR, Wellbutrin XL, Zyban
clomipramine	Anafranil
desvenlafaxine	Pristiq
doxepin	Sinequan, Silenor
duloxetine	Cymbalta
escitalopram	Cipralex
fluvoxamine maleate	Luvox
fluoxetine	Prozac
levomilnacipran	Fetzima
mirtazapine	Remeron
moclobemide	Manerix
paroxetine	Paxil
sertraline	Zoloft
trazodone	Apo-Trazodone, Teva-Trazodone
trimipramine	Apo-Trimipramine
venlafaxine	Effexor XR

Antihypertensives

Agents that control blood pressure.

Generic Name	Trade Name
acebutolol	Teva-Acebutolol
amiloride	Midamor
amlodipine	Norvasc Tab, Viacoram
atenolol	Tenormin, Tenoretic
captopril	Teva-Captopril, Apo-Capto
diltiazem	Tiazac
enalapril sodium	Vasotec
fosinopril sodium	Teva-Fosinopril, Apo-Fosinopril
furosemide	Lasix
lisinopril	Zestril
losartan potassium	Cozaar
metolazone	Zaroxolyn
metoprolol tartrate	Lopresor, Apo-Metoprolol
nifedipine	Adalat
propranolol	Inderal-LA
ramipril	Altace
sotalol hydrochloride	Apo-Sotalol, Dom-Sotalol
spironolactone	Aldactone, Aldactazide

Generic Name	Trade Name
telmisartan	Micardis
valsartan	Diovan
verapamil	Isoptin, Apo-Verap

Antilipidemics

Agents that lower lipid (fats and fatlike substances) levels in the blood.

Generic Name	Trade Name
atorvastatin	Lipitor
cholestyramine	Olestyr
ezetimibe	Ezetrol
fenofibrate	Lipidil EZ, Lipidil Supra, Fenomax
fluvastatin	Lescol
gemfibrozil	Teva-Gemfibrozil
lovastatin	Riva-Lovastatin, Apo-Lovastatin
pravastatin	Pravachol
rosuvastatin	Crestor
simvastatin	Zocor

Antiparkinsonian Agents

Drugs that treat the symptoms associated with Parkinson disease.

Generic Name	Trade Name
benserazide; levodopa	Prolopa Cap
carbidopa; levodopa	Duodopa; Sinemet, Sinemet CR
entacapone	Comtan
pramipexole	Mirapex
rasagiline	Azilect
rotigotine	Neupro

Antipsychotics

Agents effective in the management of mood control, schizophrenia, and psychosis (hallucinations and delusions).

Generic Name	Trade Name
aripiprazole	Abilify
chlorpromazine	Teva-Chlorpromazine
clozapine	Clozaril
haloperidol	Teva-Haloperidol
flupentixol	Fluanxol
fluphenazine	Modecate Concentrate
loxapine	Loxapac IM, Xylac
olanzapine	Zyprexa
paliperidone	Invega
quetiapine	Seroquel
risperidone	Risperdal
ziprasidone	Zeldox
zuclopenthixol	Clopixol

Antimanic Agents

Agents that control the manic moods associated with bipolar disorders or the mania associated with other affective disorders.

Generic Name	Trade Name
carbamazepine	Tegretol
chlorpromazine	Teva-Chlorpromazine
haloperidol	Teva-Haloperidol
lithium carbonate	Carbolith, Lithane, Lithmax
olanzapine	Zyprexa
risperidone	Risperdal
valproic acid	Depakene

Antipyretics

Agents that relieve fever.

Generic Name	Trade Name
acetaminophen	Tylenol
acetylsalicylic acid (A.S.A.)	Entrophen, Aspirin
ibuprofen	Advil, Motrin
naproxen sodium	Anaprox, Aleve

Asthma Therapy

Agents that relieve and control symptoms related to asthma.

Generic Name	Trade Name
beclomethasone dipropionate	QVAR
budesonide	Pulmicort
budesonide + formoterol	Symbicort
ciclesonide	Alvesco
fluticasone propionate	Flovent Diskus, Flovent HFA
formoterol	Oxeze
hydrocortisone sodium succinate	Solu-Cortef
ipratropium + salbutamol	Combivent UDV, Combivent Respimat
ipratropium bromide	Atrovent HFA
ketotifen fumarate	Zaditen
methylprednisolone sodium succinate	Solu-Medrol
mometasone furoate	Asmanex Twisthaler
mometasone + formoterol	Zenhale
montelukast	Singulair
omalizumab	Xolair
prednisolone	Pediapred
prednisone	Apo-Prednisone, Teva-Prednisone
salbutamol sulfate	Airomir, Ventolin, Ventolin Diskus
terbutaline sulfate	Bricanyl Turbuhaler

Continued

Generic Name	Trade Name
theophylline	Apo-Theo LA, Theo ER, Theolair
tiotropium bromide	Spiriva
salmeterol + fluticasone	Advair, Advair Diskus
salmeterol xinafoate	Serevent Diskus

Cardiac Therapy

These drugs treat heart rhythm disorders, high blood pressure, heart failure, chest pain, and coronary artery disease.

Generic Name	Trade Name
acebutolol	Teva-Acebutolol
amiodarone	Dom-Amiodarone, PMS-Amiodarone
amlodipine	Norvasc Tab, Viacoram
atenolol	Tenormin, Tenoretic
bisoprolol	Apo-Bisoprolol, Teva-Bisoprolol
captopril	Teva-Captopril, Apo-Capto
carvedilol	Auro-Carvedilol, Teva-Carvedilol
cilazapril	Inhibace
digoxin	Toloxin
diltiazem	Tiazac
disopyramide	Rythmodan
dronedarone	Multaq
enalapril sodium	Vasotec
esmolol	Brevibloc
ethacrynic acid	Edecrin
felodipine	Plendil
flecainide	Apo-Flecainide, Mar-Flecainide
fosinopril sodium	Teva-Fosinopril, Apo-Fosinopril
furosemide	Lasix
hydrochlorothiazide	Altace HCT, Apo-Hydro, Olmetec Plus
isosorbide dinitrate	ISDN
labetalol	Trandate
lisinopril	Zestril
metoprolol tartrate	Lopresor, Apo-Metoprolol
nifedipine	Adalat
perindopril	Coversyl
pindolol	Teva-Pindolol, Visken
propafenone	Rythmol
propranolol	Inderal-LA

Generic Name	Trade Name
quinapril	Accupril, Apo-Quinapril
ramipril	Altace
sotalol hydrochloride	Apo-Sotalol, Dom-Sotalol
timolol	T-Lo, Timoptic
trandolapril	PMS-Trandolapril, Mavik
verapamil	Isoptin, Apo-Verap

Cough and Cold Preparations (Over-The-Counter)

Agents that suppress cough (antitussive), thin mucus (mucolytic), and clear sinus congestion (decongestants).

Generic Name	Trade Name
dextromethorphan hydrobromide (antitussive)	Benylin DM Extra Strength Lozenges, DM Cough Syrup, Triaminic Thin Strips (Cough)
guaifenesin (expectorant; mucolytic)	Robitussin Mucus & Phlegm, Benylin Cough Plus Cold Relief, Mucinex Multi-Action Cold and Sinus
pseudoephedrine hydrochloride (decongestant)	Sudafed Sinus Complete, Allegra-D, Benadryl Total

Sedative and Hypnotic Agents

These drugs are central nervous system depressants used to treat anxiety, insomnia, and alcohol withdrawal; they are prescribed as muscle relaxants and anticonvulsants.

Generic Name	Trade Name
alprazolam	Xanax
clonazepam	Rivotril
diazepam	Valium, Diastat
lorazepam	Ativan
phenobarbital	Phenobarb
temazepam	Restoril
zolpidem	Sublinox
zopiclone	Imovane

Appendix D

Reference Sources

As a medical administrative assistant, you will endeavour to be familiar with and know how to access a wide range of reference material. In today's information age, there are several sources of information of varying types that you may choose to utilize. Some you will use on a daily basis, whereas others, only from time to time. Select standard practical sources that allow you to operate within easy reach.

Dictionaries

Of course, a standard medical dictionary is an essential tool. There are many such dictionaries available, from small pocket-size to large multi-volume editions, e-books, and mobile apps. The availability of digital media has significantly increased the choices immediately available. Some publishers of print-based dictionaries also offer a downloadable electronic or online version. Dictionaries can be sourced by medical specialty area. Another type to consider is inverted dictionaries (in which the definition is given in alphabetical order, followed by the appropriate medical term) and dictionaries of abbreviations and acronyms, syndromes, diseases, hospital terminology, and so on.

Directories

A directory is basically a list, and there are many lists available. Of relevance are physician directories, which list most doctors practising in Canada. The range of information presented in each directory varies; most contain the same core standard information, such as contact details, location, and area of specialty. The regional College of Physicians and Surgeons typically will host on its website a physician-searchable database. A database is a structured collection of data, stored and accessed electronically through a website or computer system. There are also international, national, and local directories of health organizations and institutions, hospitals, social agencies, and health care professionals. A directory can be anything from a large publication or database on a worldwide scale to a small pamphlet put out by your local association of pharmacists.

Pharmaceutical Publications

Publications dealing with pharmaceuticals come in many varieties, but the one most widely used in Canada is the *Compendium of Pharmaceuticals and Specialties* (CPS). It is published annually as a desktop reference book. The CPS is also available online. Additionally, the CPS can be accessed through the RxTx database using the RxTx mobile app. Primary access to the Canadian Pharmacists Association's CPS is included in the annual membership fee paid through the Canadian Medical Association. This reference source is a detailed listing of drugs, vaccines, and natural health products by generic name (penicillin), trade name or monograph (Valium), manufacturer, type (antihistamines, oral), indications of use, and contraindications as well as side effects. The key benefit of the CPS online and mobile app is that its content is updated weekly. The CPS can also be integrated with electronic medical record systems. Typically, you will find the desktop book or access to the CPS in every practising physician's office, hospital nursing unit, health records department, etc. Individual drugs can also be looked up on specific websites. You will want to be familiar with how to use pharmaceutical reference sources because interactions with pharmacies occur on a regular basis, so understanding how to reference key information quickly will increase your overall effectiveness in the role.

The CPS desktop is composed of six main sections plus appendices and glossary. See Table D.1 for CPS section descriptions.

Ministry of Health Fee Schedules/ Diagnostic Codes

Each provincial and territorial Ministry of Health publishes a document called *Fee Schedules and Diagnostic Code Listings*. Most are available in a downloadable format through the Ministry website.

Guidebooks for the Administrative Assistant

Every medical administrative assistant should have at least one up-to-date guidebook close at hand for quick reference. If you research in your school library, you will probably find several reliable sources. Take the time to browse through them to familiarize yourself with the type of information that is at your disposal. Also, search the medical databases available through your library to ensure you can locate current information in an efficient manner.

TABLE D.1 CPS Desktop Version Divisions by Colour

Colour	Description
Pink	Therapeutic Guide–Classification System Index
Green	Drug listing of brand and non-proprietary names
White	Glossy Pages Product Identification: A picture guide to assist in the identification of products An alphabetical list of each drug by name, including the chemical make-up of the drug; its use, indications, and contraindications; any precautions necessary when administering the drug; adverse effects; overdose symptoms and treatment; and appropriate dosages
Yellow	Manufacturers' Index
Lilac	Clinical information including the following: Poison control centres Selected resource agencies and literature Non-medicinal ingredients Clinical monitoring
Blue	Patient information

Whether you work in a one-doctor office or in a large hospital or clinic, you will be required from time to time to research certain information for your employer. The more familiar you are with the types of reference sources and the ways to access them, the more efficiently you will be able to find the information you need. A reference librarian will be pleased to show you where this material can be found. Most medical journals and handbooks are available online. Using an online database, you can source specific information you require and develop a guidebook for your personal use.

A List of Reference Sources

Canadian Medical Directory
Online available at: http://www.mdselect.com/
Compendium of Pharmaceuticals and Specialties (CPS)
Available formats: Print, online, mobile app, and data integration EMR, EHR, and DIS (drug information systems)
Publisher: Canadian Pharmacists Association (https://www.pharmacists.ca)
Dorland's Medical Dictionary
Available formats: Print, e-book, and mobile app
Publisher: Elsevier Canada (http://www.elsevier.ca)
Dorland's Dictionary of Medical Acronyms and Abbreviations
Available formats: Print and e-book
Publisher: Elsevier Canada (http://www.elsevier.ca)
Mosby's Medical Dictionary
Available formats: Hardcover and e-book
Publisher: Elsevier Canada (http://www.elsevier.ca)
Taber's Cyclopedic Medical Dictionary
Available formats: Print, e-book, and mobile app
Publisher: F.A. Davis and Company
Online available at: https://www.tabers.com/tabersonline/
Medical Language Instant Translator
Available formats: Print and e-book
Publisher: Elsevier Canada (http://www.elsevier.ca)
Sloane's Medical Word Book
Available formats: Print and e-book
Author: Ellen Drake
Publisher: Elsevier Canada (http://www.elsevier.ca)
Book of Style for Medical Transcription Available formats: Print and digital subscription
Author: Lea Sims, CHDS, AHDI-F
Publisher: Association for Healthcare Documentation Integrity

Index

Note: Page numbers followed by "f" indicate figures, "t" indicate tables, and "b" indicate boxes.